Clostridial Diseases of Animals

Clostridial Diseases of Animals

Francisco A. Uzal DVM, FRVC, MSc, PhD, Dipl. ACVP

Professor of Veterinary Diagnostic Pathology
California Animal Health and Food Safety Laboratory
San Bernardino Branch
School of Veterinary Medicine
University of California Davis
San Bernardino, California, USA

J. Glenn Songer MA, PhD, Fellow AAM, Dipl. ACVM

Professor (Emeritus) of Veterinary Science and Microbiology
College of Agriculture
The University of Arizona in Tucson
Tucson, Arizona, USA

John F. Prescott MA, VetMB, PhD, FCAHS

University Professor Emeritus
Department of Pathobiology
University of Guelph
Guelph, Ontario, Canada

Michel R. Popoff DVM, PhD

Anaerobic Bacteria and Toxins
Pasteur Institute
Paris, France

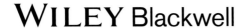

This edition first published 2016 © 2016 by John Wiley & Sons, Inc

Editorial Offices

1606 Golden Aspen Drive, Suites 103 and 104, Ames, Iowa 50010, USA

The Atrium, Southern Gate, Chichester, West Sussex, PO19 8SQ, UK

9600 Garsington Road, Oxford, OX4 2DQ, UK

For details of our global editorial offices, for customer services and for information about how to apply for permission to reuse the copyright material in this book please see our website at www.wiley.com/wiley-blackwell.

Library of Congress Cataloging-in-Publication Data

Names: Uzal, Francisco Alejandro, 1958– , editor. | Prescott, John F. (John Francis), 1949– , editor. | Songer, J. Glenn (Joseph Glenn), 1950– , editor. | Popoff, Michel R., editor.
Title: Clostridial diseases of animals / [edited by] Francisco Alejandro Uzal, John Francis Prescott, J. Glenn Songer, Michel Robert Popoff.
Description: Ames, Iowa : John Wiley & Sons, Inc., 2016. | Includes bibliographical references and index.
Identifiers: LCCN 2015047741 | ISBN 9781118728406 (cloth)
Subjects: LCSH: Clostridium diseases in animals. | Clostridium. | MESH: Clostridium Infections–veterinary | Clostridium–pathogenicity
Classification: LCC SF809.C6 C56 2016 | NLM SF 809.C6 | DDC 636.089/6931–dc23
LC record available at http://lccn.loc.gov/2015047741

A catalogue record for this book is available from the British Library.

Cover image: © Lower left courtesy of A. de Lahunta, middle left courtesy of T. Van Dreumel and upper left courtesy of E. Paredes.

Set in 9.5/12pt Meridien by SPi Global, Pondicherry, India
Printed and bound in Malaysia by Vivar Printing Sdn Bhd

1 2016

Contents

List of Contributors

Camila C. Abreu, DVM, MSc
Veterinary Pathology Laboratory
Federal University of Lavras,
Lavras, Minas Gerais, Brazil

Francisco R. Carvallo Chaigneau, DVM, DSc, Dipl. ACVP
California Animal Health and Food Safety Laboratory
San Bernardino Branch
School of Veterinary Medicine
University of California, Davis
San Bernardino, CA, USA

Kerry K. Cooper, PhD
Department of Biology
California State University, Northridge
Northridge, CA, USA

Santiago S. Diab, DVM, Dipl. ACVP
California Animal Health and Food Safety Laboratory
Davis Branch
School of Veterinary Medicine
University of California, Davis
Davis, CA, USA

Fernando Dutra Quintela, DVM, MSc, MSc, FRVCS
DILAVE "Miguel C Rubino"
Eastern Regional Laboratory
Treinta y Tres, Uruguay

Patrick Fach, PhD
ANSES
Food Safety Laboratory, IdentyPath Platform
Maisons-Alfort, Cedex, France

John W. Finnie, BVSc, MSc, PhD, FRCVS
South Australia Pathology Hanson Institute Center for Neurologic Diseases
and School of Veterinary Science
University of Adelaide
Adelaide, South Australia, Australia

Russell S. Fraser, DVM, MSc
Department of Pathobiology
University of Guelph
Guelph, Ontario, Canada

Karina C. Fresneda, DVM
California Animal Health and Food Safety Laboratory
San Bernardino Branch
School of Veterinary Medicine
University of California, Davis
San Bernardino, CA, USA

Jorge P. García, DVM
Department of Large Animal Surgical and Medical Clinics
Veterinary School
National University of the Center of Buenos Aires Province
Tandil, Buenos Aires, Argentina

Federico Giannitti, DVM
Veterinary Diagnostic Laboratory
College of Veterinary Medicine
University of Minnesota
Saint Paul, MN, USA
and
National Institute of Agricultural Research La Estanzuela
Colonia, Uruguay

Iman Mehdizadeh Gohari, DVM, MSc
Department of Pathobiology
University of Guelph
Guelph, Ontario, Canada

Ashley E. Harmon
Harmon Creative
Seattle, WA, USA

M. Kevin Keel, DVM, PhD Dipl. ACVP
Department of Pathology, Microbiology and Immunology
School of Veterinary Medicine
University of California, Davis
Davis, CA, USA

Caroline Le Maréchal, PhD
ANSES
Ploufragan-Plouzané Laboratory
Hygiene and Quality of Avian and Pig Products Unit
Ploufragan, France

Francisco C. F. Lobato, DVM, MSc, PhD
Veterinary School
Federal University of Minas
Belo Horizonte, Brazil

Janet I. MacInnes, BSc, PhD
Department of Pathobiology
University of Guelph
Guelph
Ontario, Canada

Bruce A. McClane, BSc, PhD
Department of Microbiology and Molecular Genetics
University of Pittsburgh School of Medicine
Pittsburgh, PA, USA

Paula I. Menzies, DVM, MPVM, Dipl. ECSRHM
Department of Population Medicine
Ontario Veterinary College
University of Guelph
Guelph, Ontario, Canada

Mauricio Navarro, DVM, MSc
Department of Pathology, Microbiology and Immunology
School of Veterinary Medicine
University of California, Davis
Davis, CA, USA

Carlos A. Oliveira Jr., DMV, MSc
Veterinary School
Federal University of Minas
Belo Horizonte, Brazil

Valeria R. Parreira, BSc, MSc, PhD
Department of Pathobiology
University of Guelph
Guelph, Ontario, Canada

Michel R. Popoff, DVM, PhD
Anaerobic Bacteria and Toxins
Pasteur Institute
Paris, France

John F. Prescott, MA, Vet MB, PhD, FCAHS
Department of Pathobiology
Ontario Veterinary College
University of Guelph
Guelph, Ontario, Canada

Julian I. Rood BSc(Hons), PhD, FASM, FAAM
Infection and Immunity Program, Biomedicine Discovery Institute
and
Department of Microbiology
Monash University
Clayton, Victoria, Australia

H. L. Shivaprasad, BVSc, MS, PhD, Dipl. ACPV
California Animal Health and Food Safety Laboratory
Tulare Branch
School of Veterinary Medicine
University of California, Davis
Tulare, CA, USA

Rodrigo O. S. Silva, DVM, MSc, PhD
Veterinary School
Federal University of Minas Gerais
Belo Horizonte, Brazil

J. Glenn Songer, MA, PhD, Fellow AAM, Dipl. ACVM
Professor (Emeritus) of Veterinary Science and Microbiology
College of Agriculture
The University of Arizona in Tucson
Tucson, Arizona, USA

James R. Theoret, PhD
Department of Biological Sciences
College of Southern Nevada
Las Vegas, NV, USA

Francisco A. Uzal, DVM, FRVC, MSc, PhD, Dipl. ACVP
California Animal Health and Food Safety Laboratory
San Bernardino Branch
School of Veterinary Medicine
University of California, Davis
San Bernardino, CA, USA

Cédric Woudstra, MSc
ANSES
Food Safety Laboratory
Maisons-Alfort, Cedex, France

Anson K.K. Wu, BSc, MSc
Department of Pathobiology
University of Guelph
Guelph, Ontario, Canada

Preface

Over the past 20 years or so there has been an explosion of research on clostridia. A significant part of this interest in the field is a response to the *Clostridium difficile* human pandemic and several other human diseases, including enterotoxigenic *Clostridium perfringens* food poisoning. However, there have also been important advances in all fields of clostridia, including those associated with animal diseases.

Advances in the animal field are many, and it is not our intention to mention them all in this preface, since they are the subject of this book. Amongst the most significant achievements of the past few years is the discovery of new toxins and other virulence factors, including NetB, NetF, and several others, and the fulfillment of molecular Koch postulates for several of these toxins. For instance, we know now beyond any reasonable doubt that *C. perfringens* epsilon toxin is responsible for type D enterotoxemia of ruminants, while the beta toxin of this microorganism is responsible for necrotizing enteritis of neonates of several animal species. The synergism between CPE and CPB of *C. perfringens* type C has also been demonstrated and it is possible that such interactions exist for other *C. perfringens* toxins and/or for toxins of other clostridial species.

No English-language textbook on clostridial diseases of animals has been published since Max Sterne and Irene Batty's classic *Pathogenic Clostridia*, last edited in 1975. Because understanding of clostridia and clostridial diseases has progressed so much since then, this book provides a much-needed, up-to-date reference on clostridial diseases of animals. The book was written mostly with the veterinary community in mind, including clinicians, diagnosticians, pathologists, microbiologists, and, in sum, everybody that has to deal with clostridial diseases of animals. However, we hope that all professionals and scientists working with clostridia will find something of value in these pages. An effort was made to include good-quality photographs of gross and microscopic images, which we hope will be helpful in terms of the recognition of disease patterns.

There are many things we still do not know about clostridia and clostridial diseases. In veterinary medicine the frequent lack of agreement on diagnostic criteria for several of the major clostridial diseases is particularly worrisome. For instance, what is the diagnostic value of isolating a particular clostridial species from the intestine of an animal in which this microorganism is normally found? How can we reliably define the diagnostic value of highly sensitive real-time PCR done on fecal or intestinal material and not, through this technique, over-diagnose particular diseases? The discovery of new virulence factors, such as the recently discovered NetF, which may be found in clostridia isolated from sick, but not healthy, animals, may help to resolve at least part of this dilemma. A subject we hope will receive more attention in the future is diagnostic tests for clostridial diseases, including rapid tests.

We will be pleased to receive readers' comments as well as suggestions for improvement in any future editions of this book.

Francisco A. Uzal
J. Glenn Songer
John F. Prescott
Michel R. Popoff

SECTION 1
The Pathogenic Clostridia

Taxonomic Relationships among the Clostridia

1

John F. Prescott, Janet I. MacInnes, and Anson K. K. Wu

Clostridia are prokaryotic bacteria belonging to the phylum Firmicutes, the Gram-positive (mostly), low G + C bacteria that currently contains three classes, "*Bacilli*", "*Clostridia*", and "*Erysipelotrichia*". The class "*Clostridia*" contains the order *Clostridiales*, within which the family *Clostridiaceae* contains 13 genera distributed among three paraphyletic clusters and a fourth clade represented by a single genus. The first clostridial cluster contains the genus *Clostridium* and four other genera. The genus *Clostridium* has been extensively restructured, with many species moved to other genera, but it remains phylogenetically heterogenous. The genus currently contains 204 validly described species (http://www.bacterio. net), of which approximately half are genuinely *Clostridium*.

The main pathogenic clostridial species, *Clostridium botulinum*, *Clostridium chauvoei*, *Clostridium haemolyticum*, *Clostridium novyi*, *Clostridium perfringens*, *Clostridium septicum*, and *Clostridium tetani*, clearly belong to the genus *Clostridium* because they share common ancestry with the type species *Clostridium butyricum*. These species belong to the phylogenetic group described by Collins *et al.* (1994) as "cluster I", and are *Clostridium* sensu stricto. The taxonomy of *C. botulinum* is unique since it is currently defined as *C. botulinum* only by the ability to produce one or more botulinum toxins; however, strains that can do this belong to at least four *Clostridium* species. This situation is complex and taxonomically confusing, since strains of other species, such as *C. butyricum* which may produce botulinum toxin and cause human botulism, have been given their own species designation (that is, not *C. botulinum*). To compound the inconsistency around species designation in the taxonomy of *Clostridium*, *C. novyi* type A and *Clostridium haemolyticum* belong to the same genospecies as *C. botulinum* group III (the agents of animal botulism). Many *Clostridium* species which do not belong to this genus sensu stricto, as defined by the type species *C. butyricum*, are distributed among the genera of *Clostridiaceae* but are described as "incertae sedis". These fall into different phylogenetic clusters throughout the low G +C Gram-positive phylum,

Clostridial Diseases of Animals, First Edition. Francisco A. Uzal, J. Glenn Songer, John F. Prescott and Michel R. Popoff.

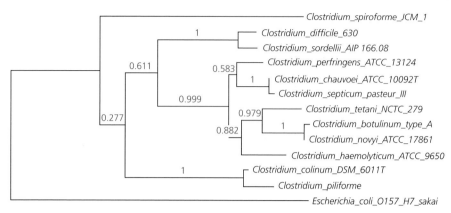

Figure 1.1 Phylogenetic tree displaying the relationship between *Clostridium* species. *Escherichia coli* from the *Enterobacteriaceae* family was used as an out group. The phylogenetic tree was constructed using the "One Click" mode with default settings in the Phylogeny.fr platform (http://phylogeny.lirmm.fr/phylo_cgi/index.cgi). The numbers above the branches are tree support values generated by PhyML using the aLRT statistical test.

and belong to distinct 16S rRNA gene-sequence-based clusters that represent different genera and different families. For example, *Clostridium difficile* and *Clostridium sordellii* fall into cluster XIa ("*Peptostreptococcaceae*"), *Clostridium colinum* falls into cluster XIVb ("*Lachnospiraceae*"), and *Clostridium spiroforme* falls into cluster XVIII, a new family. Figure 1.1 shows these relationships based on 16S rRNA sequences.

Interestingly, the genus *Sarcina* falls within the genus *Clostridium* sensu stricto, and indeed should have taxonomic preference as the genus name. This taxonomic precedence, as well as the genus attribution of the non-*Clostridium* sensu stricto animal and human pathogens currently assigned the genus name *Clostridium*, seems unlikely to change in the near future because of the chaos and the potential hazard that such otherwise justified genus name changes would engender. Future taxonomic classification based on whole-genome sequencing may help to resolve some of the complexity of clostridial classification.

Bibliography

Chevenet, F., *et al.* (2006) TreeDyn: Towards dynamic graphics and annotations for analyses of trees. *BMC Bioinfo.*, **7:** 439.

Collins, M.D., *et al.* (1994) The phylogeny of the genus *Clostridium*: Proposal of five new genera and eleven new species combinations. *Int. J. Syst. Bact.*, **44:** 812–826.

Dereeper, A., *et al.* (2008) Phylogeny.fr: Robust phylogenetic analysis for the non-specialist. *Nucl. Acids Res.*, **36:** W465.

Guindon, S. and Gascuel, O. (2003) A simple, fast, and accurate algorithm to estimate large phylogenies by maximum likelihood. *Syst. Biol.*, **52:** 696–704.

Ludwig, W., *et al.* (2009) Revised road map to the phylum *Firmicutes*. In: De Vos, P. *et al.* (eds) *Bergey's Manual of Systematic Bacteriology*, pp. 1–32. Springer Science, New York.

Skarin, H., *et al.* (2011) *Clostridium botulinum* group III: A group with dual identity shaped by plasmids, phages and mobile elements. *BMC Genetics,* **12:** 185.

Skarin, H., *et al.* (2014) Plasmidome interchange between *Clostridium botulinum, Clostridium novyi* and *Clostridium haemolyticum* converts strains of independent lineages into distinctly different pathogens. *PloS One,* **9:** e107777.

Wiegel, J., *et al.* (2006) An introduction to the Family *Clostridiaceae.* In: Dworkin, M. *et al.* (eds) *The Prokaryotes,* pp. 654–678. Springer Science, New York.

Wiegel, J. (2009) Family I. *Clostridiaceae.* In: De Vos, P. *et al.* (eds) *Bergey's Manual of Systematic Bacteriology,* p.736. Springer Science, New York.

General Physiological and Virulence Properties of the Pathogenic Clostridia

Julian I. Rood

Introduction

The key features that delineate members of the genus *Clostridium* are that they are Gram-positive rods that are anaerobic and form heat-resistant endospores. By and large these features define the genus, although there are some clostridia that stain Gram-negative and some clostridia that can grow in the presence of oxygen. Most members of this genus are commensal or soil bacteria that do not cause disease, but we tend to focus our attention on the pathogenic clostridia. The genus is extremely diverse and, by normal taxonomic criteria, should be divided into several different genera (Chapter 1). However, the established role of several clostridial species in some of the major diseases of humans and animals, including tetanus, botulism, gas gangrene, and various enteric and enterotoxemic syndromes, has precluded what would otherwise be a sensible and scientifically sound reclassification (Chapter 1). Recently, the movement of pathogens such as *Clostridium difficile* and *Clostridium sordellii* into the genera *Peptoclostridium* and *Paeniclostridium*, respectively, has been suggested, but these proposals are yet to be adopted formally.

Anaerobic metabolism

Bacterial metabolism is the process by which bacteria obtain nutrients and energy from the environment or their host, enabling them to grow and multiply. It is beyond the scope of this chapter to describe this process in detail, since entire books can and have been written on the topic. The key issue that will be discussed here is what, in general terms, distinguishes the metabolism of anaerobic bacteria from that of aerobic and facultative anaerobic bacteria. Aerobes are defined as

Clostridial Diseases of Animals, First Edition. Francisco A. Uzal, J. Glenn Songer,
John F. Prescott and Michel R. Popoff.

bacteria that are unable to grow in the absence of oxygen. Facultative anaerobes can grow in the presence or absence of oxygen, usually growing more rapidly under aerobic conditions. Anaerobic bacteria are unable to grow in the presence of oxygen, but grow very well under anaerobic conditions. Anaerobic bacteria can be divided further into two major groups: strict anaerobes, which are killed by exposure to oxygen, and aerotolerant anaerobes, which can only grow anaerobically but are not killed by exposure to oxygen.

Aerobic bacteria obtain most of their energy, in the form of ATP, in a highly efficient manner by the passage of electrons through the membrane-bound electron-transport chain, culminating in the use of oxygen as a terminal electron acceptor. This process is known as aerobic respiration. In an aerobic environment, facultative anaerobes such as *Escherichia coli* or *Salmonella* spp. use the electron-transport chain to produce ATP. In the absence of oxygen, they are reliant on the far less efficient substrate-level phosphorylation process or the use of an alternative electron acceptor.

Anaerobic bacteria may still be able to obtain their energy from the electron-transport chain by use of an alternative terminal electron acceptor, usually an inorganic compound such as a nitrate or sulfate. This process is known as anaerobic respiration. Alternatively, they may carry out anaerobic fermentation and obtain all of their ATP from substrate-level phosphorylation, with oxidized NAD regenerated by the reduction of intermediates in the glycolytic pathway to ionized carboxylic acids such as acetate, lactate, or butyrate. Such organisms may significantly increase the throughput of sugars through the glycolytic pathway and therefore do not necessarily grow at a slower rate than aerobic bacteria, even though the output from aerobic respiration (38 moles of ATP per mole of glucose catabolized to CO_2) is far greater than that from fermentation (2 moles of ATP per mole of glucose partially catabolized to a mixture of alcohols and/or organic acids).

Like many other bacteria, the clostridia are not restricted to metabolizing sugars to obtain their energy. They can ferment other compounds such as amino acids to obtain both their carbon and energy. For example, *C. difficile* uses the Stickland reaction in which pairs of amino acids are fermented in a coupled reaction, with one amino acid acting as an electron donor and the other amino acid acting as an electron acceptor.

Major clostridial diseases

Clostridial diseases and infections can be divided into three major types: neurotoxic diseases, histotoxic diseases, and enteric diseases. Although the focus of this book is clostridial diseases of animals, the clostridia are also important human pathogens. The major clostridial diseases of humans are botulism, tetanus, gas gangrene, food poisoning, pseudomembranous colitis, and antibiotic-associated diarrhea. The major clostridial diseases of animals are outlined in Chapter 3 (Table 3.1) and described in subsequent chapters.

In both humans and animals, botulism and tetanus are caused by *Clostridium botulinum* and *Clostridium tetani*, respectively. Traumatic gas gangrene or clostridial myonecrosis in humans is primarily mediated by *Clostridium perfringens* and non-traumatic gas gangrene by *Clostridium septicum*, although other clostridia such as *Clostridium novyi* and *C. sordellii* can cause severe histotoxic infections in humans and animals. Enterotoxin (CPE)-producing strains of *C. perfringens* are now the second major cause of human food poisoning in the U.S.A., and can also cause non-food-borne gastrointestinal disease. The major cause of human antibiotic-associated diarrhea and a broader range of enteric infections, including pseudomembranous colitis and toxic megacolon, is the major nosocomial pathogen, *C. difficile*.

The onset of clostridial infections

Although the pathogenesis of clostridial diseases invariably involves the production of potent protein toxins, it is important to note that, with one exception, they are true infectious diseases. The infectious bacterium needs to establish itself in the host and overcome the host's innate and acquired immune defenses so that the pathogen can grow, multiply, and elaborate its toxins. The extent of bacterial growth that occurs may be fairly limited, for example the minimal growth of *C. tetani* in the deep wounds that lead to tetanus, or very extensive, for example the rapid growth of *C. perfringens* or *C. septicum* in histotoxic infections. The exception is botulism, which is often a true toxemia, with humans or animals consuming preformed botulinum toxin in their food.

Clostridial infections invariably require predisposing conditions, either the breaking of the skin or intestinal barriers by a deep or traumatic wound, or an alteration to the gastrointestinal microbiota caused by a change in the type of feed or by treatment with antimicrobial agents. For example, *C. perfringens*-mediated avian necrotic enteritis generally involves a change to a protein-rich feed that is often coupled with a predisposing coccidial infection, which leads to overgrowth of toxigenic *C. perfringens* strains and damage to the gastrointestinal mucosa. Similarly, human *C. difficile* infections usually follow changes to the intestinal microbiota brought about by treatment of patients with antimicrobial agents.

In most enteric infections caused by other bacterial genera, we know that there is a need for the invading bacteria to adhere to the gastrointestinal epithelium if they are to cause disease. Otherwise they will be washed out of the gastrointestinal tract by the normal one-way peristaltic flow of material. In these bacteria, a considerable amount is known about the role of different fimbriae or other types of surface adhesins that mediate this process. By contrast, little is known about the adhesion process utilized by clostridial enteric pathogens, primarily because research on these pathogens has traditionally focused on their toxins. The exception is human *C. difficile* infections, where several putative cell-surface adhesins have been identified, including a lipoprotein, two sortase-anchored proteins, S-layer proteins, flagellar proteins, a fibronectin-binding protein, and a putative collagen-binding protein. Therefore, there is considerable scope to investigate and understand the numerous roles of virulence determinants other than protein toxins in the pathogenesis of clostridial diseases.

The key role of protein toxins in clostridial disease

The primary feature of clostridial infections is that cell and tissue damage are mediated by potent protein toxins that are either secreted from the cell or released upon cell lysis. These toxins fall into three major classes: enzymes that act at the cell surface, pore-forming toxins, and toxins that are taken up by their target cells and exert their effects upon release into the cytoplasm.

Alpha toxin (CPA) is an essential virulence factor in *C. perfringens*-mediated myonecrosis. It is a zinc metallophospholipase C that cleaves phosphatidylcholine in the host cell membrane to phosphorylcholine and a diacylglyceride. At low concentrations, CPA initiates an intracellular signaling cascade; at high concentrations, it disrupts the cell membrane (Chapter 5). Other *C. perfringens* toxins such as perfringolysin O, enterotoxin (CPE), beta toxin, epsilon toxin, NetB, and NetF are pore-forming toxins that oligomerize at the host cell surface and form either small or large pores in the membrane, again often inducing signaling pathways at low concentrations, but cell lysis at high concentrations (Chapter 5). These toxins have been shown to be either essential for disease or implicated in disease pathogenesis. Other clostridial pore-forming toxins include alpha toxin from *C. septicum* and toxin A from *C. chauvoei* (Chapter 4).

There are two major classes of clostridial toxins that act at the cytoplasmic level in the host cell. These toxins contain a binding component that adheres to a receptor(s) on the host cell membrane, which results in the formation of an endocytic vacuole that contains the toxin. Lysosomal fusion leads to the acidification of the vacuole, a conformation change in the toxin, and secretion of the active enzymatic component of the toxin into the cytoplasm, where it leads to cellular damage. The first class of toxins is represented by tetanus neurotoxin (TeNT) and the seven related, but distinct, botulinum neurotoxins (BoNT/A to BoNT/G) (Chapter 7). The active components of these toxins are zinc metalloproteases specific to SNARE proteins that are involved in the release of neurotransmitters at the end of the axon of neurons. The net effect is blockage of the nerve impulse at the nerve–muscle junction (BoNT) or in the relaxation pathway in the spinal cord (TeNT). The second class of intracellular toxins is the large clostridial toxins (LCTs), the best characterized of which are toxin A (TcdA, 308 kDa) and toxin B (TcdB, 270 kDa) from *C. difficile* (Chapter 6). Other toxins in this monoglycosyltransferase family include TcsH and TcsL from *C. sordellii*, TpeL from *C. perfringens,* and Tcnα from *C. novyi* (Chapter 4). TcdA and TcdB are autoproteolytic toxins whose active N-terminal domains are monoglucosyltransferases that transfer glucose moieties to the Thr-37 residue of Rho-family GTPases such as Rho and Rac, thereby irreversibly inactivating these key components of the host cell's regulatory network, which leads to alterations to the cell's cytoskeletal structure.

The key role of spores in the epidemiology of clostridial disease

The pathogenic clostridia all have the ability to undergo a cellular morphogenesis process known as sporulation, which leads to the production of resistant spores. These metabolically dormant spores are resistant to factors such as heat and desiccation and thus enable the bacteria to survive adverse environmental conditions, until such time as conditions are more conducive to bacterial growth and multiplication. The production of spores plays a crucial role in the epidemiology of most clostridial infections because they avoid the need for metabolically active vegetative bacteria to be passed from one host animal to another.

For example, both tetanus and clostridial myonecrosis result from the contamination of wounds with dormant spores present in the soil. If localized ischemic conditions are found, such as in a deep wound (tetanus) or a traumatic wound where significant damage has occurred to the vasculature (myonecrosis), then the spores will germinate into vegetative cells which subsequently produce the toxins that result in cell and tissue damage. The sporulation process itself can also play a role in toxin production. CPE-producing strains of *C. perfringens* only produce CPE when they undergo sporulation, which often occurs in the gastrointestinal tract (Chapter 5). The release of the spore from the mother cell also results in the release of CPE into the lumen of the gut, where it can cause its pathological effects. The resultant diarrhea aids in the spread of the spores into the environment.

Conclusions

The pathogenic clostridia can cause a variety of neurotoxic, histotoxic, and enterotoxic infections in humans and domestic and wild animals. The common features of these diseases are:

1 They are all mediated by potent protein toxins that act at the host cell surface, form pores in the host cell membrane, or act at the cytoplasmic level in the host cell.
2 The production of environmentally resistant spores plays an important role in the epidemiology of these diseases.

Bibliography

Jackson, S., *et al.* (2006) Analysis of proline reduction in the nosocomial pathogen *Clostridium difficile*. *J. Bacteriol.*, **188:** 8487–8495.

Keyburn, A.L., *et al.* (2008) NetB, a new toxin that is associated with avian necrotic enteritis caused by *Clostridium perfringens*. *PLoS Path.*, **4:** e26.

Kovacs-Simon, A., *et al.* (2014) Lipoprotein CD0873 is a novel adhesin of *Clostridium difficile*. *J. Infect. Dis.*, **210:** 274–284.

Leffler, D.A., *et al.* (2015) *Clostridium difficile* infection. *New Engl. J. Med.*, **372:** 1539–1548.

Lyras, D., *et al.* (2009) Toxin B is essential for virulence of *Clostridium difficile. Nature,* **458:** 1176–1179.

Mehdizadeh Gohari, I., *et al.* (2015) A novel pore-forming toxin in type A *Clostridium perfringens* is associated with both fatal canine hemorrhagic gastroenteritis and fatal foal necrotizing enterocolitis. *PLoS One,* **10:** e0122684.

Peltier, J., *et al.* (2015) Cyclic-di-GMP regulates production of sortase substrates of *Clostridium difficile* and their surface exposure through ZmpI protease-mediated cleavage. *J. Biol. Chem.* doi: 10.1074/jbc.M1115.665091.

Popoff, M.R. (2014) Clostridial pore-forming toxins: Powerful virulence factors. *Anaerobe,* **30:** 220–238.

Pruitt, R.N. and Lacy, D.B. (2012) Toward a structural understanding of *Clostridium difficile* toxins A and B. *Front. Cell. Infect. Microbiol.,* **2:** 28.

Rood, J.I. (2007) *Clostridium perfringens* and histotoxic disease. In: Dworkin, M. *et al.* (eds) *The Prokaryotes: A handbook on the biology of bacteria,* pp. 753–770. Springer, New York.

Rood, J.I. *et al.* (2002) *Clostridium perfringens:* Enterotoxaemic Diseases. In: Sussman, M. (ed.) *Molecular Medical Microbiology,* pp. 1117–1139. Academic Press, London.

Sasi Jyothsna, T.S., *et al.* (2016) *Paraclostridium benzoelyticum* gen. nov. sp. nov., isolated from marine sediment and reclassification of *Clostridium bifermentans* as *Paraclostridium bifermentans* comb. nov. Proposal of a new genus *Paeniclostridium* gen. nov. to accommodate *Clostridium sordellii* and *Clostridium ghonii. Int. J. Syst. Evol. Microbiol.* ePub 05 January, 2016 doi: 10.1099/ijsem.0.000874.

Songer, J.G. (1996) Clostridial enteric diseases of domestic animals. *Clin. Microbiol. Rev.,* **9:** 216–234.

Songer, J.G. (2005) Clostridial diseases in domestic animals. In: Durre, P. (ed.) *Handbook on Clostridia,* pp. 527–542. Taylor and Francis, Boca Raton, FL.

Stackebrandt, E., *et al.* (1999) Phylogenetic basis for a taxonomic dissection of the genus *Clostridium. FEMS Immunol. Med. Microbiol.,* **24:** 253–258.

Uzal, F.A., *et al.* (2014) Towards an understanding of the role of *Clostridium perfringens* toxins in human and animal disease. *Future Microbiol.,* **9:** 361–377.

Van Immerseel, F., *et al.* (2009) Rethinking our understanding of the pathogenesis of necrotic enteritis in chickens. *Trends Microbiol.,* **17:** 32–36.

Yutin, N., *et al.* (2013) A genomic update on clostridial phylogeny: Gram-negative spore formers and other misplaced clostridia. *Environ. Microbiol.,* **15:** 2631–2641.

3

Brief Description of Animal Pathogenic Clostridia

John F. Prescott

A brief description of the main characteristics of the major clostridial pathogens of animals is given in Table 3.1. More details of these pathogens, the diseases they cause, details of their pathogenic mechanisms, details of the epidemiology of infection, and details of diagnosis of the diseases they cause are given in relevant chapters later in this book.

Clostridial Diseases of Animals, First Edition. Francisco A. Uzal, J. Glenn Songer,
John F. Prescott and Michel R. Popoff.
© 2016 John Wiley & Sons, Inc. Published 2016 by John Wiley & Sons, Inc.

Table 3.1 Summary of the main characteristics of the major clostridial pathogens of animals

Species	Morphology, cultural and other characteristics	Types	Major toxin(s)	Main disease(s)	Main source(s)	Main hosts affected
C. botulinum	0.6–1.6 × 3–20 μm; spores oval, ST[a], colonies 2–6- mm, β-hemolytic; motile; Geographic variation in distribution of the different types; C. botulinum is defined by production of antigenically different botulinum neurotoxins (BoNTs) encoded by mobile genetic elements, but consists of four distinct species. BoNT sequencing is identifying numerous toxin subtypes, variants; other BoNT-producing species (C. baratii, C. butyricum) can also cause botulism in humans	A	Botulinum toxin (BoNT) A	Botulism in many mammalian and avian species	Vegetables, fruit (meat, fish)	Humans, mink, chickens
		B	BoNT-B		Meat, pork products. vegetables, fish	Humans, horses, cattle
		Cα	BoNT-C₁		Vegetation, invertebrates, carrion	Waterfowl
		Cβ	BoNT-C₁, D		Spoiled feed, carrion	Horses, cattle, mink humans
		D	BoNT-D		Carrion, chicken manure	Cattle, sheep, chickens, horses, humans
		E	BoNT-E		Raw fish, marine mammals	Humans, fish, fish-eating birds
		F	BoNT-F		Meat, fish	Humans
		G	BoNT-G		Soil	Humans
C. chauvoei	0.5–1.7 × 1.6–10 μm; spores oval, C to ST[a], colonies 0.5–3 mm, β-hemolytic; motile	–	CctA (toxin A)	Blackleg in cattle and rarely sheep	Soil, intestine, latent in muscle of healthy animals (endogenous)	Numerous animal species, especially domesticated ruminants; dogs, rabbits (not humans)
C. colinum	1 × 3–4 μm, single or pairs; spores (if any) oval, ST[a], colonies pinpoint–0.5 mm; most α-hemolytic; motile	–	Unknown	Ulcerative enteritis of avian species	Intestinal tract quail, chickens, grouse, partridge, pheasants, turkey	Captive bobwhite quail most susceptible; other avian species (grouse, partridge, pheasants, turkeys, other birds including pigeons) less so

Species	Description		Toxins	Disease	Reservoir/Habitat	Hosts
C. difficile	0.5–2 × 3–17 μm; sometimes short chains; spores oval, ST[a], colonies 2–5 mm, circular or rhizoid, flat; motile; chartreuse green under UV light if grown on Brucella blood agar with vitamin K–hemin; para-cresol smell (of horse manure) is characteristic; CCFA[b] selective media effective for isolation from feces	—	TcdA, TcdB, large clostridial toxins (LCTs)	Necrotizing enterocolitis (often antibiotic-associated) in several mammalian species; pseudomembranous colitis in humans	Soil, large intestine and feces of animals, including herbivores and swine, manured soil; human and animal hospital environments; possibly fecally contaminated meats; rising rates of human and possibly animal infections associated with the epidemic strain (PFGE type NAP1, ribotype 027)	Numerous species, especially humans, animals with expanded large bowels (horses, swine, guinea-pigs, rabbits, gerbils, hamsters), but also calves, dogs, elephants, ratites, etc., especially if treated orally with broad-spectrum antibiotics
C. haemolyticum	0.6–1.6 × 2–18 μm, singly or in pairs; spores oval, ST[a], colonies 1–3 mm, raised to convex, gray, scalloped margin; β-hemolytic; motile	—	PLPC (beta toxin), identical to C. novyi beta toxin but produced in larger amounts	Bacillary hemoglobinuria (a necrotizing hepatitis) of cattle and rarely sheep	Ruminant digestive tract, latent in liver of healthy animals, soil	Cattle (and other ruminants); endemic regions; correlation with liver fluke which may cause spores in liver to germinate
C. novyi[a]	0.6–1.4 × 1.6–17 μm; spores oval, C to ST[a]; colonies 1–5 mm, circular or irregular, scalloped or rhizoid margin; β-hemolytic; motile; C. novyi type A and C. haemolyticum belong to same genospecies as C. botulinum group III	A	Alpha toxin, Rho GTPase glucosylating toxin	Gas gangrene (malignant edema) in several mammalian species	Soil, manured soil, marine sediments; intestine and liver of healthy ruminants	Cattle, sheep, horses, humans, other
	1–2.5 × 3–23 μm; spores oval, C to ST[a]; colonies 1–5 mm, circular or irregular, scalloped or rhizoid margin; β-hemolytic; motile	B	Alpha toxin, Rho GTPase glucosylating toxin; PLPC[c] (beta toxin)	Infectious necrotic hepatitis ("black disease") in sheep and rarely cattle	Soil, manured soil, marine sediments; intestine and liver of healthy ruminants and possibly horses	Sheep and cattle (rarely horses, swine, other species); associated with liver fluke activation of spores

Continued

Table 3.1 (Continued)

Species	Morphology, cultural and other characteristics	Types	Major toxin(s)	Main disease(s)	Main source(s)	Main hosts affected
C. perfringens	0.6–2 × 1.3–6 μm, single or pairs; spores rarely observed; colonies 2–5 mm, circular, gray, but colonial variants common; pilus-mediated "twitching" motility; commonly produces double zone of hemolysis (inner complete PFO[c], outer partial CPA[d]); very rapid growth, broad temperature range; occasional growth in air; SFP[e] selective medium sometimes used, not especially effective in fecal isolation	A	CPA (alpha-toxin)	Gas gangrene (malignant edema) in several mammalian species; yellow lamb disease in sheep	Soil, large intestine, manured soil, widespread in nature; specific toxin types are likely also specific host-associated, found in small and large bowel	All mammalian and avian species; the full range of C. perfringens-associated enteric diseases and their toxin-mediated basis is still being characterized
			CPE (enterotoxin)	Food-poisoning in humans; possible gastroenteritis in several mammalian species		Human food poisoning; possible gastroenteritis, including antibiotic-associated diarrhea in humans and possible other mammalian species
			NetB (necrotic enteritis B-like toxin) NetF (necrotic enteritis F-like toxin)	Necrotic enteritis in poultry Necrotizing and hemorrhagic enteritis in dogs and foals		Avian, especially chickens Foal necrotizing enteritis; dog hemorrhagic gastroenteritis
		B	CPB (beta-toxin), ETX (epsilon toxin)	Lamb dysentery		Lambs
		C	CPB (CPE may be synergistic)	Hemorrhagic and necrotizing enteritis mostly in neonatal individuals of several mammalian species		Neonatal calves, foals, lambs, piglets; necrotizing enteritis in humans ("pig-bel", "Darmbrand")

Species	Morphology	Type	Toxin	Disease	Source/Epidemiology	Host species
		D	ETX	Enterotoxemia in sheep, goats and cattle possible		Sheep, goats and rarely cattle
		E	ITX (iota toxin)	Bovine hemorrhagic gastroenteritis and possible enterotoxemia in rabbits		Possibly cattle and rabbits
C. piliforme	0.5 x 3–5 μm; typically palisaded clusters of short filaments in silver stained cells; obligate intracellular pathogen, only isolated using tissue culture or other eukaryotic cells	–	–	Tyzzer's disease (enterocolitis, hepatitis, myocarditis) in several mammalian and avian species	Infected animals, spread by fecal–oral route or transplacentally; little information available	Numerous species: cats, dogs, horses, gerbils, hamsters, HIV-infected humans, hares, monkeys, muskrats, rabbits, rats, etc.
C. septicum	0.6–2 x 2–35 μm; long filaments typical; pleomorphic; spores oval, ST^a; colonies 1–5 mm, circular, irregular edges, may swarm over agar; β-hemolytic, motile	–	Csa (alpha toxin), pore-forming toxin (same family as ETX of *C perfringens*)	Gas gangrene (malignant edema) in several mammalian species; avian cellulitis and gangrenous dermatitis; necrotizing abomasitis ("braxy") in sheep and cattle	Soil, large intestine, manured soil	Cattle, sheep, horses, humans, swine, turkeys, chickens, numerous other species

Continued

Table 3.1 (*Continued*)

Species	Morphology, cultural and other characteristics	Types	Major toxin(s)	Main disease(s)	Main source(s)	Main hosts affected
C. sordellii	0.5–1.7 x 1.5–20 μm; spores oval, C or ST[a]; colonies 1–4 mm, circular or irregular, margin variable; slightly β-hemolytic; motile	–	TcsL, large clostridial glucosylating toxin; TcsH, hemorrhagic toxin, Rho GTPase glucosylating toxin is produced by some strains	Gas gangrene (malignant edema) in several mammalian species; abomasitis of sheep; gastroenteritis in several mammalian species	Soil, large bowel, manured soil	Cattle, sheep, horses, humans, swine, turkeys, chickens, numerous other species; severe enteritis described in lions, sheep, quail.
C. spiroforme	0.3–0.5 x 2–10 μm; various degrees of coiling, often long chains of tight oils; non-motile; colonies 0.7–1.5 mm, circular, non-hemolytic	–	CST, binary toxin actin-ADP-ribosylating toxin family (as C. perfringens ITX)	Typhlocolitis of rabbits	Feces humans, ceca of chickens and rabbits	Rabbits
C. tetani	0.5–1.7 x 2–18 μm; spores usually round, T[a], motile, colonies 4–6 mm, irregular edges, matt or swarming; usually narrow zone β-hemolysis	–	TeNT, tetanospasmin, a zinc endopeptidase neurotoxin closely related to botulinum toxin	Tetanus in several mammalian species	Ubiquitous in soil; feces and animal manure, especially horses	All mammalian species; humans, horses, and sheep are especially susceptible to the toxin; disease follows infection of deep wounds; navel, or post-partum uterine infection; other wounds

[a] C: central; ST: subterminal; T: terminal.
[b] CCFA: cycloserine cefoxitin fructose agar.
[c] PFO: perfringolysin.
[d] CPA: Clostridium perfringens alpha toxin.
[e] SFP: Shahadi Ferguson perfringens.
[f] PLPC: phospholipase C.
[g] C. novyi type D has been reclassified as C. haemolyticum.

Bibliography

Giovanna, F., *et al.* (2011) Identification of novel linear megaplasmids carrying a β-lactamase gene in neurotoxigenic *Clostridium butyricum* type E strains. *PloS One*, **6:** e21706.

Hunt, J.J., *et al.* (2013) Variations in virulence and molecular biology among emerging strains of *Clostridium difficile*. *Microbiol. Mol. Biol. Rev.*, **77:** 567.

Keyburn, A.L., *et al.* (2008) NetB, a new toxin that is associated with avian necrotic enteritis caused by *Clostridium perfringens*. *PloS Pathogens*, **4:** e26.

Mehdizadeh, G.I., *et al.* (2015) A novel pore-forming toxin in type A *Clostridium perfringens* is associated with both fatal canine hemorrhagic gastroenteritis and fatal foal necrotizing enterocolitis. *PloS One*, **10:** e0122684.

Prescott, J.F. (2013) Clostridial infections. In: McVey, D.S. *et al.* (eds) *Veterinary Microbiology*, 3rd edition, p. 245. Wiley-Blackwell, Ames, IA.

Smith, T., *et al.* (2014) Historical and current perspectives on *Clostridium botulinum* biodiversity. *Res. Microbiol.*, **166:** 290–302.

Stiles, B.G., *et al.* (2014) *Clostridium* and *Bacillus* binary toxins: Bad for the bowels and eukaryotic being. *Toxins*, **6:** 2626.

Vidor, C., *et al.* (2014) Antibiotic resistance, virulence factors, and genetics of *Clostridium sordellii*. *Res. Microbiol.*, **166:** 368–374.

Wiegel, J. (2009) Family I. *Clostridiaceae*. In: De Vos, P. *et al.* (eds) *Bergey's Manual of Systematic Bacteriology*, p.736. Springer Science, New York.

Toxins Produced by the Pathogenic Clostridia

4

Toxins of Histotoxic Clostridia: *Clostridium chauvoei, Clostridium septicum, Clostridium novyi,* and *Clostridium sordellii*

Michel R. Popoff

Introduction

In animals, *Clostridium chauvoei, Clostridium novyi, Clostridium septicum,* and *Clostridium sordellii* are responsible for severe toxico-infections, which result mainly from wound contamination, except for *C. chauvoei* which can induce the so-called endogenous myositis (blackleg). These clostridia produce potent toxins that are the main virulence factors involved in the generation of lesions and clinical signs. *C. chauvoei* has more invasive properties than the other clostridia in this group.

Histotoxic clostridia produce an array of different toxins with various modes of action that contribute synergistically to the local and systemic lesions and symptoms. These toxins recognize a wide range of cell types including epithelial, muscle and red blood cells, and lymphocytes. They attack the cells in different ways: disorganization of the actin cytoskeleton and intercellular junctions, and membrane damage by pore formation through the membrane and/or degradation of membrane lipid bilayers. In addition, hydrolytic enzymes secreted by these bacteria such as DNase, protease, collagenase, and hyaluronidase amplify the tissue degradation initiated by the main toxins. A remarkable feature of the lesions produced by these histotoxic clostridia is the paucity or absence of the inflammatory response because of the cytotoxic effect of the toxins on the inflammatory cells and their inhibition of migration.

The toxins produced by the histotoxic clostridia can be divided into two families:

A. Those which are active intracellularly, causing perturbation of epithelial and endothelial barriers and then cell necrosis.

B. Those which are active on cell membranes, leading to the death of various cell types (Table 4.1).

Clostridial Diseases of Animals, First Edition. Francisco A. Uzal, J. Glenn Songer, John F. Prescott and Michel R. Popoff.
© 2016 John Wiley & Sons, Inc. Published 2016 by John Wiley & Sons, Inc.

Table 4.1 Main toxins and other virulence factors of histotoxic clostridia

Clostridium	Toxin	Toxin family	Molecular size (kDa)	Biological activity	Substrate	Cellular effects
C. sordellii	Lethal toxin (LT or TcsL)	LCGT	270.26	Glucosylation	Rho/Ras (UDP glucose)	Actin cytoskeleton and intercellular junction alterations Cell necrosis
	Hemorrhagic toxin (HT or TcsH)	LCGT	298.87	Glucosylation	Rho/Ras (UDP glucose)	Actin cytoskeleton and intercellular junction alterations Cell necrosis
	Sordellilysin	CDC	55.22	Pore formation		Cell necrosis
	Phospholipase	Phospholipase	45.58	Membrane damaging	Phosphatidyl-choline	Cell necrosis
	Neuraminidase		44.61			Leucocyte proliferation, leucocytose
	Collagenase					
C. novyi	Alpha toxin (TcnA)	LCGT	249.83	Glucosylation	Rho	Actin cytoskeleton and intercellular junction alterations Cell necrosis
	Beta toxin	Phospholipase C	45.87			Inflammation, edema, increased vascular permeability, muscle contraction
	Novyilysin	CDC		Pore formation	Cholesterol	Cell necrosis Hemolysis
	Phospholipase C	Phospholipase		Membrane damaging	Phosphatidyl-choline sphingomyelin	Hemolysis
C. septicum	Alpha toxin	β-PFT	49.71	Pore formation		Cell necrosis
	Septicolysin	CDC		Pore formation		Cell necrosis Hemolysis
C. chauvoei	CctA	β-PFT	35.51			Cell necrosis
	Chauveolysin	CDC		Pore formation	Cholesterol	Hemolysis
	Neuraminidase					
	Other virulence factors: DNase, hyaluronidase					

A – Intracellularly active toxins from histotoxic clostridia

The major toxins produced by *C. novyi* and *C. sordellii* belong to the large clostridial glucosylating toxin (LCGT) family. The LCGT family encompasses *C. novyi* alpha-toxin (TcnA), *C. sordellii* lethal toxin (TcsL), and hemorrhagic toxin (TcsH), as well as *Clostridium difficile* toxins A and B (TcdA and TcdB) and TpeL (toxin *C. perfringens* large cytotoxin) from *C. perfringens*. TcdB and TcsL are highly related (76% amino acid sequence identity) and are more distantly related to TcdA and TcnA (48–60% identity). These toxins target Rho- and/or Ras-GTPases.

Most *C. sordellii* isolates are non-toxic after isolation from human or animal patients with infection by this microorganism. Toxin genes are likely on plasmid or other mobile elements which are easily lost after sub-culturing. Most toxigenic *C. sordellii* strains contain only a functional *tcsL* gene and no or a truncated *tcsH* gene. Only a few strains produce both TcsL and TcsH. *tcsH* is located downstream from the *tcsL* gene, as in *C. difficile* where *tcdA* is downstream of *tcdB*, but *tcsH* is in the opposite orientation compared to *tcsL*. In contrast to *C. difficile*, which shows numerous genetic variations in toxin genes, only two variants of TcsL have been reported (TcsL-82 from IP82 and TcsL-9048 from VPI9048).

C. novyi strains are divided into types A, B, C, and D (the latter reclassified as *Clostridium haemolyticum*) which are closely related to *C. botulinum* group III (Chapter 1, Figure 1.1). The name of *C. novyi* sensu lato has been proposed to designate this group of strains. These strains contain numerous plasmids or circular prophages, but horizontal gene transfer between these strains mainly results from phage transduction. Like botulinum neurotoxin genes type C, D, or mosaic C/D, D/C, which are harbored by phages in *C. botulinum* group III, *tcnA* is located on *C. novyi* prophages and these phages can be interchanged between *C. botulinum* and *C. novyi*. However, TcnA is highly conserved (99% identity at the amino acid level) in the different *C. novyi* strains. In contrast, *C. novyi* beta-toxin is located on the chromosome and is produced mainly by *C. haemolyticum* and also by *C. novyi* type B (Table 4.2). Gamma toxin is reported to be a phospholipase but awaits further characterization.

Structure
LCGTs are single protein chains containing at least four functional domains (receptor binding, translocation, cysteine protease, and catalytic domains). The one-third C-terminal part exhibits multiple repeated sequences (31 short repeats and 7 long repeats in TcdA), which are involved in the recognition of a cell-surface receptor. A tri-saccharide (Gal-α1-3Gal-β1-4GlcNac) has been found to be the motif recognized by TcdA, but this motif is absent in humans. Related carbohydrates could be involved as TcdA receptor. A member of the heat shock protein family, gp96, has been proposed to bind TcdA to the plasma membrane of enterocytes. The receptor for the other large clostridial toxins has not been characterized. TcdA repeats consist of a β-hairpin followed by a loop and the

Table 4.2 Toxins of *Clostridium novyi* and *Clostridium haemolyticum*

C. novyi type	Alpha toxin (TcnA)	Beta toxin	Gamma toxin[1]	Disease
A	+	−	+	Gangrene humans, animals
B	+	+	−	Gangrene animals; Necrotizing hepatitis animals
C	−	−	+?	No disease reported
D (*C. haemolyticum*)	−	++	=	Bacillary hemoglobinuria animals

[1] Gamma toxin is reported to be a phospholipase and needs further characterization. +: toxin produced; ++ large amounts of toxin produced; -: no toxin produced.

carbohydrate-binding domain adopts a β-solenoid fold. Additionally, the intermediate LCGT part harbors an alternative receptor-binding domain.

The central part contains a hydrophobic segment and probably mediates the translocation of the toxin across the membrane. The enzymatic site characterized by the DxD motif surrounded by a hydrophobic region, and the substrate recognition domain are localized within the 543 N-terminal residues corresponding to the natural cleavage site in TcdB. The N-terminal catalytic domain is cleaved off through an auto-proteolytic process stimulated by inositol hexakisphosphate and released into the cytosol. Indeed, a cysteine protease site (D587, H653, C698 in TcdB) has been identified close to the cutting site.

The overall structure of the enzymatic domains of TcsL, TcdB, TcdA, and TcnA is conserved and consists of a β-strain central core (about 235 amino acids) forming an active center pocket surrounded by numerous α-helices (Figure 4.1). The structure of the central core is similar to that of the glucosyltransferase A family. The first aspartic residue of the DxD motif binds to ribosyl and glucosyl moieties of UDP-glucose and the second aspartic residue binds to a divalent cation (mainly Mn^{2+}) which increases the hydrolase activity and/or the binding of UDP-glucose. Other amino acids in TcdB with an essential role in enzymatic activity have been identified, such as Trp102, which is involved in the binding of UDP-glucose, Asp270, Arg273, Tyr284, Asn384, Trp520, as well as Ile383 and Glu385, important for the specific recognition of UDP-glucose. Differences in α-helices, insertions–deletions, probably account for the substrate specificity of each toxin. Chimeric molecules between TcdB and TcsL have been used to identify the sites of Rho-GTPase recognition. Amino acids 408 to 468 of TcdB ensure the specificity for Rho, Rac, and Cdc42, whereas in TcsL, the recognition of Rac and Cdc42 is mediated by residues 364 to 408, and that of Ras proteins by residues 408 to 516. The four N-terminal helices which mediate the binding of TcsL to phosphatidylserine, are possibly involved in membrane interaction. Amino acids 22–27 of Rho and Ras GTPases, which are part of the transition of the α1-helix to the switch I region, are the main domain recognized by the glucosylating toxins.

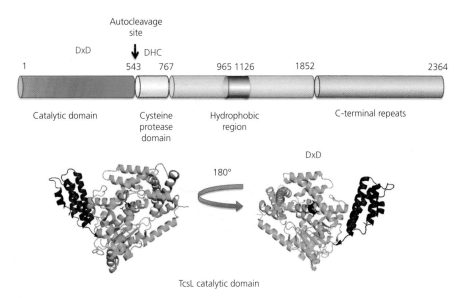

Figure 4.1 Domain organization and structure of the catalytic domain of large clostridial glucosylating toxins (LCGTs). TcsL is shown as a representative member of this toxin family. LCGTs contain C-terminal repeats involved in the recognition of the cell surface receptor and a central hydrophobic domain mediating the translocation of the N-terminal catalytic domain into the cytosol through the endosome membrane. The catalytic domain is cleaved from the rest of the molecule by an autocleavage process involving the cysteine protease domain which contains the active site DHC. The catalytic domain structure shows a compact core of β-sheet surrounded by numerous α-helices with central catalytic motif (DxD) and an extension of four N-terminal helices.

Mode of action

Large clostridial glucosylating toxins enter cells by receptor-mediated endocytosis. The cytotoxic effects are blocked by endosomal and lysosomal acidification inhibitors (monensin, bafilomycin A1, ammonium chloride) and the inhibiting effects can be bypassed by an extracellular acidic pulse. This indicates that the large glucosylating clostridial toxins translocate from early endosomes upon an acidification step. At low pH, TcdA, TcdB, and TcsL induce channel formation in cell membranes and artificial lipid bilayers, and show an increase in hydrophobicity, as determined with fluorescence methods. Membrane cholesterol seems critical for TcdA pore formation. This process probably involves a conformational change and insertion of the toxin into the membrane, possibly mediated by the hydrophobic segment of the central domain, but the exact mode of translocation remains to be determined. The N-terminal domain is then delivered into the cytosol by an auto-proteolytic activity stimulated by inositol hexakisphosphate. A cysteine protease domain has been identified close to the cutting site in TcdB (amino acids 544–955), which is conserved in all large clostridial toxins.

Large glucosylating clostridial toxins catalyze the glucosylation of Rho- and/or Ras-GTPases from UDP-glucose, except TcnA, which uses UDP-N-acetylglucosamine as co-substrate. TcdA and TcdB glucosylate Rho, Rac, and Cdc42 at Thr-37, whereas LT glucosylates Ras at Thr-35, and Rap, Ral, and Rac at Thr-37 (Table 4.3). The large glucosylating clostridial toxins cleave the co-substrate and transfer the glucose moiety to the acceptor amino acid of the Rho proteins. The conserved Thr, which is glucosylated, is located in switch I. Thr-37/35 is involved in the coordination of Mg^{2+} and subsequently in the binding of the β and γ phosphates of GTP. The hydroxyl group of Thr-37/35 is exposed to the surface of the molecule in its GDP-bound form, which is the only accessible substrate of glucosylating toxins. The nucleotide binding of glucosylated Ras by LT is not grossly altered, but the GEF activation of GDP forms is decreased. Glucosylation of Thr-35 completely prevents the recognition of the downstream effector, blocking the G-protein in the inactive form. The crystal structure of Ras modified by LT shows that glucosylation prevents the formation of the GTP conformation of the effector loop of Ras, which is required for the interaction with the effector Raf. Similar results were found with RhoA glucosylated by ToxB. In addition, glucosylation of GTPase slightly reduces the intrinsic GTPase activity, completely inhibits GAP-stimulated GTP hydrolysis, and leads to accumulation of the GTP-bound form of Rho at the membrane where it is tightly bound.

Cellular effects

Large clostridial glucosylating toxins induce cell rounding by inactivating Rho proteins, resulting in loss of actin stress fibers, reorganization of the cortical actin, disruption of the intercellular junctions, and thus an increase in cell barrier permeability. Rac inactivation is a major player in actin cytoskeleton disorganization. Indeed, TcsL and the other LCGTs induce paxilline dephosphorylation in a Rac-dependent manner, leading to disassembly of the focal adhesions, adherens junctions, and actin filament disorganization. TcdA and TcdB disrupt apical and basal actin filaments and subsequently disorganize the ultrastructure and component distribution (ZO-1, ZO-2, occludin, claudin) of tight junctions, whereas E-cadherin junctions show little alteration. In contrast, TcsL, which only modifies Rac among the Rho proteins, alters the permeability of intestinal cell monolayers, causing a redistribution of E-cadherin, whereas tight junctions are not significantly affected. *In vivo*, LT causes a marked edema in the cardio-respiratory system by altering E-cadherin junctions of lung endothelial cells.

TcdB and TcdA induce apoptosis as a consequence of Rho glucosylation and caspase activation or possibly cell necrosis. TcdB and TcsL may cause apoptosis by targeting mitochondria. In addition to the effects on the cytoskeleton, the inactivation of Rho proteins impairs many other cellular functions such as endocytosis, exocytosis, lymphocyte activation, immunoglobulin-mediated phagocytosis in macrophages, NADPH oxidase regulation, smooth muscle contraction, phospholipase D activation, activation of the pro-apoptotic RhoB, and transcriptional activation mediated by JNK, and/or p38. RhoB has been found to exhibit pro-apoptotic activity in apoptosis induced by those LCGTs that preferably glucosylate Rho-GTPases (including TcsH, TcdA, and TcdB). In contrast, RhoB exhibits cytoprotective activity in apoptosis induced by TcsL, which preferably glucosylates

Table 4.3 Substrate specificity of *Clostridium sordellii* and *Clostridium novyi* large toxins (Genth *et al.*, 2014)

Toxin	Substrate															
	RhoA	RhoB	RhoC	RhoG	Rac1	Cdc42	TC10	TCL	H-Ras	N-Ras	K-Ras	Rap2a	RalC	R-Ras1	R-Ras2	R-Ras3
TcsL-82	+	+	–	+	+++	–	+	+	+++	+++	+++	+++	++	++	++	++
TcsL-9048	+	+	+	+	+++	+	++	++	++	++	++	++	++	–	–	+
TcnA	+++	+++	+	+	+++	++	++	++	–	–	–	–	–	–	–	–
TcsH-9048	++	++	++	+	+++	++	+	+	+	+	+	++	+	–	+	–

Ras-GTPases. The effect of RhoB seems to depend on the background of the activity of other GTPases. In a background of inactive RhoA and almost active Ras (such as in cells treated with TcsH, TcdA, or TcdB), RhoB exhibits pro-apoptotic activity, whereas on a background of active RhoA but inactive Ras, RhoB exerts cytoprotective activity (such as in cells treated with TcsL).

TcdA and TcdB produce a severe inflammatory response in the mammalian intestine characterized by epithelial cell necrosis and massive infiltration with inflammatory cells. In monocytes, TcdA stimulates cytokine (TNF-α, IL-1β, IL-6, and IL-8) release and activation of p38 MAP kinase, whereas the activation of ERK and JNK is only transient. p38 activation is required for IL-8 production, IL-1β release, monocyte necrosis, and intestinal mucosa inflammation. TcdA-induced p38 activation could be mediated by toxin binding to a membrane receptor independently of Rho-GTPase glucosylation. TcdB also induces an inflammatory response including the production of Il-8 via EGF receptor and ERK activation. Other Rho-independent cellular effects induced by TcdA include the activation of NF-kB and subsequent release of IL-8 and possibly other inflammatory cytokines, mitochondrial damage, apoptosis, and activation of a neuro-immune pathway. TcsL also activates JNK independently of small GTPase glucosylation, but JNK activation facilitates target glucosylation by TcsL.

Unlike TcdA and TcdB, TcsL modifies Ras and blocks the MAP-kinase cascade and phospholipase D regulation. However, the implication of the blockade of this cellular pathway in cytotoxicity has not been demonstrated. PLD inhibition by these toxins is restored by RalA. It has been shown that RalA and ARF directly interact with PLD1, but the mode of action of RalA in PLD activity is still unknown.

B – Membrane-damaging toxins from histotoxic clostridia

Membrane-damaging toxins encompass the pore-forming toxins (PFTs) and the toxins that enzymatically cleave membrane compounds such as phospholipases. Many proteins, including toxins, are able to induce a pore through a membrane. This highly damaging action is possibly the reason why PFTs are the largest class of bacterial protein toxins. Almost one-third of bacterial protein toxins, including clostridial toxins, are PFTs. According to their structure, PFTs can be divided into two main classes: the α-PFTs and the β-PFTs. Clostridial PFTs belong mainly to the β-PFT family and are important virulence factors.

β-PFTs share a common basic mechanism of action. They are secreted as soluble monomers that diffuse in the extra-bacterial environment and recognize specific receptor(s) on the surface of target cells. Clustering of β-PFT monomers on the cell surface promotes their oligomerization and conformational change of one or two amphipathic β-sheet(s) from each monomer, which assemble and form a β-barrel, also called the pre-pore. Insertion of the pre-pore into the lipid

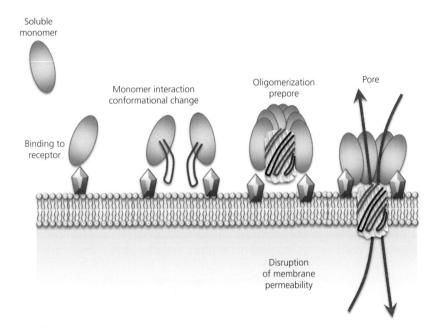

Figure 4.2 General model of β-pore-forming toxin (β-PFT) mechanism of action. The secreted soluble monomers recognize specific cell-surface receptor(s), assemble, oligomerize, unfold amphipathic β-hairpin(s), which form a pre-pore and then insert into the membrane. Reprinted with permission from Popoff (2014) *Anaerobe*, **30**: 220–238.

bilayer results in pore formation and subsequent alteration of the membrane permeability (Figure 4.2).

According to their structure, clostridial β-PFTs able to form a pore in a plasma membrane can be classified into three families:
1 Cholesterol-dependent cytolysins (CDCs);
2 Heptameric β-PFTs including the aerolysin family;
3 *Staphylococcus aureus* α-hemolysin family.

Families 1 and 2 will be discussed here. Family 3 of the β-PFT family, which includes *C. perfringens* delta, beta, and beta2 toxins, and NetB, is mainly involved in enteric diseases and is, therefore, beyond the scope of this chapter.

1 – Cholesterol-dependent cytolysins

The CDC family encompasses toxins which are produced by numerous Gram-positive bacteria such as listeriolysin O of *Listeria monocytogenes*, pneumolysin of *Streptococcus pneumoniae*, and streptolysin O (SLO) from *Streptococcus pyogenes*. Various clostridia (*C. botulinum*, *C. perfringens*, *C. tetani*) produce CDC, including all the histotoxic clostridia (Table 4.1). The members of this toxin family exhibit 40–80% identity at the primary structure and share common biological properties and structural characteristics.

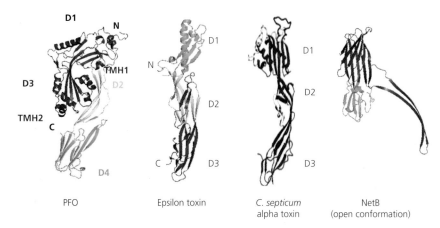

PFO   Epsilon toxin   C. septicum   NetB
                                           alpha toxin   (open conformation)

Figure 4.3 Structure of representative clostridial pore-forming toxins: *C. perfringens* perfringolysin (PFO), *C. perfringens* epsilon toxin (ETX), *C. septicum* alpha toxin (ATX, structure modeling based on sequence relatedness with epsilon toxin), and *C. perfringens* NetB. Note that PFO contains two transmembrane hairpins (TMH) shown in their helical conformation, and that ETX, ATX, and NetB contain only one TMH. Domains in green are the receptor-binding domains.

Structure of cholesterol-dependent cytolysins

The prototype of the CDC family is the perfringolysin (PFO) from *C. perfringens*. PFO is synthesized with a 27-amino-acid signal peptide, and the mature protein consists of 472 amino acids (53 kDa). PFO has an unusual elongated rod shape (Figure 4.3). The molecule is rich in β-sheets and it is hydrophilic without significant patches of hydrophobic residues on the surface. Four domains can be distinguished in the PFO molecule. Domain 1 has a seven-stranded antiparallel β-sheet and is connected to domain 4 by the elongated domain 2. Domain 3 consists of β-sheets and α-helices. The C-terminal part (domain 4) folds into a separate and compact β-sandwich domain and contains three loops (L1–L3), which are involved in the binding to cholesterol. Molecular modeling shows that cholesterol binding to this region induces a displacement of a Trp-rich loop. It is proposed that the high affinity (Kd 10–9 M) of PFO and of other CDCs for the cholesterol receptor is involved in concentrating the toxin in cholesterol molecules organized in arcs on the target membrane, thus promoting oligomerization and membrane insertion. Cholesterol is clustered in membrane microdomains enriched in certain lipids (cholesterol, sphingolipids) or rafts, and PFO is a useful tool to identify the membrane rafts.

Mode of action of cholesterol-dependent cytolysins

The proposed model of PFO pore formation includes the binding of water-soluble PFO monomers to the cholesterol of the lipid bilayer mediated by the L1–L3 loops from domain 4 (Figure 4.3). Conformational change of domain 4 on binding to cholesterol induces transition states through the molecule to the distant domains 1 and 3, thus permitting the oligomerization and unfolding of transmembrane hairpins, leading to formation of the pre-pore. The mechanism of allosteric PFO activation dependent on binding to cholesterol controls monomer interactions and pore formation when the toxin is in close contact with the cell membrane, thus avoiding formation of premature and non-productive toxin associations. A conserved undecapeptide motif among CDCs, also known as the Trp-rich loop, located at the tip of the D4 domain, plays a critical role in the allosteric coupling of membrane binding of D4 to structural change of the D3 domain. PFO monomers bound to cholesterol and orientated perpendicularly to the membrane assemble and oligomerize to form a pre-pore complex. Oligomers consist of 40 to 50 monomers forming large arcs and rings on the membrane surface. Oligomer formation results from domain 3–domain 3 interaction via hydrogen bonding between a β1-strand of one subunit and a β4-strand of a second subunit. Interaction of domain 4 with cholesterol induces a conformational change in domain 1. Thereby, PFO monomers do not oligomerize in solution even at high concentrations. In addition, conformational change in the organization of domains 2 and 3 promotes the exposure of hydrohobic residues and the insertion of a transmembrane β-barrel into the lipid bilayer. A bundle of three α-helices of domain 3 unfolds to form two amphipathic α-sheets. Each monomer uses two amphipathic β-hairpins for the formation of the transmembrane β-barrel (Figure 4.3). Monomers do not insert their transmembrane hairpins individually, but rather cooperation between PFO monomers is required to drive the insertion of the pre-pore complex, a process which appears to be all-or-nothing. The pre-pore complex remains localized above the lipid bilayer. A vertical collapse of the pre-pore of 40 Å allows the insertion of the β-barrel into the membrane and formation of a large membrane pore 300–450 Å in diameter. The charged face of domain 4 amphipathic β-hairpin forms the inner lining of the pore and the other face is protected from the hydrophobic part of the lipid bilayer by cholesterol molecules.

Role of cholesterol-dependent cytolysins in pathogenesis

Clostridial CDCs are mainly involved in gangrene lesions by contributing to tissue destruction and preventing bacterial lysis by host immune cells. It is noteworthy that clostridia responsible for gangrene produce a CDC and also other membrane-damaging toxin(s) such as another PFT or a phospholipase, as well as additional hydrolytic enzymes (Table 4.1). Thus, clostridial CDCs act synergistically with other membrane-damaging toxin(s) to generate gangrene lesions. Indeed, using *C. perfringens* mutant strains defective either on the PFO or alpha-toxin gene, a synergistic effect between PFO and alpha-toxin has been evidenced in experimental *C. perfringens* gangrene.

Among clostridial CDCs, PFO is the best characterized regarding its mode of activity. By forming large pores on the plasma membrane, PFO induces cell lysis by a colloid osmotic mechanism. Although PFO can induce or interfere with cell signaling such as the SUMOylation pathway, its main activity resides in alteration of the membrane integrity. A hallmark of clostridial gangrene lesions caused by *C. perfringens* and other histotoxic clostridia is the total absence of inflammatory cells at the site of infection. At high concentration, PFO is cytotoxic for polymorphonuclear leucocytes (PMNL) and macrophages. At lower concentrations, PFO impairs the respiratory burst, superoxide anion production, and phagocytosis of complement opsonized particles in PMNL. In addition, *C. perfringens* can survive in macrophages, and PFO has a major role in the escape of the bacteria from the phagosome by lysis of the endosome membrane and in macrophage cytotoxicity.

At the periphery of the necrotic lesions, sub-lethal concentrations of PFO reduce the migration of PMNL/macrophages and induce their adherence to endothelial cells. PFO upregulates the expression/activation of adherence molecules such as neutrophil CD11b/CD18, endothelial adherence molecules, platelet activating factor (PAF), and subsequent phospholipase A2 synthesis. Moreover, PFO prevents actin filament polymerization in leucocytes and migration of neutrophils in response to chemoattractant. Accumulation of PMNL and macrophages in the vessels around the site of infection and inhibition of their migration mostly contribute to the lack of inflammatory response. In addition, PFO synergistically with *C. perfringens* alpha toxin triggers platelet/platelet and platelet/leucocyte aggregation through activation of the platelet fibrinogen receptor gpIIb/IIIa. PFO also stimulates the expression of intercellular adherence molecule 1 (ICAM-1) in endothelial cells, but to a much lesser extent than *C. perfringens* alpha toxin. These events result in the formation of intravascular platelet/leucocyte/fibrin aggregates, leading to vessel obstruction and reduced blood flow in the microvasculature, in turn leading to necrosis. Adherence of the aggregates to the vascular endothelial cells leads to vascular injury and subsequently contributes to the impairment of leucocyte migration by diapedesis and tissue hypoxia.

The late stage of clostridial gangrene is characterized by cardiovascular collapse, tachycardia, low blood pressure, and multi-organ failure (Figure 4.4). Toxins such as PFO and alpha toxin are released into the blood circulation and act at a distance from the site of infection on the cardiovascular system. Notably, PFO reduces the systemic vascular resistance and increases the cardiac output, decreasing the heart rate without a drop in mean arterial pressure. PFO also contributes indirectly to the toxic shock (hypotension, hypoxia, reduced cardiac output) by promoting the release of inflammatory cytokines and by acting synergistically with *C. perfringens* alpha toxin.

It seems likely that the CDCs produced by *C. chauvoei*, *C. novyi*, *C. septicum*, and *C. sordellii* also share a similar synergistic role to PFO with the other tissue-damaging toxins in the pathogenesis of gangrene lesions.

2 – Heptameric β-pore-forming toxins from histotoxic clostridia

The heptameric β-PFTs are an important group of clostridial β-PFTs. In contrast to CDCs, they associate in smaller oligomers, heptamers or, to a lesser extent, hexamers or octamers, leading to the formation of small pores in the membrane. Whereas all CDCs recognize a unique cell-surface receptor, mainly cholesterol, heptameric β-PFTs bind to distinct receptor(s). Therefore, they are active on different subsets of cell types and are responsible for specific diseases. Clostridial heptameric β-PFTs are involved in myonecrosis and also in intestinal diseases.

- tegument or mucosa effraction
- Spore contamination

Clostridial proliferation
pH ↗
Redox potential ↗
Toxin and gas production

Local clostridial proliferation
continuous toxin production
extension of the local lesions

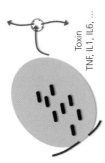

Toxin
TNF, IL1, IL6, …

Traumatic lesion
- Interruption of blood supply, hypoxia
- Drop in oxydation reduction potential
- Release of nutrients from injured cells

Spore germination
- Bacterial growth in anaerobic conditions
- Resistance to macrophages

Toxins at cytotoxic concentration
- Killing of immune cells
- Cell necrosis, tissue destruction
- Absence of inflammatory cells

Toxins at sublethal concentration
(periphery of local lesions)
- Inhibition of neutrophil/macrophage migration
- Inhibition of Phagocytosis
- leucocyte/platelet aggregation microvessel obstruction
- Endothelial cell injury
- Ischemia

Toxin in blood circulation
release of cytokines from macrophages, platelets, endothelial cells
- Cardiovascular collapse
- Multiorgan failure
- Shock

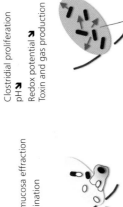

Figure 4.4 Main steps in the pathogenesis of clostridial gangrenes. Reprinted (slightly modified) with permission from Popoff (2014) *Anaerobe*, **30**: 220–238.

Based on their structure, clostridial heptameric β-PFTs are divided into two families: the aerolysin family and the *S. aureus* α-hemolysin family. Alpha toxin (ATX) from *C. septicum* is related to β-PFTs of the aerolysin family, whereas *C. chauvoei* toxin A (CctA) is part of the *S. aureus* α-hemolysin family.

ATX – a β-PFT of the aerolysin family

C. septicum alpha toxin (ATX) is the main virulence factor of this bacterium. ATX is hemolytic, dermonecrotic, and lethal, and shares a low level (27%) of amino acid sequence identity with aerolysin. ATX belongs to the aerolysin β-PFT family and it is secreted by means of an N-terminal signal peptide (31 amino acids) as an inactive prototoxin of 412 amino acids, which is proteolytically activated by removing 45 C-terminal amino acids (propeptide). Various proteases, such as trypsin and proteinase K, can activate ATX, but furin, a cell-surface protease, seems to be the main activator *in vivo*. Genetic variations have been observed in *atx* (7 patterns with 98.3–99.3% identity at the nucleotide level) according to *C. septicum* strains, but all ATX variants retain equivalent biological activity and immunogenicity.

The structure of ATX has not yet been resolved, but according to amino acid sequence homology with aerolysin, notably the high degree of similarity (72%) among domains 2–4 of aerolysin with ATX, a molecular model of ATX has been proposed.

β-PFTs from the aerolysin family exhibit a more elongated shape than PFO (Figure 4.3). They consist of three to four domains and associate mainly in heptamers, and the hallmark of this PFT family is that each monomer deploys only one β-hairpin to form the transmembrane β-barrel.

Aerolysin is an L-shaped molecule rich in β-structure with a small N-terminal lobe (domain 1) and a big, elongated lobe spilled across three more domains (2 to 4) with the characteristic feature of the presence of long β-strands (Figure 4.5). Domains 1 and 2 are involved in the recognition of GPI-anchored proteins through a double binding mechanism, leading to high affinity interaction of aerolysin with its receptor. Domain 1 binds to N-linked sugar of the protein part of GPI-anchored proteins and domain 2 to the glycan core. Domain 2, together with domain 3, is involved in the oligomerization process. Domain 4 is located on the tip of the major lobe and contains the C-terminal peptide that is released upon proteolytic cleavage. Removal of the propeptide probably induces a conformational change and reorganization of the domains that facilitates the formation of oligomers.

ATX, like the other clostridial β-PFTs of the aerolysin family including *C. perfringens* epsilon toxin (ETX), lacks the aerolysin domain 1. ATX consists of three domains (D1, D2, D3) which are homologous to the D2, D3, and D4 domains of aerolysin, respectively. The N-terminal domain 1 of ATX is involved in the interaction with the receptor. A C-terminal tryptophan motif (WDWxW) located in ATX domain 1 is critical for the binding to the GPI-anchored protein receptor. Similarly, a tryptophan-rich region has an equivalent position in domain 2 of aerolysin and is also involved in the interaction with the receptors. Although ATX and aerolysin retain the same WDWxW motif, the flanking sequences in

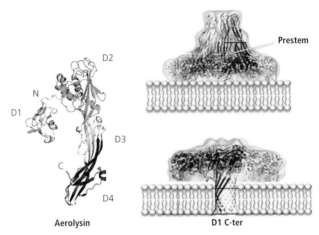

Figure 4.5 Aerolysin monomer and schematic representation of the pore formation according to Degiacomi *et al.* (2013). Binding receptor sites are localized in domains 1 and 2. The transmembrane hairpin in domain D3 is in red. Upon binding to their receptor, monomers heptamerize and form a pre-pore showing an inverted mushroom shape, of which domains 1 and 2 constitute the cap. Then the stalk, which is comprised of domains 3 and 4, rotates and completely collapses, and the β-barrel extends in the opposite orientation to that of the stalk in the pre-pore conformation. Two monomers (red and blue) are shown in the heptameric structure. Clostridial β-PFTs including *C. perfringens* epsilon toxin and *C. septicum* alpha toxin are supposed to use a similar mechanism of pore formation. Reprinted (slightly modified) with permission from Popoff (2014) *Anaerobe*, **30**: 220–238.

aerolysin (GEVKWWDWNWT) and ATX (GYSEWDWKWV) are not identical, suggesting that the two toxins recognize distinct receptors. Indeed, ATX recognizes GPI-anchored proteins as receptors, which are mostly different from those interacting with aerolysin. However, both toxins share two common receptors, Thy-1 and contactin. In contrast to aerolysin, the N-glycan of anchored proteins is not important for binding to ATX.

Domains 2 and 3 of ETX and ATX are involved in oligomerization and maintenance of the oligomers. Domain 3 of aerolysin and domain 2 of ATX contain the membrane-spanning β-hairpin. In aerolysin, the transmembrane region consists of 20 amino acids forming two amphipathic β-sheets connected by a hydrophobic 5-amino-acid-long stretch which folds in an amphipathic β-hairpin upon oligomerization and membrane insertion. The hydrophobic turn of the β-hairpin is thought to drive membrane insertion and folds back after membrane crossing in a rivet-like fashion, thereby anchoring the β-barrel in the membrane. Hydrophobic residues also lie in the interconnection between the two amphipathic β-strands in ATX.

Mode of action of ATX

The first step for β-PFTs of the aerolysin family, as for the other PFTs, is binding to the cell-surface receptor. After binding to its receptor, located by domain 1 in lipid rafts, the protoxin is cleaved to the active form (41 kDa) by furin and possibly by other cell proteases. When the toxin is activated in solution, the monomers aggregate into non-functional complexes, but when the toxin is activated after its binding to the membrane, it forms very active oligomers. The propeptide remains associated with the toxin by non-covalent interactions even after the proteolytic cleavage. The propeptide is displaced when the monomers associate in oligomers by strong interactions. Thus, the propeptide probably stabilizes an unstable conformation and facilitates the correct assembly of oligomers on the cell membrane.

The binding step to the receptor has been analyzed for ETX and ATX labeled with a photostable nanoparticle (Europiun). Toxin monomers bound to their receptor are mobile on the cell surface but only in confined areas corresponding to lipid rafts. Indeed, ETX and ATX receptors are localized in lipid rafts. The confinement seems to be mainly due to the composition and spatial organization of the lipids around the proteins and subsequent molecular interactions (local electrostatic interactions, hydrophobic interactions, lipid–protein specific and/or non-specific interactions) in the lipid rafts. Thereby, membrane depletion in cholesterol or sphingolipids results in the release of confinement, and ETX and ATX bound to their receptors move in a wider area. The actin and microtubule cytoskeleton is not directly involved in ETX and ATX mobility. However, even though the toxin receptors are not directly linked to actin filaments, other lipid raft proteins are connected to the actin cytoskeleton, which mediates the displacement of the whole lipid raft in the membrane. The mobility of toxin monomers bound to their receptors in confined areas leads to a concentration of toxin molecules and facilitates their interactions and subsequent oligomerization. Oligomerization occurs prior to the insertion of the resulting complexes into the membrane. Activated monomers bound to their GPI-anchored protein receptor diffuse laterally in the membrane, permitting interaction with other monomers and the formation of oligomers, organized in a pre-pore which inserts into the lipid membrane to form a functional pore. Important residues for monomer–monomer interaction have been identified in domains 2 and 3. The amphipathic β-hairpin (amino acids 203–232) from domain 2 has been characterized as the membrane-spanning segment, which associates with those of the other monomers to form the β-barrel. A conformational change, including a domain 2 collapse, facilitates the insertion of the β-barrel into the membrane in a similar manner to the other β-PFTs. A loop from domain 1 interacting with the membrane surface, and/or with the receptor, controls the insertion of the β-barrel. ATX forms pores in lipid bilayers estimated to be 1.3–1.6 nm in diameter, similar in size to other related toxins. ATX pores are slightly anion selective, as are aerolysin and ETX. Pore formation is absolutely required for cytotoxicity and for *in vivo C. septicum* ATX-mediated myonecrosis.

Pore formation has been resolved at the structural level with aerolysin. Aerolysin heptamer adopts a mushroom shape similar to that of α-hemolysin (see below). However, in contrast to *S. aureus* α-hemolysin, aerolysin heptamer associates with the membrane in an inverse orientation, the mushroom cap facing the membrane and the stalk in the extracellular milieu, since domains 1 and 2, which bind to the receptor, are located in the cap. Then, the heptamer undergoes a vertical collapse. Domains 3 and 4 rotate and flatten completely, and the β-hairpin from domain 3 moves through a cavity between two monomers. The β-hairpins of the seven monomers refold in a β-barrel which lies in the opposite orientation to that of the pre-pore mushroom stalk and which inserts into the membrane (Figure 4.5). In contrast, CDCs and α-hemolysin show no drastic conformational change during the pre-pore to pore conversion.

ATX is cytotoxic for a wide range of sensitive cells and induces a rapid and drastic decrease in cell monolayer integrity. ATX shares a similar mechanism of cytotoxicity to ETX, which has been investigated in more detail. The cytotoxicity is associated with pore formation and a rapid loss of intracellular potassium together with an increase in chloride and sodium ions, whereas the increase in calcium occurs later. In addition, the loss of viability also correlates with the entry of propidium iodide, indicating that ATX and ETX form pores in cell membranes. ATX and ETX cause a rapid cell death by necrosis characterized by a marked reduction in nucleus size without DNA fragmentation. Toxin-dependent cell signaling leading to cell necrosis is not yet fully understood but includes ATP depletion, AMP-activated protein kinase stimulation, mitochondrial membrane permeabilization, and mitochondrial-nuclear translocation of apoptosis-inducing factor, which is a potent caspase-independent cell death factor. The early and rapid loss of intracellular potassium induced by ETX and ATX seems to be the early event leading to cell necrosis. Change in cell membrane permeability with potassium, calcium, and ATP as the main signaling molecules is a common feature of PFTs.

In addition, ATX activates in cultured cells, such as Vero cells, the three MAPK pathways: ERK (extracellular-signal-regulated kinase), JNK (C-jun N-terminal kinase), and p38, in a pore-dependent, calcium-dependent, and Ras-c-Raf-dependent (for ERK) and -independent (for JNK and p38) manner, leading to the release of the pro-inflammatory cytokine TNF-α which contributes to the ATX-induced cell necrosis. In an *in vivo* mouse model, local infection by toxigenic or non-toxigenic *C. septicum* resulted in MAPK activation and TNF-α release at the site of infection. Other bacterial products such as peptidoglycan and lipotechoic acid can stimulate the MAPK pathways. However, MAPK activation and TNF-α release at a distance from the site of infection, such as the spleen, are only mediated by ATX which disseminates by the blood circulation. Systemic release of pro-inflammatory cytokines contributes to cell death and leucopenia as well as to the toxic shock observed in *C. septicum* infections.

Role of ATX in pathogenesis

ATX is involved in gas gangrene and also in non-traumatic myonecrosis of the intestinal mucosa, which occurs in patients with intestinal malignancy, neutropenia, leukemia, or diarrhea. This infection is accompanied by profound shock, is fulminant and often fatal. The precise mode of action of ATX in these pathologies is not well understood. ATX might target vascular endothelial cells, which could result in the extravasation of fluid from the circulatory system and subsequent shock. In animals, *C. septicum* is responsible for gas gangrene (malignant edema), necrotizing abomasitis (braxy), and possibly enterotoxemia (Chapters 17 and 20).

Other *C. septicum* toxins

C. septicum produces a hemolysin (septicolysin) from the CDC family. Septicolysin probably has a synergistic effect with ATX in the pathogenesis of the local necrotic lesions of myonecrosis and of leucopenia, similar to that observed with PFO. *C. septicum* also produces the potential virulence factors such as DNase, hyaluronidase, protease, and neuraminidase.

C. chauvoei CctA

Whole-genome sequencing of *C. chauvoei* identified a gene encoding for a protein of 317 amino acids with a signal peptide of 29 residues. The secreted protein consists of 288 amino acids with a molecular mass of 32.3 kDa and pI of 5.43. The protein named CctA shares 44% identity (60% similarity) with *C. perfringens* NetB, 33% (51% similarity) with *C. perfringens* beta toxin, and 28% (50% similarity) with *S. aureus* alpha toxin. Therefore, CctA is related to the β-PFTs of the *S. aureus* alpha toxin family, which encompasses clostridial β-PFTs (beta, beta2, delta toxins, NetB, NetF), but also staphylococcal and streptotococcal toxins (alpha-toxin, leucocidins). CctA has been found to be cytotoxic for epithelial cells and strongly hemolytic with sheep red blood cells.

CctA probably shares a similar molecular structure and mode of action with those of the *S. aureus* alpha toxin family. The structure of NetB, a representative toxin from this family, is shown in Figure 4.3.

NetB (33 kDa) (Chapter 5), like staphylococcal α-hemolysin (33 kDa), is secreted via a signal peptide. The proteins are water soluble and do not undergo further proteolytic cleavage. α-hemolysin, NetB, and delta toxin are organized in three structural domains: an N-terminal β-sandwich domain formed of two six-stranded anti-parallel β-sheets, a C-terminal rim domain that is rich in β-strands, and a central domain called a stem (Figure 4.3). A hallmark of α-hemolysin and related β-PFTs is that the central stem domain of monomers contains three short β-strands packed against the β-sandwich domain. In addition, the heptameric assembly of NetB retains a similar conformation to that of α-hemolysin pre-pore. However, the rim domain of delta toxin and NetB exhibit significant sequence and conformation differences to those of α-hemolysin. Since the α-hemolysin rim domain is involved in binding to the cell-surface receptor(s), these rim differences support the theory that NetB, delta toxin, and α-hemolysin recognize distinct receptors. Indeed, CctA interacts with a protein receptor (see below) and delta toxin uses the ganglioside GM2 as receptor. The NetB receptor is still unknown but could be membrane cholesterol.

Mode of action of *C. chauvoei* **CctA**

The mode of pore formation through a lipid bilayer has been investigated at the structural level with staphylococcal α-hemolysin. Based on their structural relatedness with α-hemolysin, clostridial β-PFTs including CctA, likely retain the same mode of activity. The first step of intoxication consists of the binding of α-hemolysin monomer to specific receptor(s) on the cell surface. Phospholipids and cholesterol were initially identified as high-affinity receptors for α-hemolysin, but it was evidenced that the membrane protein ADAM10 (A disintegrin and metalloprotease 10) is the specific receptor. When bound to its cell surface receptor via the rim domain, α-hemolysin units oligomerize into a heptameric (or hexameric) pre-pore. Upon heptamerization (or hexamerization), the stem β-strand unfolds and moves from the β-sandwich to form a β-hairpin. The β-hairpin of the stem domains associates into a 14-strand anti-parallel β-barrel that inserts into the plasma membrane and forms the transmembrane pore. The pore has a mushroom shape with an inner diameter ranging from 22 to 30 Å. Overall, α-hemolysin and related toxins share a similar mechanism of pore formation to CDCs, except that they form small pores resulting from oligomerization of 6–7 units instead of 30–50 in CDCs, and that each monomer contributes one hairpin to form the β-barrel instead of two in CDCs.

The primary activity of β-PFTs forming small pores on the cell membrane is a disruption of the membrane permeability to small molecules, leading notably to potassium and ATP efflux and influx of calcium, with subsequent deregulation of mitochondrial activity, activation of caspase 1, and the release of pro-inflammatory proteins. At high concentrations, β-PFTs generally kill cells by necrosis resulting, in particular, from mitochondria dysfunction, while at lower concentrations they induce cell death via programmed necrosis or apoptosis. At sub-lethal doses they can induce multiple effects on cells including membrane repair, changes in metabolism, activation of signaling pathways like activation of the p38 MAPK pathway, activation of caspases leading to inflammasome activation and the release of inflammatory molecules. In addition, α-hemolysin activates the ADAM10 receptor with subsequent cleavage of E-cadherin and decreased endothelial barrier integrity, which facilitates pathogen dissemination in the host.

Other virulence factors of *C. chauvoei* **and their role in pathogenesis**

CctA likely represents the major toxin of *C. chauvoei* since anti-CctA antibodies neutralize the cytotoxic and hemolytic activity of crude supernatant of *C. chauvoei* culture, and since animals vaccinated with recombinant CctA are fully protected against a challenge with virulent *C. chauvoei*.

In addition, *C. chauvoei* produces DNase, hyaluronidase, and neuraminidase, the role of which in pathogenesis is not yet understood. More importantly, *C. chauvoei* synthesizes flagella that are involved in bacterial invasion and disease pathogenesis.

Phospholipases

Certain clostridia involved in gangrene produce toxins that destabilize cell membranes through a phospholipase activity. The prototype of these toxins is the alpha toxin of *C. perfringens*. *C. perfringens* alpha toxin is a zinc-dependent phospholipase C which degrades phosphatidylcholine (PC, or lecithin) and sphingomyelin, and which is lethal in mice as well as being dermonecrotic and hemolytic. The toxin causes membrane damage to a variety of erythrocytes and cultured mammalian cells. It is the major *C. perfringens* toxin involved in gangrene, a disease process characterized by extensive local tissue destruction and necrosis without an inflammatory response and which progresses to profound shock with decreased cardiac contractility and death.

C. sordellii produces a phospholipase C which is structurally and functionally related to *C. perfringens* alpha toxin.

Beta toxin is the main toxin of *C. haemolyticum* which is responsible for bacillary hemoglobinuria. Beta toxin is a phospholipase C related to that of *C. novyi* type B but distant from that of *C. novyi* type A. The N-terminal part contains the catalytic zinc-binding motif and is highly homologous to that of *C. perfringens* alpha toxin and other clostridial phospholipases, whereas the C-terminal domain is more divergent. *C. novyi* type A synthesizes two different phospholipases, one that is specific to phosphatidylcholine and sphingomyelin like *C. perfringens* alpha toxin but phylogenetically distinct, and another that is specific to phosphatidylinositol.

The toxins produced by *C. novyi* and *C. haemolyticum* have not yet been fully investigated and the classification of these bacteria is still uncertain (Table 4.2).

Bibliography

Awad, M.M., *et al*. (2001) Synergistic effects of alpha-toxin and perfringolysin O in *Clostridium perfringens*-mediated gas gangrene. *Infect. Immun.*, **69:** 7904–7910.

Bischofberger, M., *et al*. (2012) Pathogenic pore-forming proteins: Function and host response. *Cell Host Microbe*, **12:** 266–275.

Bryant, A.E., *et al*. (2000) Clostridial gas gangrene. II. Phospholipase C-induced activation of platelet gpIIbIIIa mediates vascular occlusion and myonecrosis in *Clostridium perfringens* gas gangrene. *J. Infect. Dis.*, **182:** 808–815.

Chakravorty, A., *et al*. (2015) The pore-forming alpha-toxin from *Clostridium septicum* activates the MAPK pathway in a Ras-c-Raf-dependent and independent manner. *Toxins* (Basel), **7:** 516–534.

Degiacomi, M.T., *et al*. (2013) Molecular assembly of the aerolysin pore reveals a swirling membrane-insertion mechanism. *Nat. Chem. Biol.*, **9:** 623–629.

Dowd, K.J., *et al*. (2012) The cholesterol-dependent cytolysin signature motif: A critical element in the allosteric pathway that couples membrane binding to pore assembly. *PLoS Pathog.*, **8:** e1002787.

Dunstone, M.A., *et al*. (2012) Packing a punch: The mechanism of pore formation by cholesterol-dependent cytolysins and membrane attack complex/perforin-like proteins. *Curr. Opin. Struct. Biol.*, **22:** 342–349.

Frey, J., *et al.* (2012) Cytotoxin CctA, a major virulence factor of *Clostridium chauvoei* conferring protective immunity against myonecrosis. *Vaccine*, **30**: 5500–5505.

Genth, H., *et al.* (2014) Haemorrhagic toxin and lethal toxin from *Clostridium sordellii* strain VPI9048: Molecular characterization and comparative analysis of substrate specificity of the large clostridial glucosylating toxins. *Cell Microbiol.*, **16**: 1706–1721.

Guttenberg, G., *et al.* (2011) Inositol hexakisphosphate-dependent processing of *Clostridium sordellii* lethal toxin and *Clostridium novyi* {alpha}-toxin. *J. Biol. Chem.*, **286**: 14779–14786.

Heuck, A.P., *et al.* (2010) The cholesterol-dependent cytolysin family of gram-positive bacterial toxins. *Subcell. Biochem.*, **51**: 551–577.

Hickey, M.J., *et al.* (2008) Molecular and cellular basis of microvascular perfusion deficits induced by *Clostridium perfringens* and *Clostridium septicum*. *PLoS Pathog.*, **4**: e1000045.

Hotze, E.M., *et al.* (2012) Membrane assembly of the cholesterol-dependent cytolysin pore complex. *Biochim. Biophys. Acta*, **1818**: 1028–1038.

Iacovache, I., *et al.* (2010) Structure and assembly of pore-forming proteins. *Curr. Opin. Struct. Biol.*, **20**: 241–246.

Inoshima, I., *et al.* (2011) A *Staphylococcus aureus* pore-forming toxin subverts the activity of ADAM10 to cause lethal infection in mice. *Nat. Med.*, **17**: 1310–1314.

Kennedy, C.L., *et al.* (2009) Pore-forming activity of alpha-toxin is essential for *Clostridium septicum*-mediated myonecrosis. *Infect. Immun.*, **77**: 943–951.

Knapp, O., *et al.* (2010) The aerolysin-like toxin family of cytolytic, pore-forming toxins. *Open Toxinol. J.*, **3**: 53–68.

Mukamoto, M., *et al.* (2013) Analysis of tryptophan-rich region in *Clostridium septicum* alpha-toxin involved with binding to glycosylphosphatidylinositol-anchored proteins. *Microbiol. Immunol.*, **57**: 163–169.

Popoff, M.R., *et al.* (2013) Genetic characteristics of toxigenic Clostridia and toxin gene evolution. *Toxicon.*, **75**: 63–89.

Popoff, M.R. (2014) Clostridial pore-forming toxins: Powerful virulence factors. *Anaerobe*, **30**: 220–238.

Powers, M.E., *et al.* (2012) ADAM10 mediates vascular injury induced by *Staphylococcus aureus* alpha-hemolysin. *J. Infect. Dis.*, **206**: 352–356.

Qa'Dan, M., *et al.* (2001) pH-Enhanced Cytopathic Effects of *Clostridium sordellii* Lethal Toxin. *Infect. Immun.*, **69**: 5487–5493.

Rossjohn, J., *et al.* (2007) Structures of perfringolysin O suggest a pathway for activation of cholesterol-dependent cytolysins. *J. Mol. Biol.*, **367**: 1227–1236.

Skarin, H., *et al.* (2014) Plasmidome interchange between *Clostridium botulinum*, *Clostridium novyi* and *Clostridium haemolyticum* converts strains of independent lineages into distinctly different pathogens. *PLoS One*, **9**: e107777.

Soltani, C.E., *et al.* (2007) Structural elements of the cholesterol-dependent cytolysins that are responsible for their cholesterol-sensitive membrane interactions. *Proc. Natl Acad. Sci. USA*, **104**: 20226–20231.

Thiele, T.L., *et al.* (2013) Detection of *Clostridium sordellii* strains expressing hemorrhagic toxin (TcsH) and implications for diagnostics and regulation of veterinary vaccines. *Vaccine*, **31**: 5082–5087.

Turkcan, S., *et al.* (2013) Probing membrane protein interactions with their lipid raft environment using single-molecule tracking and Bayesian inference analysis. *PLoS One*, **8**: e53073.

Vidor, C., *et al.* (2015) Antibiotic resistance, virulence factors and genetics of *Clostridium sordellii*. *Res. Microbiol.*, **166**: 368–374.

Ziegler, M.O., *et al.* (2008) Conformational changes and reaction of clostridial glycosylating toxins. *J. Mol. Biol.*, **377**: 1346–1356.

5 | Toxins of *Clostridium perfringens*

James R. Theoret and Bruce A. McClane

Introduction

The versatile pathogenicity of *Clostridium perfringens* largely derives from the ability of this bacterium to produce a ~17 toxin armory. Four of those toxins – alpha, beta, epsilon, and iota toxins – are termed "major" toxins due to their use in a toxin-typing classification system (Table 5.1) that assigns *C. perfringens* isolates to one of five types (A–E). Although not used for this classification scheme, several of the remaining ~13 toxins are nonetheless important for the virulence of *C. perfringens*. This chapter will briefly review the biochemistry, action, and genetics of the most important *C. perfringens* toxins that have proven or suspected disease involvement.

A – Major toxins

C. perfringens alpha toxin

C. perfringens alpha toxin (CPA) is a 42.5 kDa single polypeptide with two domains. The ~250-amino-acid N-terminal domain is responsible for catalytic activity (described below), although it is not immunoprotective. The ~120-amino-acid C-terminal domain mediates host cell-binding activity in the presence of calcium and is immunoprotective. Recent studies reported that alpha toxin can bind to ganglioside GM1 on host cells.

CPA was the first bacterial toxin shown to have enzymatic properties. This toxin is a zinc metallophospholipase exhibiting both phospholipase C (lecithinase) and sphingomyelinase activities. CPA is lethal, with an LD_{50} in mice of 3 µg/kg (Table 5.2). At high concentrations, the toxin can substantially damage plasma membranes to directly lyse host cells. However, at sublytic concentrations, CPA

Clostridial Diseases of Animals, First Edition. Francisco A. Uzal, J. Glenn Songer,
John F. Prescott and Michel R. Popoff.
© 2016 John Wiley & Sons, Inc. Published 2016 by John Wiley & Sons, Inc.

Table 5.1 Toxin typing of *Clostridium perfringens*

Type	Toxin production			
	α	β	ε	ι
A	+	−	−	−
B	+	+	+	−
C	+	+	−	−
D	+	−	+	−
E	+	−	−	+

induces more limited cleavage of phosphotidylcholine and sphingomylelin, creating diacylglycerol and ceramide (Figure 5.1). Those molecules then activate several host signal transduction pathways which, via potent second messengers, induce hemolysis and a myriad of other effects, some of which are described below. An interesting recent study suggests that CPA may also be endocytosed, where it might act intracellularly.

Based on results from molecular Koch's postulate analyses, CPA is considered to be the most important toxin when *C. perfringens* causes gas gangrene (clostridial myonecrosis). During histotoxic disease, CPA impairs leukocyte migration and increases the adhesion of leukocytes to form intravascular aggregates that impair blood flow and thereby promote necrosis. Since this necrotic tissue environment is anaerobic, it favors *C. perfringens* growth. Similar analyses using alpha toxin null mutants of NetB-positive type A or type C natural intestinal disease strains suggest CPA is much less important when *C. perfringens* causes disease originating in the intestines.

CPA is encoded by the *cpa* (also referred to as *plc*) gene, which is chromosomally located. This toxin is produced by almost all *C. perfringens* strains, regardless of their type. Production of CPA is regulated by the VirS/VirR two-component regulatory system (TCRS). The *cpa* (*plc*) gene does not have VirR boxes upstream of its promoter, so this VirS/VirR regulation is indirect, involving a regulatory RNA named VR-RNA. Recently, expression of CPA was also shown to involve regulation by the Agr-like quorum-sensing (QS) system.

C. perfringens beta toxin

C. perfringens beta toxin (CPB) is expressed as a 336-amino-acid prototoxin, containing a 27-amino-acid leader sequence that is subsequently removed during secretion from the cell to generate a mature ~35 kDa polypeptide. The structure of CPB has not been resolved, but based upon its partial sequence homology with other toxins, CPB is considered a member of the β-pore-forming toxin (β-PFT) family. Like all β-PFTs, CPB is predicted to contain three functional domains: binding, oligomerization, and membrane insertion/pore formation (see below).

Table 5.2 Summary of major *C. perfringens* toxin properties

	CPA	CPB	ETX	ITX	PFO	CPE	CPB2	NetB	TpeL
Molecular weight	42.5 kDa	35 kDa	29 kDa	Ia: 47.5 kDa Ib: 71.5 kDa	54 kDa	35 kDa	28 kDa	33 kDa	~206 kDa
LD_{50} (in mice)[1]	3 µg/kg	400 ng/kg	100 ng/kg	Ia: 620 µg/kg Ib: 940 µg/kg	13–16 µg/kg	140 µg/kg	ND	ND	11 mg/kg[2]
Primary disease	Myo-necrosis	Necrotizing enteritis	Entero-toxemia	Enteritis	Synergism with CPA; no primary disease	Enteritis	Unclear; possible entero-colitis	Avian necrotic enteritis	Possible role in avian necrotic enteritis
Trypsin sensitivity	Sensitive	Sensitive	Resistant (activated)	Resistant (activated)	Susceptible	Resistant	Sensitive	Unknown	Unknown

[1] LD_{50} values determined from Gill (1982) and Uzal et al. (2010).

[2] The reported TpeL LD_{50} was determined using an unusually weak TpeL variant; the actual LD_{50} for this toxin is likely to be much lower.

ND: not determined

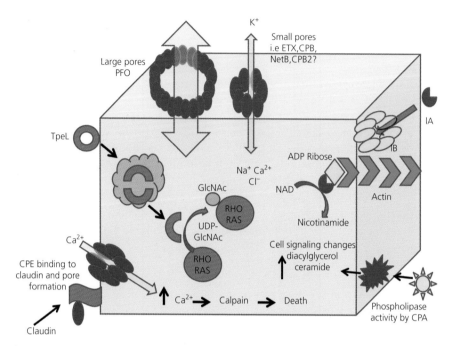

Figure 5.1 Activities of various *Clostridium perfringens* toxins on host cells. See text for a detailed explanation of their specific mechanism of action.

CPB induces cell death by creating unregulated ion channels, with a pore size of approximately 12 Å, in host cell membranes. These channels permit rapid K^+ efflux, and Na^+, Ca^{2+}, and Cl^- influx, resulting in cellular swelling and lysis (Figure 5.1). Pore formation begins with the binding of CPB to host cells using a still unidentified receptor. Recent studies showed that CPB binds to intestinal vascular endothelial cells during acute infection, leading to thrombosis and intestinal necrosis characteristic of CPB-mediated disease; whether the toxin binds to enterocytes is less clear. Once bound, CPB monomers rapidly oligomerize into hexameric or heptameric rings on the host cell surface, forming a pre-pore. Pre-pore formation is rapidly followed by toxin insertion into the membrane, presumably by an amphipathic transmembrane domain, resulting in cellular swelling and lysis. CPB is a potent toxin, with a calculated LD_{50} of 400 ng/kg (Table 5.2).

The importance of CPB in mediating intestinal disease has been demonstrated using purified toxin challenges, as well as by toxin neutralization and genetic knockout approaches. Early studies utilizing monoclonal antibodies demonstrated that neutralization of CPB was necessary and sufficient to protect mice from lethal IV challenge with culture supernatants from type C strains. Better mimicking type C disease, which originates in and involves the intestines, later studies demonstrated that challenge with highly purified CPB mixed with trypsin inhibitor caused intestinal lesions in rabbit intestinal loops. Furthermore, pre-incubation of the CPB with a CPB-neutralizing monoclonal antibody eliminated this pathological effect. More recently, compelling evidence was provided by fulfilling molecular Koch's postulates. In rabbit intestinal loops, PFO or CPA null mutants of type C strain CN3685 (a CPA/CPB/PFO positive strain) retained full pathogenicity. In contrast, a CPB null mutant was completely attenuated in this animal model. Furthermore, reversal of this CPB mutation restored virulence to wild-type levels. These findings provide solid evidence for the importance of CPB in mediating type C intestinal disease.

The *cpb* gene is present on large plasmids, ranging from 65–110 kb in size, which may also encode other clostridial toxins such as CPE or TpeL. These CPB plasmids carry a *tcp* region, indicating their potential conjugative transfer ability. *IS1151* sequences are also associated with the plasmid-borne *cpb* gene and those insertion sequences can excise the *cpb* gene from plasmids to form small circular DNAs that could be transposition intermediates. Collectively, these findings suggest that the *cpb* gene is highly mobile due to its apparent association with transposons and conjugative plasmids.

Investigations into the regulatory mechanisms controlling CPB expression have shown that the VirR/VirS TCRS system controls CPB production. This regulation has pathogenic importance, since an isogenic VirR null mutant of CN3685 was fully attenuated in rabbit intestinal loops and complementation of that mutant to regain VirS/VirR expression also restored virulence. Western blotting of intestinal fluid detected no CPB in loops treated with the VirS/VirR null mutant, confirming the role of this TCRS in *in vivo* CPB regulation. Furthermore, when tested for lethality in the mouse enterotoxemia model, a significant decrease in lethality was observed in mice challenged with the VirR null mutant.

The Agr-like quorum-sensing system also regulates CPB production, since an AgrB null mutant of CN3685 produced significantly less CPB *in vitro* compared to the wild-type parent. When tested in the rabbit model of necrotic enteritis, significant attenuation of the AgrB mutant was observed and this could be reversed by complementation to restore AgrB production. Furthermore, Western blot analysis of *in vivo* intestinal fluid samples demonstrated loss of CPB production by the AgrB null mutant, confirming that the Agr-like QS system regulates CPB production *in vivo*.

Lastly, it was also shown recently that close contact of type C strains with host cells induces a rapid upregulation of CPB production. This effect requires both a functional VirS/VirR TCRS and the Agr-like QS system.

C. perfringens epsilon toxin

C. perfringens type B and D strains secrete a relatively inactive ~33 kDa single polypeptide prototoxin that is proteolytically activated, creating the mature, ~29 kDa epsilon toxin (ETX). This activation can be caused by trypsin, chymotrypsin, or, possibly, *C. perfringens* lambda toxin in the intestine, and removes both N- and C-terminal amino acids from the prototoxin, but it is removal of the C-terminal amino acids that is critical for ETX activation. Once activated, ETX is the third most potent of all clostridial toxins, with an LD_{50} of ~100 ng/kg that ranks it behind only the botulinum and tetanus toxins.

ETX belongs structurally to the aerolysin family of pore-forming toxins. The mature ETX protein consists of three domains. Domain I is thought to be the region interacting with receptors on host cells, while Domain II contains an amphipathic loop that inserts into membranes during pore formation.

The first step in ETX action involves the binding of this toxin to a receptor. The identity of this receptor(s) is not yet clear, although hepatitis A virus cellular receptor 1 (HAVCR-1) has some properties expected of an ETX receptor. Once bound, ETX uses lipid rafts and caveolins to oligomerize into a heptameric pre-pore on the host cell membrane surface. It then extends a β-hairpin loop into the lipid bilayer to form an active pore. This pore formation results in a rapid decrease in cytoplasmic K^+ levels, with a corresponding influx of Na^+ and Cl^- into these cells (Figure 5.1).

The rapid loss of K^+ is believed to cause cellular necrosis involving a rapid decrease in nucleus size without any DNA fragmentation. This process is not yet fully understood but involves ATP depletion. However, methyl beta cyclodextrin reportedly prevents pore formation but not cell necrosis, suggesting additional processes beyond pore formation may contribute to ETX-induced cytotoxicity.

During infection, ETX prototoxin is produced by type B or D strains growing in the intestines. After its activation by intestinal proteases, as discussed earlier, or possibly *C. perfringens* lambda toxin, active ETX can affect the intestines (in goats) or it can be absorbed into the circulation (goats, sheep, and mice). The ability of ETX to traverse the intestinal epithelium even in the absence of intestinal damage suggests it may exploit paracellular permeability routes to reach the circulation. Once present in the circulation, ETX binds to internal organs, including the brain and kidneys. In the brain, ETX binds to endothelial cells and then alters the blood–brain barrier, which leads to the hallmark lesion of ETX brain effects; that is, perivascular edema that can develop rapidly. In animals with sub-acute and chronic disease, the brain lesions become necrotic and hemorrhagic and are known as focal symmetrical encephalomalacia. Another important brain effect of ETX involves increasing release of the stimulatory neurotransmitter glutamate. This effect is considered the major cause of neurologic symptoms observed during type B or D infections.

Insertion sequences are located adjacent to the *etx* gene in both type B and D strains and those sequences can excise the *etx* gene from plasmids to form small circular DNAs that could be transposition intermediates. It is possible that those putative transposons may mobilize the *etx* gene to move between plasmids in *C. perfringens*. This *etx* mobilization could help to explain the diversity of *etx* plasmids detected amongst type D strains. However, only a single *etx* plasmid is present in type B strains, which could reflect plasmid incompatibility issues – in other words, perhaps only certain combinations of *etx* plasmids and *cpb* plasmids can be stably maintained together in type B strains.

ETX is produced during log-phase growth. The regulation of ETX production is not well understood, despite some recent progress in this area. Contact with host Caco-2 cells was shown to upregulate ETX production and the Agr-like QS system is necessary for this host-cell-induced increase in ETX production by type D strain CN3718. However, ETX production is independent of the Agr-like QS system in two type B strains, indicating strain-to-strain (and perhaps type-to-type) differences in ETX regulatory control. Interestingly, the VirS/VirR TCRS does not appear to control ETX production by CN3718, suggesting there is not always regulatory cross-talk between the Agr-like QS and the VirS/VirR systems. Very recently, the CodY protein has been identified as a global regulator of virulence-associated properties of CN3718, including ETX production and bacterial adhesion to host cells.

Iota toxin

Iota toxin (ITX) has several distinguishing properties amongst *C. perfringens* toxins. First, ITX is one of only two toxins made by this bacterium (TpeL is the other) that clearly acts intracellularly. Second, ITX is the only *C. perfringens* toxin comprised of more than one polypeptide. ITX belongs to the clostridial binary toxin family because it consists of two polypeptides named IA and IB. Other members of this family include CDT of *Clostridium difficile*, the iota-like toxin of *Clostridium spiroforme*, and C2 toxin of *C. botulinum*.

Both the IA and IB components of ITX are produced as propeptides that are proteolytically activated by intestinal enzymes or, perhaps, *C. perfringens* lambda toxin. Once activated, the ~74 kDa IB binds as a monomer to receptors on host cells. Recent reports indicate that IB interacts with the lipolysis-stimulated lipoprotein (LSR), which is also a receptor for *C. difficile* and *C. spiroforme* binary toxins (although LSR is not a C2 toxin receptor). The presence of multifunctional mammalian surface protein CD44 also reportedly increases ITX binding, so CD44 could be a second receptor or a co-receptor for ITX. Once bound to host cells, IB monomers use lipid rafts to oligomerize into a heptamer. This heptamer then binds the ~48 kDa IA, followed by internalization of the entire ITX into cells by endocytosis. IA escapes from the early endosome and enters the cytoplasm, where it ADP ribosylates actin at residue Arg-177, causing a collapse of the cytoskeleton and cell death (Figure 5.1).

ITX is produced by the *iap* and *ipb* genes, which are co-transcribed in an operon and present on very large plasmids. Those plasmid-borne ITX genes are located near *IS1151* sequences and either functional or silent *cpe* gene sequences. The ITX plasmids carry a *tcp* region, suggesting that they are conjugative. In addition, *IS1151* sequences are associated with the *iap/ibp* genes, leading to the suggestion that the ITX genes have inserted onto *cpe* plasmids, converting progenitor isolates from type A to type E.

The involvement of ITX in disease remains unclear, although type E strains have been associated with enterotoxemias in calves, lambs, and, perhaps, rabbits.

B – Other toxins

C. perfringens enterotoxin

C. perfringens enterotoxin (CPE) is a 35 kDa single peptide with a unique primary amino acid sequence. Structurally, this toxin belongs to the aerolysin family of pore-forming toxins that also includes epsilon toxin. CPE consists of two major domains. The N-terminal domain functions in toxin oligomerization and also has a β-hairpin loop that inserts into membranes during pore formation. The C-terminal domain is responsible for the binding of CPE to receptors, as described below.

The action of CPE begins with the binding of this toxin to the second extracellular loop (ECL-2) in certain members of the claudin family of tight junction proteins. Of the 24 known claudins, only some (claudin-3, -4, -6, -8, and -14) can function as CPE receptors at pathophysiologically relevant toxin concentrations. An Asn residue located in the middle of ECL-2 is a key determinant of whether a claudin can function as a CPE receptor. Nearby ECL-2 residues then modulate the affinity of CPE binding, with some claudins (for example, claudin-4) possessing strong CPE-binding properties, but other claudins (for example, claudin-8) only binding CPE weakly.

Once bound to cells, CPE initially localizes in a small complex of ~90 kDa that contains CPE, receptor claudin(s), and non-receptor claudin(s), probably due to claudin:claudin interactions. Formation of the small complex is insufficient for cytotoxicity. However, CPE present in this small complex rapidly oligomerizes on the membrane surface, forming a pre-pore named CH-1. CH-1 has a molecular mass of ~450 kDa and contains six CPE molecules, receptor claudins, and non-receptor claudins. One β-hairpin from each of the six CPEs present in CH-1 then penetrates the membrane to form an active pore. Formation of the CPE pore triggers a Ca^{2+} influx that activates calpain. With low-dose CPE treatment, relatively few pores form, allowing only limited Ca^{2+} entry into cells. This effect causes modest calpain activation and cell death via a classical apoptosis involving caspase-3 activation. However, using higher CPE doses that produce many pores, Ca^{2+} floods into the cell to induce massive activation of calpain and cell death from oncosis (Figure 5.1).

In vivo, CPE-induced enterocyte death causes histologic lesions that trigger fluid secretion. This damage includes epithelial necrosis and desquamation, along with villus blunting. The toxin is active in all portions of the small intestine, but particularly the jejunum and ileum, and it also affects the colon.

CPE can be produced by all *C. perfringens* types, except type B. Only about 1–5% of type A strains produce CPE, but those CPE-producing type A strains cause:

1 *C. perfringens* type A food poisoning, which is the second most common bacterial food-borne disease in the USA;
2 Many cases of non-food-borne human gastrointestinal disease (for example, antibiotic-associated diarrhea and sporadic diarrhea); and, perhaps,
3 Some cases of diarrhea in domestic animals.

Interestingly, the enterotoxin gene (*cpe*) is chromosomal in 80% of *C. perfringens* type A food poisoning isolates but plasmid-borne in virtually all CPE-associated non-food-borne human disease and animal disease isolates. Genetic analyses have indicated that the type A food poisoning isolates with a chromosomal *cpe* gene are a separate lineage of *C. perfringens*, which also includes the CPE-positive type C strains causing some cases of human enteritis necroticans. The strong association of both those CPE-positive type A and C strains with food-borne illness is likely due to their common ability to form spores with exceptional (relative to other *C. perfringens* strains) resistance to many food environment stresses, such as heating. A key mechanism behind this extreme spore resistance phenotype is the ability to produce an unusual variant of small, acid-soluble protein-4, which binds particularly strongly to spore DNA to protect it from stresses.

CPE is produced only during *C. perfringens* sporulation, which occurs in the intestines during disease. This *in vivo* sporulation is under control of the Spo0A master regulator of sporulation. Once sporulation is initiated by phosphorylated Spo0A, the SigF alternative sigma factor directs RNA polymerase to produce two additional sporulation-associated sigma factors named SigE and SigK. Those two alternative sigma factors then target RNA polymerase to produce CPE from several SigE- or SigK-dependent promoters upstream of the *cpe* ORF. The involvement of multiple promoters leads to abundant production of CPE, which then accumulates in the cytoplasm, until the sporulating cell lyses at the end of sporulaton to release the mature endospore. Once released by mother cell lysis, CPE binds to claudins and acts on enterocytes, as already described.

C. perfringens necrotic enteritis beta-like toxin

C. perfringens necrotic enteritis beta-like toxin (NetB) is expressed as a 323-amino-acid polypeptide, containing a 30-amino-acid signal sequence that is removed prior to secretion, generating a mature 293-amino-acid protein with a molecular weight of ~33 kDa. The crystal structure of NetB was recently solved, identifying this toxin as a member of the β-PFT family that is related to CPB. Complete structure-function analysis of NetB remains to be elucidated, but several site-directed mutants generated in the proposed binding rim of the protein exhibited reduced binding to chicken hepatocellular carcinoma epithelial cells *in vitro*.

Like all β-PFTs, NetB induces cytolysis of cells by forming unregulated ion channels, with a pore diameter of ~1.4–1.6 nm, in the plasma membrane of host cells (Figure 5.1). LD_{50} determinations have not been performed at this time for NetB (Table 5.2), but doses as low as 2.5 μg/ml of the toxin cause cellular rounding and lysis of cultured LMH cells. Pore formation begins with binding of the monomeric toxin to host cells through an unknown receptor. After binding, the toxin quickly oligomerizes into a pre-pore, where the efficiency of pre-pore formation is linked to direct toxin interactions with cholesterol. The pre-pore then inserts into the host cell, presumably using an amphipathic domain identified during crystallization of the protein. Limited information exists on the ion preference of the NetB channel, but initial experiments and predictions from the modeled protein suggest it may favor cations.

In addition to lysing intestinal cells, NetB was shown to have hemolytic effects against red blood cells (RBC) *in vitro*, with stronger effects observed against avian-derived RBCs as compared to equine RBCs. The pathological significance of this RBC lysis remains to be determined *in vivo*, but considering the homology that exists between NetB and CPB, which can cause enterotoxemia, this may help to shed light on the high mortality levels observed during NE outbreaks.

Based on results from molecular Koch's postulate studies, NetB is the most important toxin involved with avian NE in poultry. Testing of NetB null mutants in poultry NE animal models failed to produce lesions in any birds tested, compared with the wild-type strain-producing lesions in 45% of the chickens tested. Further supporting the importance of NetB in causing NE, numerous studies have assayed strains isolated from poultry producers with NE outbreaks. These studies found that between 60 and 90% of strains isolated during NE outbreaks are NetB-positive.

The *netB* gene is located on a large conjugative ~85 kB plasmid in NetB positive type A strains, where it is part of a recently identified pathogenicity locus. Production of NetB is under control of the VirR/VirS TCRS. The transcriptional regulator VirR controls NetB expression by binding to two repeated sequences named VirR boxes that are located directly upstream of the NetB promoter. It remains to be determined if NetB expression is also regulated by the Agr-like QS system.

Perfringolysin O

Perfringolysin O (PFO) is a 54 kDa single polypeptide that belongs to the cholesterol-dependent cytolysin (CDC) toxin family. PFO consists of four domains, two of which are of particular functional importance. Domain 4 mediates membrane binding and contains an undecapeptide that couples membrane binding with the initiation of structural changes that begin pore formation (see next paragraph). Domain 3 contains two transmembrane hairpin regions that penetrate the membrane during pore formation.

Like all CDCs, PFO acts by forming large pores with a >10-fold larger diameter than the pores formed by other pore-forming toxins such as *C. perfringens* enterotoxin (Figure 5.1). The action of PFO begins with its binding, via a region of domain 4, to cholesterol on host cell plasma membranes. Approximately 40 bound PFO monomers then oligomerize on the plasma membrane surface to form a pre-pore. Upon structural changes to PFO, each monomer in the pre-pore then inserts two transmembrane hairpins into the membrane lipid bilayer to form the active pore. This pore formation can result in cell lysis, but PFO is also active at sublytic effects, as described below. PFO is weakly lethal, with an LD_{50} of ~15 µg/kg (Table 5.2).

Use of PFO null mutants provided insights into the role of this toxin in gas gangrene. While CPA is clearly the most important toxin in the *C. perfringens* gas gangrene mouse infection model, PFO does act synergistically with CPA to inhibit leukocyte infiltration and reduce blood supply into *C. perfringens* infected tissue, thus enhancing damage. There appears to be a more limited role for PFO in intestinal disease. Studies with PFO null mutants of type C strain CN3685 indicated that this toxin makes only minor, if any, contributions to necrotic enteritis or enterotoxemia, at least in laboratory animal models. Furthermore, many type A and type C strains causing human intestinal disease naturally lack the *pfoA* gene.

When present, the *pfoA* gene encoding this toxin is located on the chromosome. Expression of PFO is directly regulated by the VirS/VirR TCRS, via VirR boxes located upstream of the *pfoA* open reading frame. Recent studies have shown that PFO expression is also regulated by the Agr-like QS system of *C. perfringens*.

Toxin perfringens Large (TpeL)

TpeL is by far the largest of the *C. perfringens* toxins; this single-polypeptide toxin is ~206 kDa in size, although a much less active TpeL variant has been identified that is ~15 kDa smaller. TpeL is a member of the large clostridial glucosylating toxin (LCGT) toxin family. It possesses 30–40% homology with *Clostridium difficile* toxins A and B, which are also LCGTs. As is typical of LCGTs, TpeL possesses a glucosyltransferase domain in the N-terminal half of the protein. Adjacent to that enzymatic domain is a cysteine protease domain which, in the presence of inositol hexakisphosphate, autocatalytically processes TpeL inside host cells. Interestingly, even the full-length, 206-kDa form of TpeL lacks the C-terminal CROPS region of other LCGTs, which is interesting since this CROPS domain has been thought to target LCGTs to host cells; in other words, TpeL must have another receptor-binding domain.

The action of TpeL begins with its binding to a still unidentified cellular receptor, followed by clathrin-mediated endocytosis. In the low pH of the endosome, TpeL probably undergoes a conformational change, facilitating its insertion into the endosomal membrane, and translocation of the toxin begins. After proteolytic cleavage by the intrinsic cysteine protease activity of TpeL, the N-terminal domain containing glucosyltransferase activity is released into the cytoplasm. In this location, TpeL uses a UDP-glucose or, preferentially, UDP-N-acetylglucosamine to monoglucosylate host Rho/Ras proteins. Ras is the preferred protein substrate for this modification, which inactivates the Ras signaling pathway. This blockage results in cytotoxicity via apoptosis (Figure 5.1).

TpeL is encoded by large plasmids. Thus far, TpeL-producing type A, B, and C strains of *C. perfringens* have been identified. This large toxin can be produced during sporulation, where it is under the control of the master sporulation regulator Spo0A and the alternative sigma factor SigE.

The contribution of TpeL to virulence is not yet clear, however, this toxin has been associated with type A avian necrotic enteritis strains (Table 5.2).

C. perfringens beta 2 toxin

C. perfringens beta 2 toxin (CPB2) has perhaps the most unclear etiological role of the major clostridial toxins. CPB2 is expressed as a 31 kDa polypeptide which is cleaved post-translationally to the biologically active 28 kDa form. Despite its name, CPB2 shares little sequence homology with CPB. *In vitro* cellular modeling with CHO and I407 cell lines demonstrated CPB2 causes cellular rounding and death at toxin concentrations $\geq 20\,\mu g/ml$. The mechanism by which CPB2 elicits this cytotoxicity is not currently known, but it has been proposed that pore formation is the most plausible explanation.

Currently, there are no reports in the literature describing the experimental fulfillment of molecular Koch's postulates using CPB2. Indeed, the vast majority of the evidence in support of CPB2 having a role in disease comes from *cpb2*-positive strains isolated from diseased animals. However, CPB2 or *cpb2*-positive strains are not found in all diseased animals, and *cpb2*-positive strains are often found in healthy animals, making it difficult to draw conclusions about its role in disease. CPB2 has been reported to cause lethality in mice when administered IV (3 µg minimum lethal dose), as well as hemorrhagic necrosis of the intestinal wall in the guinea pig ligated loop model. Additionally, one study comparing type A *C. perfringens* reported more pronounced disease in bovine ligated intestinal loops when inoculated with a *cpa+/cpb2+* strain as compared to *cpa+/cpe+* and *cpa+* strains, suggesting that CPB2 and CPA may have synergistic effects *in vivo*.

CPB2 is encoded on plasmids ranging in size from 50 to 95 kB that are distinct from plasmids carrying CPB. This toxin has been detected in strains from toxinotypes A, B, C, and D. Regulation of expression of CPB2 has been tested using *C. perfringens* strain 13 (type A), where it was found to be under the control of the VirS/VirR system. Furthermore, like CPA, this regulation appears to be indirect, involving the sRNA VR-RNA. In addition to regulation by VirS/VirR, recent work has also shown positive regulation of CPB2 production by the Agr-like QS system in type A, but not in type B *C. perfringens* strains.

Binary enterotoxin of *C. perfringens*

A novel *C. perfringens* toxin called binary enterotoxin of *C. perfringens* (BEC) has been recently linked to two food-borne outbreaks in Japan. This plasmid-encoded toxin shares 43% identity with iota toxin and is a member of the ADP-ribosylating binary toxin family since it consists of BecA and BecB. Three lines of evidence suggest a role for BEC in disease:

1 rBEC demonstrated cytotoxicity to Vero cells *in vitro*;
2 rBEC caused significant fluid accumulation in a suckling mouse model;
3 Culture supernatants from a *becB* null mutant lost fluid accumulation activity in the suckling mouse model.

Bibliography

Aktories, K., *et al.* (2012) Bidirectional attack on the actin cytoskeleton. Bacterial protein toxins causing polymerization or depolymerization of actin. *Toxicon*, **60**: 572–581.

Animoto, K., *et al.* (2007) A novel toxin homologous to large clostridial cytotoxins found in culture supernatant of *Clostridium perfringens* type C. *Microbiol.* **153**: 1198–1206.

Awad, M.M. (1995) Virulence studies on chromosomal alpha-toxin and theta-toxin mutants constructed by allelic exchange provide genetic evidence for the essential role of alpha-toxin in *Clostridium perfringens*-mediated gas gangrene. *Molec. Microbiol.*, **15**: 191–202.

Awad, M.M., *et al.* (2001) Synergistic effects of alpha-toxin and perfringolysin O in *Clostridium perfringens*-mediated gas gangrene. *Infect. Immun.*, **69**: 7904–7910.

Ba-Thein, W., *et al.* (1996) The *virR/virS* locus regulates the transcription of genes encoding extracellular toxin production in *Clostridium perfringens*. *J. Bacteriol.*, **178**: 2514–2520.

Billington, S.J., *et al.* (1998) *Clostridium perfringens* type E animal enteritis isolates with highly conserved, silent enterotoxin sequences. *Infect. Immun.*, **66**: 4531–4536.

Briggs, D.C., *et al.* (2011) Structure of the food-poisoning *Clostridium perfringens* enterotoxin reveals similarity to the aerolysin-like pore-forming toxins. *J. Molec. Biol.*, **413**: 138–149.

Chakrabarti, G., *et al.* (2003) Death pathways activated in CaCo-2 cells by *Clostridium perfringens* enterotoxin. *Infect. Immun.*, **71**: 4260–4270.

Chakrabarti, G., *et al.* (2005) The importance of calcium influx, calpain, and calmodulin for the activation of CaCo-2 cell death pathways by *Clostridium perfringens* enterotoxin. *Cell Microbiol.*, **7**: 129–146.

Chalmers, G., *et al.* (2008) Multilocus sequence typing analysis of *Clostridium perfringens* isolates from necrotic enteritis outbreaks in broiler chicken populations. *J. Clin. Microbiol.*, **46:** 3957–3964.

Chen, J., *et al.* (2012) Cysteine scanning mutagenesis supports the importance of *Clostridium perfringens* enterotoxin amino acids 80–106 for membrane insertion and pore formation. *Infect. Immun.*, **80:** 4078–4088.

Chen, J., *et al.* (2012) Role of the Agr-like quorum-sensing system in regulating toxin production by *Clostridium perfringens* type B strains CN1793 and CN1795. *Infect. Immun.*, **80:** 3008–3017.

Chen, J., *et al.* (2013) Host cell-induced signaling causes *Clostridium perfringens* to upregulate production of toxins important for intestinal infections. *Gut Microbes*, **5**.

Cheung, J.K., *et al.* (2004) The spatial organization of the VirR boxes is critical for VirR-mediated expression of the perfringolysin O gene, *pfoA*, from *Clostridium perfringens*. *J. Bacteriol.*, **186:** 3321–3330.

Cheung, J.K., *et al.* (2010) The VirSR two-component signal transduction system regulates NetB toxin production in *Clostridium perfringens*. *Infect. Immun.*, **78:** 3064–3072.

Cole, A.R., *et al.* (2004) *Clostridium perfringens* epsilon-toxin shows structural similarity to the pore-forming toxin aerolysin. *Nat. Struct. Mol. Biol.*, **11:** 797–798.

Deguchi, A., *et al.* (2009) Genetic characterization of type A entertoxigenic *Clostridium perfringens* strains. *PLoS One*, **4:** e5598.

Dunstone, M.A., *et al.* (2012) Packing a punch: The mechanism of pore formation by cholesterol dependent cytolysins and membrane attack complex/perforin-like proteins. *Curr. Opin. Struct. Biol.*, **22:** 342–349.

Fisher, D.J., *et al.* (2006) Dissecting the contributions of *Clostridium perfringens* type C toxins to lethality in the mouse intravenous injection model. *Infect. Immun.*, **74:** 5200–5210.

Gao, Z., *et al.* (2012) Use of *Clostridium perfringens* enterotoxin and the enterotoxin receptor-binding domain (C-CPE) for cancer treatment: Opportunities and challenges. *J. Toxicol.*, article ID: 981626.

Gibert, M., *et al.* (1997) Beta2 toxin, a novel toxin produced by *Clostridium perfringens*. *Gene*, **203:** 65–73.

Gill, D.M. (1982) Bacterial toxins: A table of lethal amounts. *Microbiol. Rev.*, **46:** 86–94.

Gurjar, A., *et al.* (2010) Characterization of toxin plasmids in *Clostridium perfringens* type C isolates. *Infect. Immun.*, **78:** 4860–4869.

Guttenberg, G., *et al.* (2012) Molecular characteristics of *Clostridium perfringens* TpeL toxin and consequences of mono-O-GlcNAcylation of Ras in living cells. *J. Biol. Chem.*, **287:** 24929–24940.

Hanna, P.C., *et al.* (1991) Localization of the receptor-binding region of *Clostridium perfringens* enterotoxin utilizing cloned toxin fragments and synthetic peptides. The 30 C-terminal amino acids define a functional binding region. *J. Biol. Chem.*, **266:** 11037–11043.

Harry, K.H., *et al.* (2009) Sporulation and enterotoxin (CPE) synthesis are controlled by the sporulation-specific factors SigE and SigK in *Clostridium perfringens*. *J. Bacteriol.*, **191:** 2728–2742.

Hickey, M.J., *et al.* (2008) Molecular and cellular basis of microvascular perfusion deficits induced by *Clostridium perfringens* and *Clostridium septicum*. *PLoS Pathogens*, **11:** e1000045.

Hotze, E.M., *et al.* (2012) Membrane assembly of the cholesterol-dependent cytolysin pore complex. *Biochim. Biophys. Acta*, **1818:** 1028–1038.

Huang, I.H., *et al.* (2004) Disruption of the gene (*spo0A*) encoding sporulation transcription factor blocks endospore formation and enterotoxin productioin in enterotoxigenic *Clostridium perfringens* type A. *FEMS Microbiol. Lett.*, **233:** 233–240.

Hunter, S.E.C., *et al.* (1993) Molecular genetic analysis of beta-toxin of *Clostridium perfringens* reveals sequence homology with alpha-toxin, gamma-toxin, and leukocidin of *Staphylococcus aureus*. *Infect. Immun.*, **61:** 3958–3965.

Ivie, S.E., *et al.* (2011) Gene-trap mutagenesis identifies mammalian genes contributing to intoxication by *Clostridium perfringens* epsilon-toxin. *PLoS One*, **6:** e17787.

Johansson, A., *et al.* (2010) Genetic diversity and prevalence of *netB* in *Clostridium perfringens* isolated from a broiler flock affected by mild necrotic enteritis. *Vet. Microbiol.*, **144:** 87–92.

Keyburn, A.L., *et al.* (2006) Alpha-toxin of *Clostridium perfringens* is not an essential virulence factor in necrotic enteritis in chickens. *Infect. Immun.*, **74:** 6496–6500.

Keyburn, A.L., *et al.* (2008) NetB, a new toxin that is associated with avian necrotic enteritis caused by *Clostridium perfringens*. *PLoS Pathogens*, **4:** e26.

Keyburn, A.L., *et al.* (2010) Association between avian necrotic enteritis and *Clostridium perfringens* strains expressing NetB toxin. *Vet. Res.*, **41:** 21.

Kokai-Kun, J.F., *et al.* (1994) Comparison of Western immunoblots and gene detection assays for identification of potentially enterotoxigenic isolates of *Clostridium perfringens*. *J. Clin. Microbiol.*, **32:** 2533–2539.

Lepp, D., *et al.* (2010) Identification of novel pathogenicity loci in *Clostridium perfringens* strains that cause avian necrotic enteritis. *PLoS One*, **5:** e10795.

Li, J., *et al.* (2007) Comparison of virulence plasmids among *Clostridium perfringens* type E isolates. *Infect. Immun.*, **75:** 1811–1819.

Li, J., *et al.* (2008) A novel small acid soluble protein variant is important for spore resistance of most *Clostridium perfringens* food poisoning isolates. *PLoS Pathogens*, **4:** e1000056.

Li, J., *et al.* (2010) Evaluating the involvement of alternative sigma factors SigF and SigG in *Clostridium perfringens* sporulation and enterotoxin synthesis. *Infect. Immun.*, **78:** 4286–4293.

Li, J., *et al.* (2011) The Agr-like quorum-sensing system regulates sporulation and production of enterotoxin and beta2 toxin by *Clostridium perfringens* type A non-food-borne human gastro-intestinal disease strain F5603. *Infect. Immun.*, **79:** 2451–2459.

Li, J., *et al.* (2013) CodY is a global regulator of virulence-associated properties for *Clostridium perfringens* type D strain CN3718. MBio **4:** e00770–00713.

Ma, M., *et al.* (2011) The VirS/VirR two-component system regulates the anaerobic cytotoxicity, intestinal pathogenicity, and enterotoxemic lethality of *Clostridium perfringens* type C isolate CN3685. mBio 2: e00338-00310.

Ma, M., *et al.* (2012) Genotypic and phenotypic characterization of *Clostridium perfringens* isolates from Darmbrand cases in post-World War II Germany. *Infect. Immun.*, **80:** 4354–4363.

Macfarlane, M.G., *et al.* (1941) The biochemistry of bacterial toxins: The lecithinase activity of *Cl. welchii* toxins. *Biochem. J.*, **35:** 884–902.

Manteca, C., *et al.* (2002) The role of *Clostridium perfringens* beta2-toxin in bovine enterotoxaemia. *Vet. Microbiol.*, **86:** 191–202.

Marks, S.L., *et al.* (2002) Genotypic and phenotypic characterization of *Clostridium perfringens* and *Clostridium difficile* in diarrheic and healthy dogs. *J. Vet. Intern. Med.*, **16:** 533–540.

Martin, T.G., *et al.* (2009) Prevalence of NetB among some clinical isolates of *Clostridium perfringens* from animals in the United States. *Vet. Microbiol.*, **136:** 202–205.

McClane, B.A., *et al.* (2006) The Enterotoxic Clostridia. In: Dworkin, M. *et al.* (eds) *The Prokaryotes*, pp. 688–752. Springer NY Press, New York.

McClane, B.A., *et al.* (2013) *Clostridium perfringens*. In: Doyle, M.P. *et al.* (eds) *Food Microbiology: Fundamentals and Frontiers*, pp.465–489. ASM Press, Washington DC.

Miclard, J., *et al.* (2009) *Clostridium perfringens* beta-toxin targets endothelial cells in necrotizing enteritis in piglets. *Vet. Microbiol.*, **137:** 320–325.

Miyamoto, K., *et al.* (2008) Sequencing and diversity analyses reveal extensive similarities between some epsilon-toxin-encoding plasmids and the pCPF5603 *Clostridium perfringens* enterotoxin plasmid. *J. Bacteriol.*, **190:** 7178–7188.

Miyamoto, K., *et al.* (2011) Identification of novel *Clostridium perfringens* type E strains that carry an iota toxin plasmid with a functional enterotoxin gene. *PLoS One*, **6:** e20376.

Miyata, S., *et al.* (2001) Cleavage of a C-terminal peptide is essential for heptamerization of *Clostridium perfringens* epsilon-toxin in the synaptosomal membrane. *J. Biol. Chem.*, **276:** 13778–13783.

Miyata, S., *et al.* (2002) *Clostridium perfringens* epsilon-toxin forms a heptameric pore within the detergent-insoluble microdomains of Madin–Darby canine kidney cells and rat synaptosomes. *J. Biol. Chem.*, **277:** 39463–39468.

Monturiol-Gross, L., *et al.* (2013) Internalization of *Clostridium perfringens* alpha-toxin leads to ERK activation and is involved in its cytotoxic effect. *Cell Microbiol.*, **16:** 535–547.

Nagahama, M., *et al.* (2003) Biological activities and pore formation of *Clostridium perfringens* beta toxin in HL 60 cells. *J. Biol. Chem.*, **278**: 36934–36941.

Nagahama, M., *et al.* (2011) *Clostridium perfringens* TpeL glycosylates the Rac and Ras subfamily proteins. *Infect. Immun.*, **79**: 905–910.

Oda, M., *et al.* (2012) *Clostridium perfringens* alpha-toxin recognizes the GM1a-TrkA complex. *J. Biol. Chem.*, **287**: 33070–33079.

Ohtani, K., *et al.* (2003) The *VirR/VirS* regulatory cascade affects transcription of plasmid-encoded putative virulence genes in *Clostridium perfringens*. *FEMS Microbiol. Lett.*, **222**: 137–141.

Ohtani, K., *et al.* (2009) Virulence gene regulation by the agr system in *Clostridium perfringens*. *J. Bacteriol.*, **191**: 3919–3927.

Papatheodorou, P., *et al.* (2011) Lipolysis-stimulated lipoprotein receptor (LSR) is the host receptor for the binary toxin *Clostridium difficile* transferase (CDT). *Proc. Natl Acad. Sci. USA*, **108**: 16422–16427.

Papatheodorou, P., *et al.* (2012) Identification of the cellular receptor of *Clostridium spiroforme* toxin. *Infect. Immun.*, **80**: 1418–1423.

Paredes-Sabja, D., *et al.* (2011) *Clostridium perfringens* tpeL is expressed during sporulation. *Microbial Pathogen.*, **51**: 384–388.

Petit, L., *et al.* (1999) *Clostridium perfringens*: Toxinotype and genotype. *Trends Microbiol.*, **7**: 104–110.

Popoff, M.R. (2011) Epsilon toxin: A fascinating pore-forming toxin. *FEBS J.*, **278**: 4602–4615.

Robertson, S.L., *et al.* (2007) Compositional and stoichiometric analysis of *Clostridium perfringens* enterotoxin complexes in Caco-2 cells and claudin 4 fibroblast transfectants. *Cell Microbiol.*, **9**: 2734–2755.

Robertson, S., *et al.* (2010) Identification of a claudin-4 residue important for mediating the host cell binding and action of *Clostridium perfringens* enterotoxin. *Infect. Immun.*, **78**: 505–517.

Sakurai, J., *et al.* (2004) *Clostridium perfringens* alpha-toxin: Characterization and mode of action. *J. Biochem.* (Tokyo), **136**: 569–574.

Sakurai, J., *et al.* (2009) *Clostridium perfringens* iota-toxin: Structure and function. *Toxins*, **1**: 208–228.

Savva, C.G., *et al.* (2012) Molecular architecture and functional analysis of NetB, a pore-forming toxin from *Clostridium perfringens*. *J. Biol. Chem.*, **288**: 3512–3522.

Sayeed, S., *et al.* (2005) Epsilon-toxin is required for most *Clostridium perfringens* type D vegetative culture supernatants to cause lethality in the mouse intravenous injection model. *Infect. Immun.*, **73**: 7413–7421.

Sayeed, S., *et al.* (2007) Virulence plasmid diversity in *Clostridium perfringens* type D isolates. *Infect. Immun.*, **75**: 2391–2398.

Sayeed, S., *et al.* (2008) Beta toxin is essential for the intestinal virulence of *Clostridium perfringens* type C disease isolate CN3685 in a rabbit ileal loop model. *Mol. Microbiol.*, **67**: 15–30.

Sayeed, S., *et al.* (2010) Characterization of virulence plasmid diversity among *Clostridium perfringens* type B isolates. *Infect. Immun.*, **78**: 495–504.

Shatursky, O., *et al.* (2000) *Clostridium perfringens* beta-toxin forms potential-dependent, cation-selective channels in lipid bilayers. *Infect. Immun.*, **68**: 5546–5551.

Shimizu, T., *et al.* (2002) Clostridial VirR/VirS regulon involves a regulatory RNA molecule for expression of toxins. *Mol. Microbiol.*, **43**: 257–265.

Shimizu, T., *et al.* (2002) Complete genome sequence of *Clostridium perfringens*, an anaerobic flesh-eater. *Proc. Natl Acad. Sci. USA*, **99**: 996–1001.

Shrestha, A., *et al.* (2013) Human claudin-8 and -14 are receptors capable of conveying the cytotoxic effects of *Clostridium perfringens* enterotoxin. mBio 4.

Smedley, J.G. 3rd, *et al.* (2008) Noncytotoxic *Clostridium perfringens* enterotoxin (CPE) variants localize CPE intestinal binding and demonstrate a relationship between CPE-induced cytotoxicity and enterotoxicity. *Infect. Immun.*, **76**: 3793–3800.

Steinthorsdottir, V., *et al.* (2000) *Clostridium perfringens* beta-toxin forms multimeric transmembrane pores in human endothelial cells. *Microb. Pathogen.*, **28**: 45–50.

Stevens, D.L., *et al.* (2006) Gram-positive pathogens. In: Fischetti, V.A. *et al.* (eds) *Histotoxic Clostridia.* ASM Press, Washington, DC.

Uzal, F.A., *et al.* (2010) Toxins involved in mammalian veterinary diseases. *Open Toxinol. J.,* **2:** 24–42.

Vidal, J.E., *et al.* (2008) Effects of *Clostridium perfringens* beta-toxin on the rabbit small intestine and colon. *Infect. Immun.,* **76:** 4396–4404.

Vidal, J.E., *et al.* (2009) Contact with enterocyte-like Caco-2 cells induces rapid upregulation of toxin production by *Clostridium perfringens* type C isolates. *Cell Microbiol.,* **11:** 363–369.

Vidal, J.E., *et al.* (2009) Use of an EZ-Tn5-based random mutagenesis system to identify a novel toxin regulatory locus in *Clostridium perfringens* strain 13. *PLoS One,* **4:** e6232.

Vidal, J.E., *et al.* (2012) Evidence that the Agr-like quorum sensing system regulates the toxin production, cytotoxicity and pathogenicity of *Clostridium perfringens* type C isolate CN3685. *Mol. Microbiol.,* **83:** 179–194.

Wigelsworth, D.J., *et al.* (2012) CD44 promotes intoxication by the clostridial iota-family toxins. *PLoS One,* **7:** e51356.

Yan, X., *et al.* (2013) Structural and functional analysis of the pore-forming toxin NetB from *Clostridium perfringens.* mBIO 4: e00019–00013.

Yonogi, S., *et al.* (2014) BEC, a novel enterotoxin of *Clostridium perfringens* found in human clinical isolates from acute gastroenteritis outbreaks. *Infect. Immun.,* **82:** 2390–2399.

6 Toxins of *Clostridium difficile*

J. Glenn Songer, Ashley E. Harmon, and M. Kevin Keel

Introduction

The virulence of *C. difficile* is mediated by two members of the large clostridial cytotoxin family, toxin A (TcdA) and toxin B (TcdB). An enormous amount is known about these toxins and their variants, as well as about their regulation and the possible effects of accessory toxins and strain differences in the occurrence and severity of *C. difficile* infection (CDI), but many questions remain. To date, understanding toxin function and the role in pathogenesis has formed the basis for numerous advances in prevention and therapy. With time, it seems likely that abrogating the effects of these toxins will be the major key in allowing prevention and control of CDI.

Toxins A and B

Introduction
Toxins A (TcdA) and B (TcdB) are the essential virulence factors of *C. difficile*. The genes, *tcd*A and *tcd*B, respectively, are located on a large pathogenicity locus (PALoc) in the bacterial chromosome. Molecular mechanisms regulating toxin production are, in a sense, directly responsible for disease. The toxin region of the PALoc containing the *tcd*A and *tcd*B, and accessory genes, is shown in Figure 6.1.

General features
TcdA is an enterotoxin, and TcdB is a potent cytotoxin *in vitro;* for many years it was thought, based on hamster studies, that TcdB had little activity *in vivo* unless there was prior damage to mucosal epithelium. The toxins were thought to act synergistically, with TcdA creating widespread damage to the mucosa that

Clostridial Diseases of Animals, First Edition. Francisco A. Uzal, J. Glenn Songer,
John F. Prescott and Michel R. Popoff.
© 2016 John Wiley & Sons, Inc. Published 2016 by John Wiley & Sons, Inc.

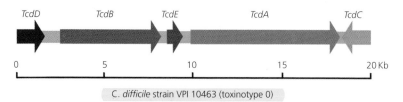

C. difficile strain VPI 10463 (toxinotype 0)

Figure 6.1 Genetic organization of the PALoc toxin region of *C. difficile* showing the *tcdA* and *tcdB* genes, and accessory *tcd* genes. *tcdC* and *tcdR* are genes involved in regulating toxin production, and *tcdE* encodes a holin protein involved in toxin secretion. Sequence differences in the *tcdA* and *tcdB* genes are used in PCR-based "toxinotyping", of which over 30 types are recognized. These differences can have profound effects on toxin production and potency.

permitted TcdB to affect epithelial cells. There are numerous reports of CDI in patients infected by TcdA-negative, TcdB-positive strains of *C. difficile*. The long-held paradigm belief that TcdA was the major toxin virulence determinant in CDI, based on the activity of purified toxins and on immunoprotection in hamsters, has been challenged by recent *tcdA* and *tcdB* mutation studies, supported by clinical observations.

TcdA⁺ TcdB⁻ mutants do not occur naturally, whereas TcdA⁻ TcdB⁺ mutants are both fairly common and fully virulent. Strains producing TcdB alone are associated in CDI with both severe, localized intestinal damage and systemic organ damage. Disease associated with *tcdB* only strains is equally, and sometimes more, severe than disease produced by *tcdA⁺ tcdB⁺* strains. Thus, TcdB may be responsible for the onset of multiple organ dysfunction syndrome (MODS), an often fatal complication of CDI. TcdB is also primarily responsible for induction of the innate immune and inflammatory responses. Gene mutation studies, supported by clinical observation, have thus changed the paradigm to suggest that TcdB is the major virulence factor of *C. difficile*. These mutation studies have not involved gene complementation and the conclusions are based on a very specific animal model, which does not fully represent human CDI. Nevertheless, these studies and clinical observations importantly focus possible preventive strategies on TcdB and not on TcdA. Further work is, however, required to understand the relative roles of these toxins in CDI.

Genetic regulation of toxin production

Toxin synthesis is regulated by an accessory gene regulator quorum-signaling system, mediated via a small thiolactone that can be detected in stools of CDI patients. Interfering with toxin regulation may form the basis for future development of quorum-signaling-based non-antibiotic therapies to combat CDI.

Toxin secretion mechanism

TcdA and TcdB consist of single, large polypeptide chains with folds stabilized by disulfide bonds (Figure 6.2). They have no export signature. The mechanism by which these large toxins are secreted from bacterial cells is not yet clear but involves TcdE (Figure 6.1), a holin-like protein. A TcdE mutant was restored to

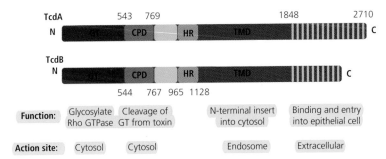

Figure 6.2 Schematic of the functional domain structure of TcdA and TcdB. The four major domains have N-terminal glucosyltransferase activity (GT), autocatalytic cysteine protease activity (CPD), central translocation (TMD), and C-terminal receptor binding (C) (see text).

full ability to secrete toxins by complementation with functional TcdE. Three possible translation start sites have been identified, and it has been suggested that each isoform may play a specific role in toxin release by the TcdE-mediated process. The different functional domains of TcdA and TcdB (Figure 6.2) are involved in binding and entry into epithelial cells, glycosylation of Rho GTPase in the cytosol, and N-terminal insertion into the endosome.

Toxin receptors

The carboxy-termini of both toxins include the receptor-binding domain (Figure 6.2); that for TcdA apparently differs significantly from that for TcdB. Carbohydrate receptors for TcdA include Galα1-3β1-4GlcNAc-R (α-Gal epitope), Galβ1-4{Fuβ1-3}GlcNAc (Lewis X), Galβ1-4GlcNAcβ1 (Lewis Y), Galβ1-14GlcNAcβ1-3Galβ1-4(Glc) (Lewis I), and sucrose-isomaltase. These receptors are on the brush border of susceptible intestinal epithelial cells and may occur elsewhere as well. A receptor for TcdB has not been identified, but may be present on the basolateral aspect of epithelial cells. Physical trauma, or the effects of TcdA, may compromise cell–cell contacts, providing TcdB access to receptors that are normally unavailable.

Receptor binding: subsequent activity

The toxin amino-termini are catalytic (Figure 6.2) and are highly conserved; both function in the target cell cytoplasm by similar mechanisms. Receptor binding by TcdA initiates endocytosis by coated pits and the resulting vesicles fuse with lysosomes. The mechanism of TcdB attachment and endocytosis has not been described. Acidification of the endolysosome produces a toxin conformational change, which is followed by its activation and escape into the cytoplasm. In the cytoplasm, the toxins specifically inactivate Rho, and other Rho-subtype GTPases, by glycosylation of threonine. This class of GTPases comprises signal transduction molecules associated with apoptosis and maintenance/regulation of actin filaments. Actin filaments are a necessary part of some cell adhesion molecules (for example, zonula adherens, tight junctions, and focal adhesions) and their disruption results in the loss of cell–cell contacts, in increased paracellular permeability of mucosal surfaces, in cell rounding, and, eventually, in cell death.

Toxin effects: beyond cytotoxicity

TcdA and TcdB amplify the disease process beyond simple disruption of function and death of mucosal epithelial cells. Initiation of an inflammatory cascade that can damage host tissues is particularly important. TcdA causes mitochondrial dysfunction, with depletion of ATP and intracellular generation of reactive oxygen intermediates. Degradation of IκB follows degradation and nuclear translocation of NF-κB, with elaboration of IL-8 and possibly other pro-inflammatory mediators. Factors regulating disease severity are poorly understood. Secretion of toxins A and B causes inflammation and tissue damage, and a portion of this tissue damage may be due to an inappropriate host immune response. Toxins A and B, in combination with both bacterium- and host-derived danger signals, can induce expression of pro-inflammatory cytokines IL-1β and IL-23. Studies have shown that IL-1β signaling enhances IL-23 production and could lead to increased inflammation during CDI.

IκB is degraded before glycosylation of Rho and is inhibited by antioxidant pretreatment of TcdA-exposed cells. IL-8 is a chemokine associated with mobilization, activation, and degranulation of neutrophils, as well as chemotaxis of basophils and T-cells. Another potent chemotaxin of neutrophils, macrophage inhibitory protein-2 (MIP-2), is elaborated by rat ileal epithelial cells within 30 minutes of exposure to TcdA. TcdA can also directly stimulate neutrophil migration *in vitro*. Neutrophils play a prominent role in the pathophysiology of CDI by directly contributing to necrosis of host tissues. Inhibition of neutrophil infiltration by blocking the activity of CD18 or MIP-2 reduces lesion severity.

Macrophages and monocytes also participate in the inflammatory cascade associated with CDI. TcdA causes lamina propria macrophages to express cyclooxygenase-2 (Cox-2), with subsequent production of prostaglandin E_2 (PGE_2). The effect is probably by direct action of TcdA on intestinal macrophages, as opposed to the indirect influence of intermediary cytokines released by some other cell type. Circulating monocytes produce IL-1, IL-6, IL-8, and tumor necrosis factor-α (TNFα) in response to application of TcdA. PGE_2 inhibits sodium chloride and water absorption in the intestine and induces chloride secretion by enterocytes. In addition, TcdA induces vasodilation that may contribute to effusion across the intestinal mucosa. The secretory effects of TcdA have been inhibited by administration of a Cox-2 inhibitor.

Mucosal mast cells may also be involved in the development of CDI. Administration of TcdA causes degranulation of mast cells within 15 to 30 minutes. Mast-cell-deficient mice have reduced infiltration of neutrophils and intestinal secretion in response to TcdA challenge, but reconstitution of the mice fully restores their susceptibility.

The disease and lesions of CDI also have a neural component. Release of substance P results from direct stimulation of primary sensory neurons by TcdA; this, in turn, stimulates mast-cell degranulation. Substance P is also associated with mast-cell-independent pathways of inflammation, through its potent vascular effects and its ability to increase vascular permeability by directing formation of endothelial gaps in venules. TcdA inhibits the release of norepinephrine from sympathetic postganglionic nerve fibers in the small intestine and directly causes excitation of enteric secretomotor neurons in the submucosal plexus. The net result is increased secretion of water and electrolytes into the intestinal lumen. Denervation of ileal loops greatly reduces both secretion and inflammation due to TcdA, but the protective effect is overcome by higher doses of toxin.

Severe and fulminant disease outcomes often result from toxemia. Circumstantial evidence suggests that toxemia may occur in patients with CDI, but a positive diagnosis is extremely rare. Critical variation in the 1753–1851 region of TcdB affects exposure of neutralizing epitopes in the toxin. Biochemical, analytical, and mutagenesis experiments have revealed that this region promotes protein–protein interactions, which may shield neutralizing epitopes that would otherwise be exposed in the toxin.

Neutralization experiments suggest that the amino terminus of TcdB interacts with an upstream region and affects the exposure of neutralizing epitopes in the carboxyl terminus. These data suggest that variations in this upstream region affect molecular interactions within TcdB and that these interactions affect the exposure of neutralizing epitopes.

Pathogenesis of apoptosis associated with TcdA and TcdB

Apoptosis is one mechanism of cell death that is directly induced by *C. difficile* toxins. Apoptosis is generally utilized to eliminate irreversibly damaged cells with minimal tissue reaction. Two distinct apoptotic cell death pathways exist, both ultimately dependent upon caspase activation. The intrinsic pathway is associated with increased mitochondrial outer membrane permeabilization (MOMP) whereas the extrinsic pathway is initiated by activation of cell-membrane-associated death receptors. Both mechanisms seem to be involved with TcdA, but only the intrinsic pathway seems to be implicated as a mechanism for TcdB-induced apoptosis.

The ability of TcdA to initiate apoptosis has been demonstrated to be dependent upon Rho glucosylation and involves caspases associated with both the intrinsic and extrinsic pathways of apoptosis. However, some studies indicate a caspase-independent pathway of cell death dependent upon increased mitochondrial outer membrane permeability. Necroptosis, another mechanism of programmed cell death, is caspase independent but shares some of the intracellular signaling mechanisms of apoptosis and can be associated with mito-chondrial outer membrane permeability.

Since both TcdA and TcdB have glucosyltransferase activity, it is not surprising that there are some similarities in the mechanisms by which they induce apoptosis. Inactivation of Rho by TcdB seems to be, at least in part, responsible for apoptosis by reduced expression of the anti-apoptotic factors Bcl-2 and Mcl-1 with increased expression of Bid, a pro-apoptotic factor. Some research, however, suggests a TcdB-associated mechanism of apoptosis independent of Rho glucosylation. In fact, TcdB is known to induce calcium-dependent swelling of isolated mitochondria, with subsequent release of cytochrome c, another pro-apoptogenic factor. TcdB is also able to increase endoplasmic reticulum stress, another mechanism for involving the intrinsic pathway of apoptosis in a glucosylation-independent manner.

C. difficile ADP-ribosylating toxin (CDT)

A small percentage of *C. difficile* strains produce an actin-specific ADP-ribosyltransferase, CDT. This toxin can be detected in 17–23% of strains, but its role, if any, in spontaneous CDI in humans and animals has not been clearly defined. CDT is consistently produced by those strains associated with hyper-virulence, including ribotypes 027, 028, and 244 (see below), but historically it has been uncommon among endemic strains of *C. difficile*.

CDT is a binary toxin, formed from separate, unlinked polypeptides, and a member of the clostridial iota-like toxins, all of which are characterized by two separate components, an ADP-ribosyltransferase subunit and a binding subunit responsible for translocation of the holotoxin. CDTa is the enzymatic (ADP-ribosyltransferase) component of CDT and CDTb is the binding component. CDTb binds to a cell-surface receptor and mediates translocation to the cytosol of enzymatic component CDTa. In the cytosol, CDTa ADP-ribosylates actin, leading to depolymerization of actin filaments and disruption of the cytoskeleton. The ultimate effect of CDT on the host cell is to cause the formation of microtubule-based protrusions at the apical surfaces of cells and to redirect extracellular matrix proteins from the basolateral surface to the apical surface, both of which are associated with increased adherence of *C. difficile*. CDT is directly toxic to Chinese hamster ovary cells and may serve as a virulence factor. In hypervirulent, *cdt*-positive-strains, strain differences in toxin B composition give the toxin broader tropism and cytotoxicity than TcdB from conventional strains (see below).

Hypervirulence of C. difficile and its potential mechanisms

Certain strains of *C. difficile* have recently been associated with widespread epidemics and significantly increased morbidity and mortality attributed to hypervirulence. This trend was first recognized among patients in Quebec in 2002 and was attributed to PCR ribotype 027, also identified as toxinotype III and pulsotype NAP1 (North American Pulsotype 1). The incidence in Quebec increased from 35.6 cases per 100,000 people in 1991 to 156.3 cases per 100,000 in 2003. Similar increases have been observed in the United States and in many European countries. Phylogenetic analysis suggests that the most common epidemic strains emerged in North America with subsequent dispersal to the United Kingdom, continental Europe, and Australia. The complete explanation for the emergence of hypervirulent strains remains elusive but a number of important differences from historic strains are recognized. It seems likely that the emergence of hypervirulent strains is the additive result of multiple genetic changes.

Although ribotype 027 is the strain most commonly associated with hypervirulence, increased mortality rates associated with ribotype 078 and ribotype 244 have also been reported. Although some researchers have suggested that biased study design and other factors have contributed to an apparent but spurious increase in virulence of a given ribotype, and that that ribotype is not predictive of disease severity, the increased incidence of disease due to those strains is generally not disputed.

Comparative phylogenomic analyses of diverse human and animal isolates indicate that isolates defined as hypervirulent in the context of human disease form a distinct clade. In addition, several genetic islands identified in that clade could be related to virulence and niche adaptation; these elements are related to antibiotic resistance, motility, adhesion, and enteric metabolism. More targeted studies have also identified a number of specific features attributed to increased virulence of epidemic strains.

TcdA and TcdB are the principal virulence factors for both endemic and epidemic (that is, hypervirulent) strains of *C. difficile* and have dose-dependent effects on the intestinal epithelium. Recent evidence indicates that both increased production and increased potency of toxins are associated with a hypervirulent strain of ribotype 027, and may, in part, explain the severity of disease in the associated infections. In one study, the median production of TcdA and TcdB by ribotype 027 was 16 and 23 times higher, respectively, than the median quantities produced by diverse endemic isolates of *C. difficile*. Not only do hypervirulent strains seem to produce more toxin but they also may produce toxins that act upon their cellular targets with greater efficiency. TcdB has a demonstrable increase in potency when produced by hypervirulent isolates, an increased potency that is apparently due to more efficient activation within the host cell. TcdB is internalized by receptor-mediated endocytosis; acidification of the resultant endosomes causes conformational changes in TcdB necessary for its entry into the cytoplasm. In one study, TcdB from a hypervirulent isolate was found to be processed in the endosome 20% more efficiently than TcdB from a well-studied endemic strain of *C. difficile*, which could account for its increased toxicity. Hypervirulent strains also have a nonsense mutation in *tcdC*, an anti-sigma factor regulatory gene, which has the effect of increasing toxin production.

A number of other strain attributes such as production of the CDT binary toxin, variation in cell-wall-associated proteins, dysregulation of TcdA and TcdB by alterations in the anti-sigma factor, TcdC, increased sporulation efficiency, and antibiotic resistance have also been presented as possible virulence factors associated with the recently emerged hypervirulent strains. Such factors have been systematically and comprehensively reviewed by multiple authors.

Immunotherapy of *C. difficile* infections

An approach to the prevention of CDI (in domestic animals, if not in humans) is the use of monoclonal antibodies with selective activity against TcdA and TcdB. In theory, systemically administered human IgG monoclonal antibodies reach the gut mucosa during the course of disease, protecting the host against systemic intoxication. Leakage of antibody from the circulation into the damaged colon probably also protects the mucosa from further damage, facilitating the initiation of repair and recovery.

In a small clinical trial, a monoclonal antibody infusion, with vancomycin or metronidazole, was more effective than antibiotics alone in preventing relapses. In another study, an efficacious cocktail contained one mAb against the receptor-binding domain of TcdA and two mAbs with specificity against the non-overlapping regions of the glucosyltransferase domain of TcdB.

A novel chimeric protein, mTcd138, has been developed that comprised the glucosyltransferase and cysteine protease domains of TcdB and the receptor-binding domain of TcdA (Figure 6.2) (see below). It was further engineered to insure non-toxicity. Immunization of mice and hamsters with mTcd138 induced neutralizing, and thus protective, antibodies to both toxins; immunized animals were protected against challenge with a hypervirulent *C. difficile* strain.

The most important step in toxin:cell interaction is receptor-mediated uptake of toxins. If antibodies against the toxin carboxy terminus block endocytosis of toxins, lesions do not develop. This and multiple other approaches to target these toxins, including IV immunoglobulin and vaccines, have been explored, with various degrees of success.

Conclusion

Knowledge of the toxins produced by *C. difficile* is extensive, and, to date, understanding toxin function and the role in pathogenesis has formed the basis for numerous advances in prevention and therapy. With time, it seems likely that abrogating the effects of toxins will be the major key in allowing prevention and control of CDI.

Bibliography

Alcantara, C., *et al.* (2001) Role of inducible cyclooxygenase and prostaglandins in *Clostridium difficile* toxin A induced secretion and inflammation in an animal model. *J. Infect. Dis.*, **184:** 648–652.

Anosova, N.G., *et al.* (2015) A combination of three fully human toxin A- and toxin B-specific monoclonal antibodies protects against challenge with highly virulent epidemic strains of *Clostridium difficile* in the hamster model. *Clin. Vaccine Immunol.*, **22:** 711–725.

Carter, G.P., *et al.* (2012) The role of toxin A and toxin B in the virulence of *Clostridum difficile*. *Trends Microbiol.*, **20:** 21–29.

Carter, G.P., *et al.* (2015) Defining the roles of TcdA and TcdB in localized gastrointestinal disease, systemic organ damage, and the host response during *Clostridium difficile* infections. *MBio.* **6:** e00551.

Castagliuolo, I., *et al.* (1998) *Clostridium difficile* toxin A stimulates macrophage-inflammatory protein-2 production in rat intestinal epithelial cells. *J. Immunol.*, **160:** 6039–6045.

Cohen, O.R., *et al.* (2014) Systemically administered IgG anti-toxin antibodies protect the colonic mucosa during infection with *Clostridium difficile* in the piglet model. *PLoS One*, **9:** e111075.

Cowardin, C.A., *et al.* (2015) Inflammasome activation contributes to interleukin-23 production in response to *Clostridium difficile*. *MBio.* **6:** e02386–14.

D'Auria, K.M., *et al.* (2015) High temporal resolution of glucosyltransferase dependent and independent effects of *Clostridium difficile* toxins across multiple cell types. *BMC Microbiol.*, **15:** 7.

Darkoh, C., *et al.* (2015) Toxin synthesis by *Clostridium difficile* is regulated through quorum signaling. *MBio* **6:** e02569.

Eckert, C., *et al.* (2015) Prevalence and pathogenicity of binary toxin-positive *Clostridium difficile* strains that do not produce toxins A and B. *New Microbes New Infect.*, **3:** 12–17.

Engevik, M.A., *et al.* (2015) Human *Clostridium difficile* infection: Inhibition of NHE3 and microbiota profile. *Am. J. Physiol. Gastrointest. Liver Physiol.*, **308:** G497–G509.

Goldberg, E.J., *et al.* (2015) *Clostridium difficile* infection: A brief update on emerging therapies. *Am. J. Health Syst. Pharm.*, **72:** 1007–1012.

Gonçalves, C., *et al.* (2004) Prevalence and characterization of a binary toxin (actin-specific ADP-ribosyltransferase) from *Clostridium difficile*. *J. Clin. Microbiol.*, **42:** 1933–1939.

Govind, R., *et al.* (2015) Observations on the role of TcdE isoforms in *Clostridium difficile* toxin secretion. *J. Bacteriol.*, **197:** 2600–2609.

He, D., *et al.* (2002) *Clostridium difficile* toxin A triggers human colonocyte IL-8 release via mitochondrial oxygen radical generation. *Gastroenterology*, **122:** 1048–1057.

Kink, J.A., *et al.* (1998) Antibodies to recombinant *Clostridium difficile* toxins A and B are an effective treatment and prevent relapse of *C. difficile*-associated disease in a hamster model of infection. *Infect. Immun.*, **66:** 2018–2025.

Larabee, J.L., *et al.* (2015) Exposure of neutralizing epitopes in the carboxyl-terminal domain of TcdB is altered by a proximal hypervariable region. *J. Biol. Chem.*, **290:** 6975–6985.

Leslie, J.L., *et al.* (2015) Persistence and toxin production by *Clostridium difficile* within human intestinal organoids result in disruption of epithelial paracellular barrier function. *Infect. Immun.*, **83:** 138–145.

Mantyh, C.R., *et al.* (2000) Extrinsic surgical denervation inhibits *Clostridium difficile* toxin A induced enteritis in rats. *Neurosci. Lett.*, **292:** 95–98.

McVey, D.C., *et al.* (2001) The capsaicin VR1 receptor mediates substance P release in toxin A-induced enteritis in rats. *Peptides*, **22:** 1439–1446.

Perelle, S., *et al.* (1997) Production of a complete binary toxin (actin-specific ADP-ribosyltransferase) by *Clostridium difficile* CD196. *Infect. Immun.*, **65:** 1402–1407.

Pothoulakis, C., *et al.* (2001) Microbes and microbial toxins: Paradigms for microbial–mucosal interactions II. The integrated response of the intestine to *Clostridium difficile* toxins. *Am. J. Physiol. Gastrointest. Liver Physiol.*, **280:** G178–G183.

Qa'Dan, M., *et al.* (2000) pH-induced conformational changes in *Clostridium difficile* toxin B. *Infect. Immun.*, **68:** 2470–2474.

Shah, P.J., *et al.* (2015) Role of intravenous immune globulin in streptococcal toxic shock syndrome and *Clostridium difficile* infection. *Am. J. Health Syst. Pharm.*, **72:** 1013–1019.

Sörensson, J., *et al.* (2001) Involvement of nerves and calcium channels in the intestinal response to *Clostridium difficile* toxin A: An experimental study in rats *in vivo*. *Gut*, **49:** 56–65.

Varela Chavez, C. *et al.* (2015) The catalytic domains of *Clostridium sordellii* lethal toxin and related large clostridial glucosylating toxins specifically recognize the negatively charged phospholipids phosphatidylserine and phosphatidic acid. *Cell Microbiol.*, **17:** 1477–1493.

Wang, Y.K., *et al.* (2015) A chimeric protein comprising the glucosyltransferase and cysteine proteinase domains of toxin B and the receptor binding domain of toxin A induces protective immunity against *Clostridium difficile* infection in mice and hamsters. *Cell Microbiol.,* **11:** 2212–2215.

Yang, Z., *et al.* (2015) Mechanisms of protection against *Clostridium difficile* infection by the monoclonal antitoxin antibodies actoxumab and bezlotoxumab. *Infect. Immun.,* **83:** 822–831.

Yu, H., *et al.* (2015) Identification of toxemia in patients with *Clostridium difficile* infection. *PLoS One,* **10:** e0124235.

7   Clostridium botulinum and Clostridium tetani Neurotoxins

Michel R. Popoff

Introduction

Clostridium botulinum is defined as a *Clostridium* sp. that produces one or several neurotoxins inducing flaccid paralysis. These are termed botulinum neurotoxins (BoNTs) and are responsible for botulism, a rare but often severe disease with a high lethality rate. In contrast, *Clostridium tetani* synthesizes a related neurotoxin called tetanus toxin (TeNT), which causes a dramatic spastic paralysis. Both BoNTs and TeNT exert neurotoxicity by blocking the release of neurotransmitters. While BoNTs inhibit the evoked release of acetylcholine at the neuromuscular junctions causing the aforementioned flaccid paralysis, TeNT impairs neuroexocytosis at central inhibitory interneurons, resulting in prevention of the inhibitory pathways and, thus, inducing the noted spastic paralysis. BoNTs and TeNT are the most potent toxic compounds and are responsible for severe, often-fatal paralysis in humans and domestic animals.

Clostridia producing botulinum neurotoxins

Clostridia capable of producing BoNTs display heterogeneous bacteriological characters and are divided into several species and groups. The taxonomic position of the *C. botulinum* species was originally based on only one phenotype; the BoNT non-toxic variant strains, genetically related to *C. botulinum*, were assigned to different species, such as *Clostridium sporogenes* and *Clostridium subterminale*. It soon transpired that BoNTs are, in fact, seven different protein neurotoxins that are immunologically distinct and have been designated by the letters A to G. A novel type, BoNT/H, which seems to be a hybrid between BoNT/F and BoNT/A, has been reported but awaits further characterization. More recently,

Clostridial Diseases of Animals, First Edition. Francisco A. Uzal, J. Glenn Songer, John F. Prescott and Michel R. Popoff.
© 2016 John Wiley & Sons, Inc. Published 2016 by John Wiley & Sons, Inc.

sequence analysis has permitted scientists to distinguish subtypes within the BoNT types (see below and Table 7.1). However, all of them cause the typical flaccid paralysis of botulism in experimental animals, similar to that observed in humans and domestic and wild animals suffering from botulism. Physiological differences among *C. botulinum* strains have been identified, but the production of the different BoNT types does not necessarily correlate with *C. botulinum* strain phenotypes. The species has been divided into six physiological groups (Table 7.1):

- Group I: *C. botulinum* A and proteolytic strains of *C. botulinum* B and F;
- Group II: *C. botulinum* E and glucidolytic strains of *C. botulinum* B and F;
- Group III: *C. botulinum* C and D;
- Group IV: *C. botulinum* G (or *C. argentinense*);
- Group V: *C. butyricum;*
- Group VI: *C. baratii.*

Group IV, which also includes non-toxic strains previously identified as *C. subterminale* and *C. hastiforme*, is metabolically distinct from the other groups and has been assigned to a different species called *C. argentinense.*

Genetic analysis using various techniques (23s and 16S rRNA gene sequencing, amplified fragment length polymorphism (AFLP), pulse-field gel electrophoresis (PFGE), multilocus sequence typing (MLST)) supports the view that the different groups of botulinum neurotoxin-producing clostridia correspond to distinct species. Phenotypic properties, DNA/DNA homology, and 16S rRNA analysis of all strains in each group, regardless of toxin type, are closely related but not strictly identical. Atypical toxigenic *C. butyricum* and *C. baratii* strains are phenotypically and genetically related to the type strains of these species and not to the other BoNT-producing clostridia. The genetic diversity of the botulinum-neurotoxin-producing clostridia versus non-neurotoxigenic clostridia is well illustrated by the analysis of 16S rRNA gene sequences. The six groups of botulinum-neurotoxin-producing clostridia are located on distinct phylogenetic branches as individual *Clostridium* spp.

Whole genome sequences of representative *Clostridium botulinum* strains are available and confirm the distribution of botulinum-neurotoxin-producing clostridia in various genetic groups. An overall comparison between complete *C. botulinum* genomes revealed strong similarity between genomes from group I strains, and their great distance from group II strains. Most proteins (81–86%) of group I strains share a protein identity of over 90%, but only 2–3% of proteins from group II genomes have orthologs encoded by group I genomes with such a high protein identity. However, several lineages can be differentiated among group I strains which likely represent strain adaptation to environmental or clinical niches. Indeed, nordic *C. botulinum* type B strains from group I belong to two homogeneous clusters, which differ by their resistance to toxic compounds such as cadmium and arsenic. Since a 100-fold higher concentration of arsenic occurs in certain areas of Finland compared to other European sites, the acquisition of arsenic resistance possibly represents an adaptive response to growing in specific environments. Moreover, whole-genome phylogenic single-nucleotide-polymorphism

Table 7.1 Groups and main properties of botulinum neurotoxin producing Clostridia, *botulinum* neurotoxin types and subtypes according to (Peck 2006, Peck 2009, Peck *et al.* 2011, Mazuet *et al.* 2012, Raphael *et al.* 2012, Hill and Smith 2013, Diao *et al.* 2014, Raphael *et al.* 2014, Weedmark *et al.* 2014, Kull *et al.* 2015, Mazuet *et al.* 2015)

Neurotoxin producing-*Clostridium*	Group I	Group II	Group III	Group IV	Group V	Group VI
Toxin type	A, proteolytic B, F	E, non proteolytic B, F	C, D	G	E	F
Sub type	A1, A2, A3, A5, A6, A7, A8 B1, B2, B3, B6, B7 F1, F3, F4, F5 bivalent A1(B), B5a4, Bf2, A2f4, A2f5 trivalent A2f4f5	B4 (or Bnp) E1, E2, E3, E6, E7, E8, E9, E10, E11, E12 F6	C, D, C/D, D/C	G	E4, E5	F7
Proteolysis	+	−	−	+	−	−
Lipase production	+	+	+	−	−	−
Growth temperature[a] Optimum	30–40°C	25–37°C	37–40°C	30–37°C	30–37°C	30–45°C
Minimum	10–12°C	2.5–3°C	15°C		12°C	10–15°C
Minimum pH for growth[a]	4.6	5	5.1	ND	4.8	3.7
Minimum water activity for growth[a]	0.96	0.97	0.97	0.94	ND	ND
NaCl concentration preventing growth[a]	10%	5%	ND	6.50%	ND	8.5
Spore thermoresistance[a]	$D_{121°C} = 0.21\,min^a$ $D_{121°C} = 0.19\,min^b$	$D_{82.2°C} = 2.4–231\,min$	$D_{104°C} = 0.1–0.9\,min$	$D_{104°C} = 0.8–1.12\,min$	$D_{100°C} < 0.1\,min$	ND
Botulism	Human Animal (rare)	Human Animal (rare)	Animal Human (very rare)	ND	Human Animal?	Human Animal?
Related non botulinum toxin producing *Clostridium*	*C. sporogenes*	ND	*C. novyi* *C. haemolyticum*	*C. subterminale* *C. proteolyticus* *C. schimacherense*	*C. butyricum*	*C. baratii*

[a] Thermoresistance of spores in phosphate buffer at pH7 according to (Peck *et al.* 2011).
[b] Thermoresistance of spores in liquid medium at pH7 according to (Diao *et al.* 2014).
ND: no data available.

(SNP) analysis revealed five distinct lineages among *C. botulinum* strains of group I according to type/subtype and/or botulinum locus organization with *ha* or *orfX* operon (see below). Although monitoring with a DNA microarray shows that group II *C. botulinum* strains are genetically closely related, two subsets can be individualized, one encompassing type B and F strains and a second containing the type E strains. The strains of the two subsets share common physiological properties such as minimal growth temperature and inhibitory NaCl concentration, but differ by their profile of carbohydrate metabolism.

Physiological properties

Group I (*C. botulinum* A and proteolytic strains of types B and F)

The strains of this group are characterized by proteolytic and lipase activity and by no or weak acidification of carbohydrates (Table 7.1). Glucose is acidified weakly. The cell wall contains glucose as sugar. The optimal temperature for growth is 37 °C. The strains of group I usually do not grow and do not form toxins at 10 °C or below. However, a large inoculum and long incubation period might result in sufficient growth and toxin formation at low temperatures such as 12 °C within 3–4 weeks. Growth of group I strains is inhibited by acid pH (< 4.6) and NaCl concentrations ≥ 10%. The thermoresistance of the spores is usually high (above 120 °C), but varies according to strain and the heating of the buffer and recovery culture medium.

Botulism was a major problem in the early days of the canning industry and, since its inception, the thermotolerance of *C. botulinum* strains has been extensively investigated in order to recommend safety rules for heat treatment. The most heat-resistant strains require heating at 121 °C for 0.21 min to reduce the number of viable spores by a factor of 10^{12} (12-D or *D* value). Therefore, for commercial and low-acid canned foods, heating at 121 °C for 3 min has been recommended.

Group II (*C. botulinum* E and glucidolytic strains of types B and F)

Group II strains acidify various carbohydrate substrates (amygdalin, dextrin, fructose, galactose, glucose, glycogen, maltose, ribose, sorbitol, sucrose, and trehalose but not lactose, mannitol, melibiose, or salicin). They mainly produce butyric and acetic acids from trypticase–yeast extract–glucose broth. They hydrolyze gelatin, but are non-proteolytic. The strains within this group contain glucose and galactose as cell-wall sugars. They have a lower optimal temperature of growth (around 25–30 °C) and can grow and produce toxins at very low temperatures (Table 7.1). Growth and toxin production have been reported to occur at temperatures as low as 3.0–3.3 °C in 5–7 weeks. However, most of the strains grow poorly below 5 °C. Spores are only moderately resistant to heat and do not survive 10 min at 90 °C. The highest temperature resistance of these spores in a phosphate buffer was reported to be 82.2 °C. Spores of group II strains are lysozyme-dependent for their germination. Lysozyme diffuses in the spore coat and induces peptidoglycan hydrolysis in the cortex, permitting the first step of germination. Lysozyme also increases spore recovery after heat treatment and thus increases heat resistance. In the presence of lysozyme, the heat resistance time at 82.2 °C is increased by a hundred-fold, from 2.31 min to 231 min. BoNT produced by group II strains, mainly type E, is not fully activated by endogenous protease. Trypsinization enhances the toxicity of these cultures. In addition, strains from group II are more sensitive than proteolytic *C. botulinum* strains to NaCl (inhibitory concentration 5% and above) and to low pH, with no growth below pH 5.

Group III (*C. botulinum* C and D)
The organisms within this group are either non-proteolytic or only very slightly so. They ferment glucose, glycerol, inositol, ribose, and xylose. Their cell wall does not generally contain sugar but may contain traces of glucose. The main end products of metabolism are acetate and butyrate. They grow at higher temperatures than the other *C. botulinum* strains, with the optimal temperature for growth being 37–40 °C. Most strains within this group grow well at 45 °C, with the minimal growth temperature being approximately 15 °C.

This group is heterogeneous according to some biochemical properties (the fermentation of several sugars and production of indole and hydrogen sulfide). Division into four subgroups has been proposed.

Group IV (*C. botulinum* G, also referred to as *C. argentinense*)
The strains of this species are proteolytic, hydrolyze gelatin, and do not ferment any of the usual carbohydrates. Unlike strains within the other *C. botulinum* groups, *C. argentinense* strains do not produce a lipase. They do, however, produce acetate, butyrate, iso-butyrate, iso-valerate, and phenylacetate as end products of metabolism. The optimal temperature of growth is 30–37 °C. The spores exhibit a similar heat resistance to group III strains.

Phenotypic differences have been observed between toxigenic and non-toxigenic *C. argentinense* strains by using cellular fatty analysis and multilocus enzyme electrophoresis. *C. argentinense* strains are phenotypically and genetically closely related to *C. subterminale* strains that are non-neurotoxigenic.

Group V (*C. butyricum*)
Toxigenic *C. butyricum* strains are phenotypically and genetically related to the typical strains of the *C. butyricum* species. They are non-proteolytic nor do they hydrolyze gelatin, but they strongly acidify various carbohydrates including glucose, cellobiose, fructose, galactose, glycogen, lactose, maltose, mannose, melibiose, raffinose, ribose, salicin, starch, sucrose, trehalose, xylose, and pectin. They do not produce lipase or lecithinase. They are mesophilic bacteria with an optimal growth temperature of 30–37 °C. The lowest pH for growth and toxin synthesis was found to be 4.8. Spores of neurotoxigenic *C. butyricum* are less resistant to heat ($D_{100\,°C} < 0.1$ min) than non-toxigenic strains ($D_{100\,°C} = 4.7$ min) .

C. butyricum strains producing type E neurotoxin have been isolated from cases of infant botulism and from young people in Italy, as well as from cases associated with the consumption of fermented soybean in China and in India and Japan. Based on the toxin gene sequence, toxigenic *C. butyricum* strains from Italy and China are divided into two distinct subtypes, termed E4 and E5, respectively, indicating independent evolution of *bont/E* after transfer into *C. butyricum*.

Group VI (*C. baratii*)

Toxigenic and non-toxigenic *C. baratii* strains display similar morphological and biochemical characteristics. *C. baratii* is phenotypically closely related to *C. perfringens*. Both species are non-motile and appear as thick, straight rods (0.5–1.9 x 1.6–15 μm). Strains sporulate poorly in an anaerobic culture medium. They produce lecithinase but not lipase.

C. baratii is readily differentiated from *C. perfringens* by the inability of *C. baratii* to hydrolyze gelatin. The optimal growth temperature is around 30–45 °C, with a minimum at around 10–15 °C. *C. baratii* acidifies culture medium containing various carbohydrates.

Neurotoxigenic *C. baratii* strains are genetically related to their non-toxigenic counterparts. Botulinum neurotoxin type F gene sequences from *C. baratii* form a cluster distinct from that containing strains of *C. botulinum* type F. Neurotoxigenic *C. baratii* type F is involved in a limited number of human cases, mainly due to intestinal colonization of infants or adults.

Geographical distribution of botulinum-neurotoxin-producing clostridia

C. botulinum is widespread in soils as well as in lake and sea sediments in most parts of the world. However, the different toxinotypes of *C. botulinum* are not equally distributed, some of them being restricted to particular ecological areas. The factors responsible for the geographical distribution of the different toxinotypes are poorly understood. In general, toxinotypes A, B, E, F, and G seem to have their principal habitat in soil, and sea- and fresh-water sediments. Toxinotypes A and B occur more frequently in soil, and the regional distribution of these two toxinotypes is different. Toxinotype E is more predominant in sea or lake sediments and fish than in soil. Toxinotypes C and D appear to be obligate parasites of birds and of other animals. Cadavers of animals or birds dead from botulism, or healthy carriers are the main sources of these organisms. They are seldom encountered in soil samples, except in the areas where the incidence of animal botulism is high. *C. botulinum* is not usually found in the digestive tract of healthy humans, but it can be found in that of animals, particularly *C. botulinum* C and D in regions where botulism is frequent.

C. botulinum A and B

Numerous investigations have surveyed the prevalence of *C. botulinum*, particularly in the USA. Types A and B were generally found in neutral to alkaline soil samples poor in organic matter, and much more rarely in aquatic sediment. *C. botulinum* type A is predominant in the western part of the United States (west of the Missouri and Mississippi rivers), in soil that is neutral to alkaline (average pH 7.5) with a lower than average organic content. In contrast, type B prevails largely in the eastern part of the USA. This toxinotype was recovered in slightly more acidic soil samples (average pH 6.25) with a higher level of organic matter and mainly from cultivated soils (pastures and fields). Other investigations reported the prevalence of type B in cultivated soil samples, but noted that this type is rare in soils contaminated with manure or animal feces. Fertilization was not considered a significant factor responsible for the frequent presence of *C. botulinum* type B in cultivated soils.

The incidence of *C. botulinum* A and B is very low in aquatic (sea- or freshwater) sediments and soil samples in the northern part of North America (Alaska, Canada).

Fewer investigations have been performed in Central and South America. Surveys of soil samples from Argentina, Brazil, and Paraguay demonstrated the presence of *C. botulinum* A and B, with a greater prevalence of type A.

C. botulinum type B is the most common type from soil and sediment samples in central and southern Europe (Great Britain, Ireland, Netherlands, France, Switzerland, and Italy), and from soil samples in Denmark. In Great Britain and Ireland, *C. botulinum* is much more frequent in lake and loch sediments than in soil samples, and type B is predominant.

C. botulinum A and B occur broadly in Asia, including the countries of the former USSR, China, and Taiwan. Contamination levels and type detection vary from region to region and depend upon factors including temperature, moisture, organic substance content, and other unidentified factors. Soil from southern regions with warm climates or subtropical and tropical areas showed the highest incidence of *C. botulinum* A and B. Highly populated regions are much more contaminated than desert areas. Distribution of types A and B varies locally and does not correspond to large geographical areas, as in North America.

There are few reports on the incidence of *C. botulinum* in Africa. In Kenya, soil samples seemed to be heavily contaminated, with a predominance of type A. In contrast, the contamination in South Africa was low, with *C. botulinum* B identified in three soil samples out of 102.

In Australia and New Zealand, *C. botulinum* A and B have been found, but their presence in the environment is low, consistent with a low incidence of human botulism in these areas.

C. botulinum E

The distribution of type E is more regional than other types. Type E is mainly found in northern areas of the Northern Hemisphere. This includes the northern part of North America (Alaska, Canada, northern United States), northern Europe (Ireland, Greenland, Denmark, Norway, Sweden, and the coast of the Baltic Sea), and North Asia (northern part of the countries of the former USSR, the Caspian Sea, and northern Japanese islands, including Hokkaido and the northern part of Honshu).

The ability of *C. botulinum* E to grow at a very low temperature is reflected in its prevalence in areas with cold temperatures. Its frequency decreases considerably in southern areas with warm weather. This type is mainly found in the aquatic environment (sediment and soil from the shores of lakes, seas, and rivers). Other factors such as organic matter content, salinity, and other unidentified factors influence the distribution of type E, which varies greatly from one region to another. Thus, this organism is commonly found in the Great Lakes in the northern United States, but more frequently in Lake Michigan than in any of the other lakes, and in Lake Michigan it was found more frequently in Green Bay than elsewhere. Type E is also very common in the Pacific Northwest of North America. Sediment samples of Lake Washington near Seattle contained 18 to 25 *C. botulinum* E per g. These particular areas seem to represent the principal habitat of *C. botulinum* E, where it can grow and multiply. A particularly high prevalence of *C. botulinum* E occurs in the Baltic Sea. This bacterium is most frequent and spore counting more abundant in sea- than in fresh-water sediment samples. Low oxygen content, low salinity, the presence of biomass, and depth seem to be more important factors than temperature controlling the propagation of type E in the aquatic environment. Contamination of raw fish in Finland ranges from 10 to 40% depending on the fish species. Type E has also been detected in fish roe (4–14% of the samples), vacuum-packed (5%) and air-packed (3%) fishery products, and vacuum-packed hot-smoked whitefish (10%). Investigations on Finnish trout farms revealed *C. botulinum* type E in farm sediment samples (68%), fish intestinal contents (15%), and fish skin samples (5%). A recent investigation in northern France showed a prevalence of *C. botulinum* of 16.5% from 175 sea fish samples, but the predominant toxinotype was type B (72%) followed by types A (24%) and E (4%). Only one sediment sample in 25 contained *C. botulinum* E.

C. botulinum C and D

C. botulinum types C and D are widespread throughout the world. *C. botulinum* C is mainly found in mud and sediments of marshes, ponds, and seashore where botulism in waterfowl is endemic. Outbreaks of botulism in birds and the presence of *C. botulinum* C in their environment have been reported in the United States, Great Britain, Denmark, Netherlands, France, and Japan. Intestinal contents and cadavers of susceptible birds seem to be the principal habitat of *C. botulinum* C. This type has also been detected in soil from warm areas such as in Indonesia, Bangladesh, and Thailand.

   C. botulinum D is more frequently associated with botulism in animals (ruminants, horses, and others). Carcasses of these animals and also from small animals (rodents and others) constitute the most common source of this organism. *C. botulinum* D can also be identified in soil samples where animal botulism is common (south and central Africa, Australia, America, and Europe).

C. botulinum F and G

Types F and G are much less frequently encountered than other types. Since the first identification of *C. botulinum* type F from a homemade liver paste responsible for a human botulism outbreak on the Danish island Langeland, this type has been demonstrated in marine sediment of the west coast of the United States, and in marine and fresh-water sediments in Brazil, Venezuela, and Indonesia.

C. botulinum G was first isolated from a soil sample in Argentina, and was identified from necropsy specimens in cases of unexplained death in adults and infants, and from five soil samples out of 41 in close association with cultivated land in Switzerland.

C. butyricum

C. butyricum is a widespread bacterium in the environment, including soil, fresh-water and marine sediments, cheese, the rumen of healthy calves, animal and human feces, and more rarely in clinical specimens (blood, urine, respiratory tract, pleural cavity, abdomen, wounds, and abscesses). *C. butyricum* has been involved in cases of necrotizing enterocolitis in newborns. Artificial feeding and intestinal stasis support abundant proliferation of *C. butyricum* in the intestinal content. Bacterial overgrowth is accompanied by large-scale production of hydrogen and organic acids (mainly butyric acid) which have been recognized as the main virulence factors of *C. butyricum* in neonatal necrotizing enterocolitis.

The first two neurotoxigenic *C. butyricum* strains were isolated from infant botulism in 1985–1986 in Rome (Italy). Extensive studies have been carried out in the vicinity of Rome, and no strains producing BoNT/E were isolated; only *C. botulinum* A and B strains were found in 9.6% of 52 soil samples. Ten years later, two additional cases of toxico-infection with neurotoxigenic *C. butyricum* strains were described in young people in Italy. These isolates were genotypically and phenotypically identical to the former Italian strains. In 1994, several cases of food-borne botulism were reported in China. The implicated food consisted of salted and fermented paste made of soybeans and wax gourds. *C. butyricum* type E was isolated from soil samples around the patients' houses. The *bont*/E gene sequences from 11 Chinese *C. butyricum* strains were identical and differ from those of *C. botulinum* E (96.9% identity at the amino acid level) and the Italian *C. butyricum* strain BL6340 (95% identity). PFGE, Southern blot hybridization, and randomly amplified polymorphic DNA permitted distinction of three clones among the neurotoxigenic *C. butyricum* strains: two corresponding to the Chinese isolates, one of which was responsible for the food-borne botulism outbreak, and one to the Italian strains. This indicates that the neurotoxigenic *C. butyricum* strains are clonally distributed across vast areas. In contrast, *C. botulinum* type E strains from fish and fish products showed a wide biodiversity (62 different subtypes among 92 isolates).

C. baratii

C. baratii is isolated from soil, sediments, normal human and rat feces, and occasionally from war wounds, peritoneal fluid, and infection of the eyes, ear, and prostate. The source of the toxigenic *C. baratii* producing a BoNT/F responsible for one case of infant botulism and cases of adult botulism in the United States, Spain, and France has not been elucidated.

The botulinum locus

BoNTs are produced by neurotoxigenic strains of clostridia, together with several associated non-toxic proteins (ANTPs). BoNTs and ANTPs associate to form large complexes of various sizes, also known as progenitor toxins. ANTPs encompass a non-toxic, non-hemagglutinin component (NTNH) and several hemagglutinin components (HAs) or OrfX proteins.

The genes encoding the neurotoxins and ANTPs, which associate with BoNT to form the botulinum complexes, have been cloned and sequenced in representative clostridial strains of each BoNT type. The BoNT and ANTP genes are clustered in close vicinity and constitute the botulinum locus. They are organized into two operons. The operon localized in the 3′ part of the *botulinum* locus contains *bont*, which is immediately preceded by *ntnh*, which encodes the NTNH component. The *ntnh–bont* operon is conserved in all *C. botulinum* strains. In *C. botulinum* types E and F and certain *C. botulinum* A strains, this operon contains an additional gene called *p47*, encoding a 47 kDa protein. The second operon consists of the hemagglutinin (HA) genes or OrfX genes and is localized upstream of the *ntnh–bont* operon. The *ha* or *orfX* operon is transcribed in the opposite orientation to that of the *ntnh–bont* operon and shows more strain variation than the *ntnh–bont* operon, which is highly conserved in all *C. botulinum* strains. The *ha* operon consists of three genes (*ha70, ha17,* and *ha33*) in *C. botulinum* B, C, D, and some A strains. The *ha* genes of *C. botulinum* G only comprise *ha17* and *ha70*. The *ha* genes are missing in the non-hemagglutinating toxinotypes A1, A2, A3, A4, E, and F and an *orfX* operon (*orfX1, orfX2, orfX3*) instead of an *ha* operon lies upstream of the *ntnh–bont* operon. It is noteworthy that a *bont* gene can be inserted into an HA or OrfX locus. However, *bont/A1* is the only gene that has been found in either of the two types of botulinum locus.

A gene (*bontR*, previously called *orf21* or *orf22*), encoding an alternative sigma factor involved in the regulation of botulinum locus gene expression, is present in different positions in *C. botulinum* strains except in *C. botulinum* E and toxigenic *C. butyricum*.

Usually, one clostridial strain produces only one type of neurotoxin and the botulinum locus is present in a single copy in the genome, as suggested by Southern blotting of DNA fragments separated by pulsed-field gel electrophoresis. However, some rare strains synthesize two different BoNTs: BoNT/A–BoNT/B, BoNT/A–BoNT/F, and BoNT/B–BoNT/F producing strains have been isolated. The A–B strain contains two *bont* genes related to those of *C. botulinum* A2 and proteolytic *C. botulinum* B, respectively. In such strains, the two BoNTs are usually produced in different proportions. Thus, in Ba and Bf strains, BoNT/B is produced ten times more than BoNT/A and BoNT/F. Some clostridial strains contain silent neurotoxin genes. Several *C. botulinum* A strains isolated from food-borne and infant botulism contain a silent *bontB* gene. These strains are denoted A(b). The characterization of strain NCTC2916 shows that it has two loci, A and B, which are 40 kbp distant within the chromosome. The botulinum B locus consists of *bont/B, ntnh, bontR/B, ha33,* and *ha11* genes. *bont/A* is identical to the gene in *C. botulinum* A1 strains, but the organization of the botulinum A locus is similar to that of *C. botulinum* A2 and F strains. The BoNT/B nucleotide sequence is related to that of *C. botulinum* B strains (97% identity), but it has a stop mutation in position 128 and two base deletions (positions 2839 and 2944), resulting in reading frameshifts and multiple stop codons. Silent *bont/B* is also evidenced in non-toxigenic *C. subterminale* strains. The strain *C. botulinum* 667 also contains two loci, A and B, 40 kbp distant within the chromosome. The genetic organization is the same as that in strain NCTC2916 and the *bont/B* gene is silenced by mutations and deletions.

Genomic localization of the botulinum locus

The genes encoding for the different types of BoNT are on different genetic elements, including chromosomes, plasmids or phages depending on the species and strain of clostridia. In *C. tetani* and *C. argentinense*, the neurotoxin genes are present on a large plasmid (51 and 76 MDa respectively). Plasmids of various sizes and bacteriophages have been found in *C. botulinum* A, B, E, and F and previous works have shown that toxigenicity was not associated with the presence of these genetic elements. Therefore, the genes encoding for these neurotoxins were assumed to be located on the chromosome. However, it has been found that in some strains such as Loch Maree strain (subtype A3), 657Ba (type Ba and subtype A4), Okra (subtype B1), and Eklund 17B (type Bnp or B4), the botulinum neurotoxin genes are harbored by large plasmids (47 to 270 kb) (Table 7.2). Plasmid location of neurotoxin genes is common in *C. botulinum* type B strains, mainly in subtype B1, bivalent, and non-proteolytic strains. In the bivalent strain Ba657, the two botulinum loci, locus A and locus B, are located on the same plasmid and are separated by approximately 97 kbp. Similarly, the neurotoxin genes, *bontB* and *bont/f*, from one Bf strain are located on the same plasmid (pBf), which is closely related to pCLJ from the Ba657 strain. Interestingly, none of the botulinum plasmids show synteny to *C. tetani* plasmid pE88, which contains the *tent* gene. In *C. botulinum* type E and neurotoxigenic *C. butyricum* strains, *bont/E* is located mainly on the chromosome (Table 7.2). In three of 36 *C. botulinum* E strains, *bont/E1* is located on a large plasmid. In *C. botulinum* C and D, it has been clearly evidenced that BoNT is encoded by genes on bacteriophages.

The location of the botulinum locus within a chromosome or plasmid seems to occur not at random but at specific sites. Indeed, five specific sites of botulinum locus integration have been identified in strains from group I or II, whose genome sequencing is available. *orfX–bont/A2*, *orfX–bont/A1*, and *orfX–bont/F* loci are located in the *ars* operon, which contains three to five genes involved in arsenic reduction. *orfX–bont/A1* and *orfX–bont/F* loci share a similar integration site at the 5′ end of the *ars* operon, whereas the *orfx–bont/A2* locus is inserted between two copies of *arsC*. The *ha–bont/A1* and *ha–bont/B* loci, which contain a recombinant *ntnh* gene from type A and type B strains, are found in the *oppA/ brnQ* operon encoding for extracellular solute-binding protein and branched-chain amino acid transport proteins, respectively. This operon is lacking in non-proteolytic *C. botulinum* type B and *C. butyricum* type E strains. The third

Table 7.2 Genomic localization of botulinum loci in *botulinum* neurotoxin-producing Clostridia according to (Sakaguchi *et al.* 2005, Hill *et al.* 2009, Skarin *et al.* 2011, Hill and Smith 2013) (Franciosa *et al.* 2009, Brüggemann *et al.* 2011, Dover *et al.* 2013, Zhang *et al.* 2013, Hosomi *et al.* 2014, Raphael et al. 2014)

Chromosome			
Group	**Type/Subtype**	**Botulinum locus**	**Insertion site**
Group I	A1(B)	*orfX-bont/A1*	*arsC* operon
	A2	*orfX-bont/A2*	ND
	F	*orfX-bont/F*	ND
	A1	*ha-bont/A1*	*oppA/brnQ* operon
	A1(B)	*ha-bont/B*	ND
	A5(B)		*oppA/brnQ* operon
	B1, B2	*ha-bont/B*	ND
	A2f4f5	*orfX-bont/A2*	*arsC* operon
		orfX-bont/F4	*pulE* gene
	F4	*orfX-bont/F4*	*pulE* gene
Group II	E1, E3, E9	*orfX-bont/E1, 3*	*rarA* operon
	F6	*orfX-bont/F6*	*topB*
Group V	E4	*orfX-bont/E4*	*rarA* operon

Plasmid			
Group	**Type/Subtype**	**Botulinum locus**	**Plasmid**	**Size (bp)**
Group I	A3	*orfX-bont/A3*	pCLK	266785
	B5A4	*ha-bont/B5*	pCLJ	270346
		orfX-bont/A4		
	B1	*ha-bont/B1*	pCLD	148780
	B5f2	*ha-bont/B5*	pBf	ND
		orfX-bont/F2		
	A2b5	ND	plasmid strain CDC1436	ND
	A2f4f5	*orfX-bont/F5*	pCLQ	246124
	B2	*ha-bont/B2*	pCB111	265575
	F5	*orfX-bont/F5*	plasmid	~242000
Group II	B4 (or npB)	*ha-bont/B4*	pCLL	47642
	B4 (or npB)	*ha-bont/B4*	pCB17B	47689
	B4 (or npB)	*ha-bont/B4*	pCDC3875	58175
	B4 (or npB)	*ha-bont/B4*	pIFR05/025	60574
	E1	*orfX-bont/E1*	plasmid (strainCB11/1-1)	ND
	E1	*orfX-bont/E1*	plasmid	~146000

Phage			
Group	**Type/Subtype**	**Botulinum locus**	**Plasmid**	**Size (bp)**
Group III	C	*ha-bont/C*	C-st	185683
	D, C/D, D/C	*ha-bont/D, C/D, D/C*	D-phage, other phages	ND

ND: no data available

integration site is the *rarA* gene in group II and V strains, which contains the *orfX–bont/E* locus in *C. botulinum* type E and *C. butyricum* type E strains. *rarA* encodes a resolvase protein involved in recombination or insertion events of transposons. Interestingly, the botulinum E locus is inserted in the same codon (102) of *rarA* in both *C. botulinum* type E and *C. butyricum* type E strains, and the inserted botulinum locus contains an additional intact *rarA* gene. The trivalent strain A2f4f5 contains the *orfX–bont/A2* and *orfX–bont/F4* loci located in the chromosome at *arsC* and *pulE* (type II secretion system protein E), respectively. In *C. botulinum* F, the *orfX–bont/F6* locus has been found in a new chromosomal integration site, *topE*.

Two specific sites of botulinum locus location have been identified on plasmids from group I strains: one contains *orfX–bont/A3*, *orfX–bontT/A4* from the Ba strain, or *orfX–bontF* from the Bf strain, and the second harbors the *ha–bont/B* locus from *C. botulinum* B1 strains or bivalent Ba4 or Bf strains. The *ha–bont/B4* locus in non-proteolytic strains is located on a plasmid different from those of group I strains. However, the downstream flanking region of the HA–*npB* locus contains an IS element, a transposon-associated resolvase, and a site-specific recombinase. It is noteworthy that *C. botulinum* plasmids harboring *bont* genes such as pCLJ, pCLL, and pCDC-A3 (related to pCLK) are transferable by conjugation into a group I *C. botulinum* strain.

Genetic diversity of *Clostridium botulinum* strains and botulinum neurotoxin gene variation

Genetic analysis by 16S RNA gene sequence comparison or DNA/DNA homology has shown that *C. botulinum* strains form four distinct clusters which correspond to the physiological groups I to IV. AFLP and PFGE analysis also confirm the classification of proteolytic types A, B, and F strains in group I and the non-proteolytic types B, E, and F strains in group II, but can differentiate individual strains into each group. These methods have been used in epidemiological studies and are useful tools to investigate relatedness between strains isolated from patients and food. For example, among proteolytic *C. botulinum* strains, PFGE analysis differentiates the toxinotypes A, B, and F at an 83–86% similarity level, and enables discrimination of most individual strains. A greater diversity was observed among type A strains than among type B strains. These studies also indicate that each *C. botulinum* group is heterogeneous at the genome level.

A high level of similarity was observed between strains from group I by using DNA hybridization with a DNA microarray including 94% of the coding sequences from strain Hall. Two type A strains share 95–96% of the strain Hall coding sequences, and seven other proteolytic strains have 87–91% common coding sequences. A larger investigation reported that 58 *C. botulinum* strains from group I share 63% of coding sequences with those of strain ATCC3502. Interestingly, two *C. sporogenes* strains (physiologically related to *C. botulinum* group I but non-toxigenic) are significantly similar to strain Hall and share 84–87% of the coding sequences. In another microarray study, three *C. sporogenes* strains show approximately 63% common coding sequences with *C. botulinum* A ATCC3502.

The BoNT gene has been sequenced from a large number of strains, and sequence comparison has permitted identification of sequence variations in each toxinotype. Thereby, botulinum toxinotypes are divided into subtypes, which are defined as toxin sequences differing by at least 2.6% at the amino acid identity level. BoNT genes from type A strains show 92–95% nucleotide identities, corresponding to 84–90% amino acid identities, and are divided into subtypes termed A1 to A8 (Table 7.1). Subtypes A1 to A8 also differ in the botulinum locus composition. Type B genes differ from 2 to 4% at the nucleotide level and 3 to 6% at the amino acid level. They are classified into several subtypes: B1, B2, B3, B5, B6, B7, bivalent B, and non-proteolytic B. BoNT genes from non-proteolytic type B strains form only one subtype, whereas those from proteolytic strains show a greater variation, leading to a four-subtype division (Table 7.1). Sequences of neurotoxin genes in type B show less variation overall than those of type A, but a greater sequence variation is observed within members of each type B subtype compared to *bont/A*. BoNT/E sequences from *C. botulinum* type E (group II) fit into ten subtypes (E1, E2, E3, E6, E7, E8, E9, E10, E11, E12) sharing 99% nucleotide identity and 97–99% amino acid identity; they are more distantly related to BoNT/E sequences from *C. butyricum* strains which fall into two subtypes (E4, E5) with 97–98% nucleotide and 95–96% amino acid identities between sequences from both *Clostridium* species. Gene diversity has also been evidenced in the other parts of the genome, as tested by MLST and AFLP analysis, but most strains of *C. botulinum* E are conserved in the same clade. Subtype variation in *C. botulinum* E strains seems to result from recombination events rather than random mutations. Large differences (up to 25%) have been found in nucleotide sequences of BoNT/F, mainly in the region encoding the light chain, and five subtypes have been identified in proteolytic *C. botulinum* F versus one subtype in non-proteolytic *C. botulinum* F. The BoNT/F sequence from *C. baratii* (F7) forms a different cluster of those from *C. botulinum* F. The low number of strains of types C, D, F, and G that were analyzed does not permit significant evaluation of neurotoxin gene diversity. In group III, mosaic genes between BoNT genes of types C and D can be distinguished from classical strains of types C and D.

The significance of sequence diversity in each toxinotype is not yet well known, but could be important in the development of diagnostic tests and therapeutic agents such as those based on immunotherapy. Therefore, BoNT/A1 and BoNT/A2, which differ by 10% at the amino acid sequence level, have large differences in monoclonal-antibody-binding affinity. Among six monoclonal antibodies that bind to BoNT/A1 with high affinity, three show a marked decrease in binding affinity (500 to more than 1000 fold) to BoNT/A2. Only combinations of monoclonal antibodies that bind tightly to toxin subtypes potently neutralize the corresponding toxin *in vivo*. Association of the three monoclonal antibodies with high affinity binding to subtypes A1 and A2 completely neutralizes A1 or A2 toxin, while replacement of two of the three monoclonal antibodies by two with a low binding affinity to BoNT/A2 induces a decrease in BoNT/A2 neutralization (50-fold less). The impact of subtype variation in binding and neutralization potency of polyclonal antibodies remains to be determined. Thus, the development of therapeutic polyclonal or monoclonal antibodies as well as vaccines based on single-toxin subtypes, needs to be evaluated in terms of their ability to protect against the other, related subtypes. Two toxins with little variation can be markedly different in activity if amino acid variations are in strategic toxin sites. Subtypes A1, A2, A3, and A4 of BoNT/A have been analyzed by sequence comparison, as well as by molecular modeling and structure comparison with the crystal structure of subtypes, the impact of which is not known. The ganglioside-binding site is conserved in all subtypes of BoNT/A. The greatest variability was found in the light (L) chain, mainly between subtypes A3 and A4 (76% identity). The enzymatic site of the L chain is conserved, but non-conservative mutations are observed in domains involved in substrate (SNAP-25) recognition. When compared to subtypes A1 and A2, subtypes A3 and A4 show sequence variation in a-exosite and S1′ subsite recognition, respectively, suggesting that these subtypes have a decreased affinity and catalytic efficiency for their substrate. Indeed, L chains from subtypes A3 and A4 show different catalytic properties toward the substrate SNAP-25 compared to L chains from subtypes A1 and A2, which show the same catalytic activity, although all L chain isoforms bind SNAP-25 with similar affinity. An L chain from subtype A4 and, to a lower extent from subtype A3, cleaves SNAP-25 less efficiently than an L chain from subtype A1 (2- and 23-fold less, respectively).

Another example of gene variation and toxin activity difference is found in neurotoxins of type B. BoNT/B from infant botulism strain 111 (subtype B2) differs from that produced by strain Okra/NT (associated with food-borne botulism in Japan) by 56 amino acid changes (95.7% identity), which mostly occur in the C-terminal part of the toxin. BoNT/B from strain 111 shows an approximate 10-fold lower specific activity than that of strain Okra/NT, and most of the monoclonal antibodies that recognize the C-terminus of Okra/NT BoNT/B do not react with BoNT/B of strain 111. The binding affinity of BoNT/B of strain 111 to the receptor synaptotagmin II in the presence of ganglioside GT1b is 4.2-fold lower than that of Okra/NT BoNT/B. Mutations of 23 residues in the C-terminus of strain 111 BoNT/B have been attributed to the lower binding affinity of the toxin to its receptor and thus to the lower specific toxicity.

Sequence comparison of *bont* genes suggests that they have evolved separately in different genomic backgrounds. BoNT genetic diversity could also reflect a different geographical distribution of strains or their involvement in different epidemiological situations. *C. botulinum* subtype A2 was first identified in infant botulism in Japan and was found to differ from strains involved in food-borne botulism in adults, referred to as subtype A1. However, no correlation was evidenced between strains of subtypes A1 and A2 isolated from the United States and the UK and their clinical origin – food-borne or infant botulism. But, strains of subtype A1 are more prevalent in the United States, whereas subtype A2 strains are commonly isolated in Europe. Indeed, all the strains from food-borne botulism in the United States which have been analyzed fall into subtype A1, and all 33 *C. botulinum* type A isolated from Italy belong to subtype A2 as well as two strains from infant botulism in the United Kingdom. However,

18 *C. botulinum* type A strains isolated in France or elsewhere in Europe by Prevot during the period approximately 1950–1960 are of subtype A1. Divergent strains of subtype A2 characterized by five amino acid differences in BoNT/A2 as well as by a slightly different botulinum locus organization (locus A2–OrfX') with a shorter intergenic region between *orfX1* and *bontR/A* genes (77 versus 1228 nucleotides) when compared to strain A2 Kyoto-F, have been identified in Italy, such as strains associated with consumption of contaminated cheese (Mascarpone). Organization of the botulinum locus of strain Mascarpone is closely related to that of the locus containing *bont/A1* in strain type A(B) NCTC2916. Strains Mascarpone and Kyoto-F probably have a common origin and then a distinct evolution including a gene rearrangement in strain Mascarpone with an ancestor of strain NCTC2916. Four *C. botulinum* A5 (B) strains isolated from wound botulism in heroin users in the UK and one from infant botulism in California (USA) support *bont* gene evolution independent of the geographical location and epidemiological situation.

Genetic diversity is also observed in the two flagellar glycosylation island (FGI) regions. Six profiles have been evidenced in 58 proteolytic strains from group I by DNA microarray that correlate with the diversity of flagellin glycan composition, as determined by mass spectrometry. The FGI genetic diversity does not match with that of the botulinum locus, indicating an independent evolution of FGI and botulinum locus genes in a relatively stable genomic background of group I *C. botulinum* strains. In addition to cell-wall and surface-structure variations, a marked difference in proteolytic strains of group I consists of resistance to toxic compounds. Thereby, group I *C. botulinum* type B strains representative of strains found in northern Europe are divided into two clusters (BI and BII), which differ by 413 coding sequences but contain the same neurotoxin gene of B2 subtype in an HA locus. In contrast to cluster BI strains, cluster BII strains are more resistant to arsenic and more sensitive to cadmium. Moreover, strains from the two clusters show other differences in metabolism, such as cluster BII strains growing at lower temperatures than cluster BI strains. This suggests a differential evolution of these environmental clostridia in response to adaptation to distinct ecological niches.

Differential genetic evolution is also illustrated by neurotoxigenic *C. butyricum* strains. *C. butyricum* strains producing type E neurotoxin have been isolated from infant botulism and from young people in Italy, as well as from botulism associated with consumption of fermented soybean in China. Based on the toxin gene sequence, toxigenic *C. butyricum* strains from Italy and China are divided into two distinct subtypes, called E4 and E5, respectively, indicating an independent evolution of the *bont/E* gene after transfer to *C. butyricum*.

Clostridium tetani

Tetanus neurotoxin (TeNT) is produced by a uniform group of bacteria belonging to the species *Clostridium tetani*.

Morphological and cultural characteristics

The cells of *C. tetani* are usually 0.3 to 0.6 μm in width and may vary considerably in length between 3 and 12 μm. They are Gram-positive in young cultures, but they lose the Gram coloration upon prolonged incubation. *C. tetani* is usually highly motile by peritrichous flagella, this property being responsible for its swarming growth on agar medium. However, some strains are non-motile and non-flagellated. These bacteria form spores, which appear as translucid terminal enlargements and give the typical appearance of drumsticks. The sporulation rate is variable according to strain. At pH 7 or above and at temperatures near 37 °C, sporulation starts within 24 hours of culture and continues for 4–12 days or more. Sporulation does not occur above 41 °C and it is slow at pH < 6. The sporulation process depends on the nature of the culture medium. Spores generally survive moderate heating (75 to 80 °C for 10 min) but usually are destroyed within one hour at 100 °C.

Germination of *C. tetani* spores occurs both under anaerobic and aerobic conditions, but the outgrowth of *C. tetani* following germination is strictly dependent upon a low oxidation–reduction potential. *C. tetani* forms colonies on the surface of agar medium only in anaerobiosis. Motile strains swarm over the entire surface of the agar, yielding a transparent film. Discrete colonies (2 to 5 mm) can be obtained by cultivation on media containing 3–4% agar. On blood agar, colonies are slightly raised, semi-translucent, and gray, with an irregular margin and surrounded by a narrow zone of hemolysis. *C. tetani* grows fairly well on the usual media containing peptones or tissue extracts.

Most of the usual biochemical tests used for identification of *Clostridium* spp. are negative, as no carbohydrates are acidified, and there is neither proteolysis nor production of lipase and lecithinase. Gelatin is liquefied slowly (2 to 7 days). The peptone used in the basal medium is of considerable importance when evaluating the ability of *C. tetani* to liquefy the gelatin. H_2S and indole are usually produced.

C. tetani strains are sensitive to penicillin and metronidazole. However, intravenous administration of penicillin can be inefficient due to impaired transport of the antibiotic in the wound, and wound debridement is a required step in the treatment of tetanus.

Genetic characteristics of *C. tetani*

The G + C content of *C. tetani* is 25–26%. This species has been classified in *Clostridium* group II by using 23S rRNA homology. The *Clostridium* genus encompasses more than 100 species which display a wide range of phenotypes and genotypes. Recently, phylogenetic analysis using 16S rRNA comparison indicates that the *Clostridium* genus should be restricted to the homology group I, as defined by Johnson and Francis. According to these data, *C. tetani* should be classified in a different genus. However, a study based on restriction maps of 16S rRNA showed that *C. tetani* belongs to the same cluster as *C. perfringens*, *C. sporogenes*, and *C. botulinum* C and G, which are members of the homology group I of Johnson and Francis.

Ten neurotoxigenic and three non-toxigenic *C. tetani* strains studied by Nakamura *et al.* in 1979 were homogeneous in DNA/DNA hybridization (85–93% similarity). *C. tetani* is similar culturally and biochemically to *C. cochlearium* and *C. tetanomorphum*, but it can be distinguished from the two latter species by DNA comparison. *C. cochlearium* and *C. tetanomorphum* are non-toxic and they are difficult to differentiate from the non-toxic *C. tetani* strains according to the bacteriological characteristics, as they do not, or weakly, liquefy gelatin. In contrast to *C. tetani*, *C. tetanomorphum* acidifies glucose and maltose.

The complete genome sequence of a toxigenic *C. tetani* strain has been determined. It consists of a 2,799,250 bp chromosome containing 2372 putative genes, and of a 74,082 bp plasmid containing 61 genes. *C. tetani* possesses many genes encoding peptidases and for products involved in amino acid and lipid degradation, whereas genes for sugar utilization are lacking. It contains numerous transport-related genes, in particular 35 genes for sodium-ion-dependent systems indicate that the Na$^+$ gradient is a major driving force in membrane transport. The TeNT-encoding gene and seven putative regulatory genes are localized on the plasmid, whereas the tetanolysin (a hemolysin) gene and putative adhesin genes are located on the chromosome. Many genes encoding putative adhesins have been identified: 2 fibronectin-binding proteins, 11 related surface-layer proteins (SLPs), 19 homologues to a *Clostridium difficile* adhesin, and 2 proteins with multiple leucine-rich repeat domains similar to the *Listeria monocytogenes* internalin A. SLP-A shows important size variation from strain to strain. Genome analysis has revealed different sets of surface-associated protein genes in pathogenic clostridia, which probably mediate their interactions with the environment or host and account for the fact that some clostridial species such as *C. tetani* and, to a lesser extent some *C. botulinum* strains of group I, can develop in wounds.

Distribution of *C. tetani* in the environment

C. tetani is a ubiquitous organism that is commonly found in soil samples in all parts of the world. The frequency of its isolation is variable according to the different investigations. Surveys in Japan, Canada, Brazil, and the United States have yielded 30–42% positive samples. Several factors influence the different frequencies of *C. tetani* isolation from soil, including pH, temperature, moisture, and the amount and type of organic materials. Thus, germination and multiplication of *C. tetani* have been observed preferentially in neutral or alkaline soil, with temperatures > 20 °C and humidity reaching 15%.

The geographical distribution of *C. tetani* shows a higher presence in southern regions, and accordingly, the incidence of tetanus is higher in warmer countries (western and central Africa, south-east Asia, India, the Pacific islands, and south of the United States) than in the cooler parts of the world (Canada, Norway, the UK, Finland, Sweden, and others). This bacterium can be found in the intestines of animals, but it does not represent a significant part of the normal digestive flora. Different surfaces and objects contaminated with soil particles, dust, or feces may contain *C. tetani*. Toxigenic strains have also been isolated within hospitals from catgut, cotton wool, dust and air samples, human skin, and wounds.

Susceptibility of animal species to clostridial neurotoxins

Susceptibility to botulinum neurotoxins
Naturally occurring botulism is found in all animals. However, the susceptibility to the different BoNT types varies according to the animal species. The sensitivity of several animal species to crude preparations of BoNT types has been determined experimentally in comparison with the toxicity in mice (Table 7.3). These data are only an estimation, since great individual variations are observed. Globally, small rodents such as mice are highly susceptible to all BoNT types. Cattle are highly susceptible to type D and, to a lesser extent, to type C. Botulism has rarely been reported in sheep, although type C outbreaks have been described in Australia and, more recently, type C and D outbreaks have occurred in South Africa and the United Kingdom. Botulism in cattle and sheep is commonly associated with feeding of broiler or poultry litter, although this is no longer allowed in the US. Horses are susceptible to types A, B, and E, but under natural conditions botulism types C and D are the most frequent. Carnivores (cats, dogs) and, to a greater extent, swine are more resistant to BoNT. However, mink are highly susceptible to types A and C. Among birds, ducks and other waterfowl are susceptible to types A, C, D, and E. Outbreaks frequently involve type C or D. In contrast, gallinaceous birds (chickens, peafowl, pheasants, turkeys) are more resistant to type D. Severe outbreaks of botulism type E with multiple genetically distinct strains of *C. botulinum* E have occurred in wild birds in North America and in northern Europe.

The more recent identification of mosaic BoNT C/D and D/C shows that *C. botulinum* C/D is preferentially associated with botulism in farmed and wild birds, and *C. botulinum* D/C with botulism in cattle. The toxin activity of *C. botulinum* D/C is completely neutralized by anti-BoNT/D antibodies and partially with anti-BoNT/C antibodies, whereas toxic sera from birds with botulism type D/C are neutralized by both anti-BoNT/C and anti-BoNT/D antibodies. However, the mosaic *C. botulinum* C/D and D/C strains seem to be widely distributed in mammals, birds, and the environment. Toxigenic *C. botulinum* is not a normal inhabitant of the digestive tract of birds, indicating that botulism is exogenously acquired.

Susceptibility to BoNT types also depends on the route of administration. Experimentally, the oral route is much less efficient than the parenteral route. Some examples are shown in Table 7.4.

Susceptibility to tetanus neurotoxin
All mammalian species are susceptible to TeNT, but the minimum lethal dose varies greatly from one species to another. Relative doses according to animal species based on the lethal dose in the most susceptible species are shown in Table 7.5. These

Table 7.3 Toxicity of botulinum toxin types according to the animal species and injected intraperitoneally or as indicated. The toxicity titers are expressed as intra-peritoneal mouse lethal doses (MLD) per kg of body weight, according to (Smith 1977) and [a] from (Wright 1955)

Animal species	BoNT type					
	A	B	C	D	E	F
Monkey	400 650 (Oral)	180 (Oral)	> 9,000 > 100,000 (Oral)	> 70,000 > 600,000 (Oral)	1,500–2,500 (Oral)	50,000–75,000 (Oral)
Horse	1800 (SC)	ND	> 8,000 (SC)	20,000 (Oral)	Animal species	Animal species
Mice	1	1	1	1	1	1
Rat	10–25	ND	ND	ND	ND	ND
Guinea pig	5	4	1.6–30	4	34	ND
Rabbit	25–40	ND	20	12 (SC)	ND	ND
Cattle	ND	ND	ND	2.2	ND	ND
Swine	20,000 (IV)	ND	> 18,000 (IV)	> 67,000 (IV)	ND	ND
Cat	12,000	ND	40,000 (SC)	7.5×10^7 (SC)	ND	ND
Dog	18,000	ND	1,000[a]	100,000[a]	100[a]	ND
Mink	1,000–24,000	100,000	1,000 40–167 (SC)	10^7	10,000	10^6
Ferret	ND	ND	10^6 (Oral)	ND	ND	ND
Chicken	10 (IV)	20,000 (IV)	16,000 (IV)	> 320,000 (IV)	100 (IV)	640,000 (IV)
Duck	ND	ND	500–76,000 45–80,000 (Oral)	ND	ND	ND
Peafowl	170 (IV)	33,000 (IV)	2,700 (IV)	> 320,000 (IV)	170 (IV)	640,000 (IV)
Pheasant	44–170 (IV)	88,000 (IV)	70 (IV)	> 320,000 (IV)	440 (IV)	640,000 (IV)
Turkey	20 (IV)	40,000 (IV)	320 (IV)	> 320,000 (IV)	200 (IV)	640,000 (IV)

SC: subcutaneous
IV: intravenous
ND: no data available

Table 7.4 Susceptibility to crude preparations of BoNT types according to intraperitoneal or intravenous administration versus oral administration. The BoNT toxic activity is expressed as intra-peritoneal mouse lethal doses per kg of body weight (Smith 1977)

BoNT type	Animal species	Intraperitoneal administration	Intravenous administration	Oral administration
A	Monkey	400	40	650–1,700
	Guinea pig	5.2	ND	717
	Rabbit	25–40	ND	25,000–40,000
	Rat	10–25	ND	420,000–>10^7
	Mink	1,000	ND	10^7
	Swine	ND	20,000	> 10^6
	Chicken	ND	10	10^6
	Peafowl	ND	170	500,000
	Pheasant	ND	170	500,000
	Turkey	ND	20	200,000
Type B	Mink	100,000	ND	10^6
	Swine	ND	180	3×10^6
Type C	Monkey	> 9,000	ND	200,000
	Guinea pig	1.6–30	ND	177
	Rabbit	20	ND	37,500
	Mink	1,000	ND	100,000
	Swine	ND	> 18,000	> 320,000
	Chicken	ND	16,000	160,000
	Peafowl	ND	2,700	270,000
	Pheasant	ND	70	7,000
	Turkey	ND	320	3,000
	Swine	ND	180	3×10^6
Type D	Guinea pig	4.1	ND	436
	Mink	10^7	ND	> 10^8
	Swine	ND	> 67,000	> 780,000
Type E	Guinea pig	34	ND	178,000
	Mink	10,000	ND	10^7
	Swine	ND	14,000	> 1.4×10^6
	Chicken	ND	100	100,000
	Pheasant	ND	440	440,000
	Turkey	ND	200	200,000
Type F	Mink	10^6	ND	> 10^6
	Swine	ND	4,000	> 170,000
	Chicken	ND	> 64,000	100,000
	Pheasant	ND	> 64,000	440,000
	turkey	ND	> 64,000	200,000

ND: no data available

values are only indicative and reflect that some animal species are highly susceptible to TeNT and others are rather resistant. The species most susceptible to tetanus include horses, guinea pigs, monkeys, sheep, mice, and goats, whereas cats and dogs are less vulnerable, and birds are resistant. Humans are among the most susceptible

Table 7.5 Lethal amounts of tetanus neurotoxin

Species	Relative minimum lethal dose[a]	Lethal dose per Kg body weight
Human	ND	10 MLD100[b] < 2.5 ng
Horse	0.5–1	ND
Guinea pig	1	0.3 ng[c]
Monkey	2	ND
Sheep	2–4	ND
Mouse	2–20	1 ng[c]
Goat	12	ND
Rabbit	12–900	0.05 – 5[c]
Dog	300–480	ND
Cat	1,200–960	ND
Goose	6,000	ND
Pigeon	6,000–24,000	ND
Hen	180,000	ND

[a] The relative minimum lethal doses are reviewed in (Wright 1955). The differences depend on the different studies performed with different toxin preparations, the breeds, sex, and age of the animals, and distinct experimental conditions. These values are only a broad estimation and have been estimated from intramuscular or subcutaneous injection.
[b] from (Rethy et al. 1997) (MLD, mouse lethal dose)
[c] from (Gill 1982)
ND: no data available

species. In the natural-occurring tetanus, the mortality rate is about 90–95% in sheep and goats, 75% in horses and pigs, and 50% in cattle and dogs.

Structure of clostridial neurotoxins

BoNTs and TeNT share a common structure. They are synthesized as a precursor protein (about 150 kDa), which is inactive or weakly active. The precursor, which does not contain a signal peptide, is released from the bacteria possibly by an as-yet-misunderstood cell-wall exfoliation mechanism. The precursor is proteolytically activated in the extra-bacterial medium either by clostridial proteases or by exogenous proteases such as digestive proteases in the intestinal content. The active neurotoxin consists of a light chain (L, about 50 kDa) and a heavy chain (H, about 100 kDa), which remain linked by a disulfide bridge. The structure of BoNTs shows three distinct domains: an L chain containing α-helices and β-strands and including the catalytic zinc-binding motif, the N-terminal part of the H chain forming two unusually long and twisted α-helices, and the C-terminal part of the H chain consisting of two distinct subdomains (H_{CN} and H_{CC}) involved in the recognition of the receptor. While the three domains are arranged in a linear manner in BoNT/A and BoNT/B, both the catalytic domain and the binding domain are on the same side of the translocation domain in BoNT/E. This domain organization in BoNT/E might facilitate a rapid translocation process.

The overall sequence identity at the amino acid level between BoNTs and TeNT ranges from 34 to 97%. Several highly conserved domains account for the common mode of action of these toxins. Thereby, the central domains of L chains are closely related in all the clostridial neurotoxins and contain the consensus sequence (His-Glu-X-X-His) characteristic of a zinc-metalloprotease active site. The N-terminal half of the H chains is also highly conserved, and it is involved in the translocation of the L chain into the cytosol. Thus, a similar mechanism of internalization of the intracellular active domain into target cells is shared by all the clostridial neurotoxins. In contrast, the C-terminal half of the H chain, mainly the H_{CC} subdomain, is the most divergent. This accounts for the different receptors recognized by the clostridial neurotoxins (see below).

Mode of action of clostridial neurotoxins

Although BoNTs and TeNT use different routes to enter their final neuronal targets, they display a similar intracellular mechanism of action. BoNTs enter by the oral route (food-borne botulism) or are produced directly in the intestine (infant or intestinal botulism) subsequent to *C. botulinum* intestinal colonization and then undergo a transcytosis across the digestive mucosa. After diffusion into the extracellular fluid and bloodstream, BoNTs target motor neuron endings. In contrast, TeNT is formed in wounds colonized by *C. tetani*. A similar situation is encountered during wound botulism. TeNT diffuses in the extracellular fluid and can target all types of nerve endings (sensory, adrenergic neurons, and motor neurons), but it is mainly transported retrogradely through the motor neurons (see below).

Each type of BoNT and TeNT recognizes specific receptors on demyelinated terminal nerve endings, mainly through the H_{CC} subdomain. BoNT/A, /C, /E, and /F exploit the three isoforms of the vesicle protein SV2 as specific receptors, while BoNT/B and /G bind to synaptotagmin I or II. The GPI-anchored membrane protein Thy-1 has been proposed to act as a TeNT receptor, but this has not been confirmed. A subunit of a neurotrophin receptor has been proposed as well. Although SV2 has not been defined as a receptor for TeNT, SV2A and SV2B are involved in the uptake of TeNT into central neurons. Ganglioside-binding sites have been characterized in the H_{CC} subdomain. Interestingly, TeNT and BoNT/D exhibit two carbohydrate-binding sites, whereas BoNT/A and BoNT/B show only one. Accordingly, TeNT can bind simultaneously to two gangliosides. BoNT/C and BoNT/D interact with gangliosides (GD_{1b}, GT_{1b}) and phosphatidylethanolamine, respectively by their H_{CC} subdomain. Gangliosides (GD_{1b}, GT_{1b}, and GD_2) and SV2A/B/C also mediate the entry of BoNT/D into neurons, but by a different mechanism than that used by BoNT/A and BoNT/E. The role of the H_{CN} subdomain, which may interact with phosphatidylinositol phosphates, is still unclear. Overall, whatever the considered clostridial neurotoxin, the identified protein receptors are not neurospecific and are expressed on several cell types including intestinal crypt epithelial cells in the intestine. The distribution of the gangliosides recognized by BoNTs differs from that of the protein receptors. Thus, the high affinity of BoNTs and TeNT for presynaptic membranes probably results from multiple and synergistic interactions with the ganglioside and protein parts of the receptor, and binding to gangliosides which induces conformational changes in the Hc domain, probably facilitates subsequent binding to protein receptors. Co-presence of the *ad hoc* ganglioside(s) and protein receptors likely facilitates the identification of the cell subset targeted by TeNT or BoNTs at the very low concentrations encountered in the physiological medium during the disease. At higher concentrations, binding to the protein receptor is likely sufficient for mediating toxin binding. Indeed, the number of cell types affected by these toxins expands with increasing toxin concentrations. Therefore, BoNTs can target numerous (but not all) neurons, as well as non-neuronal cells at high concentrations, inhibiting the release of various compounds.

A neurotoxin bound to its receptor is internalized by receptor-mediated endocytosis. An essential difference between the two types of neurotoxins is that BoNTs are directly endocytosed in recycling synaptic vesicles or clathrin-coated vesicles, which, when acidified, trigger the translocation of the L chain into the cytosol. Therefore, the BoNT L chain is delivered to the peripheral nervous system, specifically to neuromuscular junctions where it blocks the release of acetylcholine, leading to a flaccid paralysis. In contrast, TeNT enters different endocytic vesicles, which are not acidified. Retroaxonal ascent of these cargos in a microtubule-dependent manner mediates retrograde transport of the toxin to the cell body of neurons in the spinal cord. The tubulo-vesicular organelles involved in TeNT transport are characterized by the presence of neurotrophin receptor such as p75[NTR]. The C-terminal fragment of TeNT drives the retrograde transport of the toxin, and can be used to transport heterologous protein in the same way. When released into the extracellular space, TeNT carries out a transsynaptic migration and reaches its final target neurons, which are inhibitory interneurons involved in the regulation of the motor neuron activity. TeNT enters target inhibitory interneurons via vesicles that are acidified, thus permitting the delivery of the L chain into the cytosol, where it inhibits the regulated release of glycine and GABA. Overall, the mechanism of translocation is not completely understood for BoNT and TeNT. Acidification of the vesicle lumen triggers a conformational change in the neurotoxin and subsequent translocation of the L chain into the cytosol. It remains unclear whether a single H chain or a tetramer of it inserts into lipid membranes to form a channel, allowing transmembrane passage of the defolded L chain. These channels appear to be cation selective and permeable to small molecules (< 700 Da). The N-terminal part of the H chain mediates the translocation of the L chain into the cytosol at acidic endosomal pH by modifying the electrostatic interactions with the phospholipids without detectable conformational changes. In addition, the disulfide bond between the two chains has a crucial role in the translocation process. Then, the L chain refolds in the neutral pH of the cytosol. Cytosolic translocation factors such as β-COPI may be involved in this mechanism, as has been found for diphtheria toxin.

L chains of all clostridial neurotoxins are zinc-metalloproteases that cleave one of the three members of the SNARE proteins. TeNT and BoNT/B, D, F, and G attack synaptobrevin (or VAMP), BoNT/A and E cleave SNAP-25, and BoNT/C1 cuts both SNAP-25 and syntaxin. The cleavage sites are different for each neurotoxin except BoNT/B and TeNT, which proteolyse synaptobrevin at the same amino acid bound. Cleavage of SNARE proteins occurs only when disassembled. Since VAMP, SNAP-25, and syntaxin play a major role in the regulated fusion of synaptic vesicles with the plasma membrane at the release sites, their cleavage induces a blockade of the neurotransmitter exocytosis.

SNAP-25 cleavage by BoNT/A or BoNT/E alters SNAP-25 and synaptotagmin interaction, thus strongly reducing the responsiveness to Ca^{++} of exocytotic machinery. Indeed, removal of the nine C-terminal amino acids of SNAP-25 by BoNT/A deeply disrupts the coupling between Ca^{++} sensing and the final step in exocytosis. Truncated SNAP-25 can behave as a dominant negative mutant upon the exocytotic process, suggesting that after BoNT/A treatment, the block of release is due to both functional elimination of SNAP-25 and accumulation of the cleavage product which competitively inhibits exocytosis. In contrast, blockade of exocytosis by BoNT/E is only due to the elimination of functional SNAP-25, not to the production of competitive antagonists of SNARE complex formation. Indeed, inhibition of exocytosis by BoNT/E can be rescued by supplementing the C-terminal portion of SNAP-25 removed by the toxin. Truncation of SNAP-25 by BoNT/E destabilizes the four-helix bundle of the SNARE complex, and SNAP-25 truncated by BoNT/E is not retained by syntaxin.

VAMP cleavage abolishes its interaction with the adaptor protein AP3 and affects synaptic vesicle recycling *via* early endosomes. The SNARE cleavage products also have the potential to interfere with fusion processes. Consistent with synaptophysin-1 controlling specifically the targeting of VAMP2 but not VAMP1 to synaptic vesicles, is the observation that the cytosolic cleavage product of VAMP2 but not VAMP1, released upon TeNT or BoNT/B activity, blocks neurotransmitter release. This result suggests an alteration of the exocytosis due to a disturbance of synaptophysin-1/VAMP2 interaction and of coupling between detecting Ca^{++} and synaptic vesicle triggering. Since the synaptic vesicles docked with unproductive complexes cannot fuse or undock, they stay at the fusion sites (with slightly increased numbers) irreversibly plugging the fusion sites that would normally accommodate intact vesicles. This progressively reduces the number of active release sites to which exocytosis can occur, as recently demonstrated for TeNT at identified *Aplysia* cholinergic synapses. When VAMP is cleaved by TeNT, BoNT/B or /G, the VAMP portion (~20 amino acids) remaining in the synaptic vesicle membrane does not contain interaction sites for the other SNAREs. Therefore, the synaptic vesicle membrane is no longer linked to a SNARE complex, and fusion with the plasma membrane cannot occur. When VAMP is cleaved by BoNT/D or /F, the C-terminal fragment remaining in the vesicle membrane is long enough to anchor the synaptic vesicle to the SNARE complex, but fusion cannot occur because the SNARE complex cannot transit into the thermally stable four-helix bundle.

BoNT/C cleaves both syntaxin-1 and SNAP-25, but *in vitro* cleavage of SNAP-25 by BoNT/C occurs with low efficiency (~1000-fold difference) versus cleavage by BoNT/A or /E. This raises a question as to which of the two targets is involved in BoNT/C neuroexocytosis blockade. In squid giant synapses, BoNT/C cleaves syntaxin-1, but not SNAP-25, whereas in cultured hippocampal slices or spinal neurons from mammals, BoNT/C efficiently removes nearly all SNAP-25. Thus, depending on the cell type, the secretory blockade is likely due to syntaxin and/or SNAP-25 cleavage. In addition, a BoNT/C mutant, able to cleave only syntaxin, blocks neurotransmitter release, further supporting the role of syntaxin in Ca^{++} triggered neuroexocytosis. Upon syntaxin cleavage, SNARE complexes are formed, but are loosely docked to the plasma membrane. Thus, synaptic vesicles remain tethered to the plasma membrane and cannot fuse.

Although the physiological properties induced by the cleavage of VAMP, SNAP-25, or syntaxin are not equivalent at the neuromuscular junctions, all the clostridial neurotoxins cause a blockade of the regulated neurotransmission, which varies in intensity and duration according to each neurotoxin type. TeNT and BoNT/B share the same molecular mechanism. They are translocated in different subsets of neurons (excitatory neuron: BoNTs >> TeNT; inhibitory neurons: TeNT >> BoNTs), producing strongly different symptoms. This induces different clinical signs (TeNT: spastic paralysis; BoNTs: flaccid paralysis). Indeed, the peripheral dysautonomia and flaccid paralysis caused by BoNTs result from preferential inhibition of acetylcholine release. In the spinal cord or facial motor nuclei, TeNT-mediated blockade of glycine or GABA release disrupts the negative controls exerted by the inhibitory interneurons onto the motor neurons, turning on excessive firing of the motor neurons and ensuing muscle contraction.

Concluding remarks

During their evolution, bacteria of the *Clostridium* genus have developed protein toxins that affect the central and peripheral nervous system of various vertebrates. Numerous other clostridial toxins utilize a similar strategy. They first bind to receptors on the plasma membrane of susceptible host cells, undergo endocytosis and translocate their enzymatically active domains/subunits into the cytosol, where, finally, they elicit the deleterious effects commonly associated with the holotoxins. Two unique classes of clostridial toxins, the BoNTs and TeNT, have evolved as specific inhibitors of the exocytosis machinery. Because this machinery mediates the release of transmitters, the BoNTs and

TeNT disrupt synaptic transmission which is indispensable for life in higher organisms. It is intriguing that toxins produced by environmental bacteria, which are not normally adapted for a commensal life with higher organisms and only interact accidentally with them, possess such specific and highly sophisticated tools. What is the underlying selective pressure for such evolution from a bacterial protease to a neurotoxin? What is the inherent benefit derived by an environmental bacterium to produce a neurotoxin, which apparently does not recognize other bacterial or environmental substrates? The benefit for an environmental bacterium to produce such potent toxins leading to rapid killing of the host is still speculative. Cadavers are appropriate substrates for these neurotoxigenic clostridia. They are able to invade the whole cadaver and thus to multiply at high levels. However, an adaptive and non-lethal growth in certain host compartments, such as the digestive tract, all through the life of the host would allow a more dense bacterial proliferation than during a unique cadaver invasion. On the other hand, bacterial multiplication in a cadaver increases the environmental contamination locally, facilitating the transmission to additional hosts and subsequent killing and bacterial propagation. Neurotoxigenic clostridia seem to have selected a brutal strategy rather than a long-term adaptive interaction with the host, unless disease associated with these bacteria only results from accidental events.

Bibliography

Abe, Y., *et al.* (2008) Infantile botulism caused by *Clostridium butyricum* type E toxin. *Pediatr. Neurol.*, **38**: 55–57.

Ahmed, S.A., *et al.* (2001) Enzymatic autocatalysis of botulinum A neurotoxin light chain. *J. Protein. Chem.*, **20**: 221–231.

Ahsan, C.R., *et al.* (2005) Visualization of binding and transcytosis of botulinum toxin by human intestinal epithelial cells. *J. Pharmacol. Exp. Ther.*, **315**: 1028–1035.

Altwegg, M., *et al.* (1988) Multilocus enzyme electrophoresis of *Clostridium argentinense* (*Clostridium botulinum* toxin type G) and phenotypically similar asaccharolytic Clostridia. *J. Clin. Microbiol.*, **26**: 2447–2449.

Anniballi, F., *et al.* (2002) Influence of pH and temperature on the growth of and toxin production by neurotoxigenic strains of *Clostridium butyricum* type E. *J. Food Prot.*, **65**: 1267–1270.

Anza, I., *et al.* (2014) The same clade of *Clostridium botulinum* strains is causing avian botulism in southern and northern Europe. *Anaerobe*, **26**: 20–23.

Apland, J.P., *et al.* (2003) Inhibition of neurotransmitter release by peptides that mimic the N-terminal domain of SNAP-25. *J. Protein Chem.*, **22**: 147–153.

Arndt, E.R., *et al.* (2006) A structural perspective of the sequence variability within botulinum neurotoxin subtypes A1–A4. *J. Mol. Biol.*, **362**: 733–742.

Aureli, P., *et al.* (1986) Two cases of type E infant botulism caused by neurotoxigenic *Clostridium butyricum* in Italy. *J. Infect. Dis.*, **154**: 207–211.

Bajohrs, M., *et al.* (2004) A molecular basis underlying differences in the toxicity of botulinum serotypes A and E. *EMBO Rep.*, **5**: 1090–1095.

Barash, J.R., *et al.* (2005) First case of infant botulism caused by *Clostridium baratii* type F in California. *J. Clin. Microbiol.*, **43**: 4280–4282.

Barash, J.R., *et al.* (2014) A Novel Strain of *Clostridium botulinum* That Produces Type B and Type H Botulinum Toxins. *J. Infect. Dis.*, **209**: 183–191.

Bohnert, S., *et al.* (2005) Tetanus toxin is transported in a novel neuronal compartment characterized by a specialized pH regulation. *J. Biol. Chem.*, **280**: 42336–42344.

Bohnert, S., *et al.* (2006) Uptake and transport of clostridium neurotoxins. In: Alouf, J.E. and Popoff, M.R. (eds) *The Comprehensive Sourcebook of Comprehensive Bacterial Protein Toxins*, 3rd edition, pp. 390–408. Elsevier Academic Press, Oxford, UK.

Breidenbach, M.A., *et al.* (2005) 2.3 A crystal structure of tetanus neurotoxin light chain. *Biochemistry*, **44**: 7450–7457.

Brüggemann, H., *et al.* (2003) The genome sequence of *Clostridium tetani*, the causative agent of tetanus disease. *Proc. Natl Acad. Sci. (USA)*, **100**: 1316–1321.

Bruggemann, H., *et al.* (2008) Comparative genomics of clostridia: Link between the ecological niche and cell surface properties. *Ann. NY Acad. Sci.*, **1125**: 73–81.

Brüggemann, H., *et al.* (2011) *Clostridium botulinum*. In: Fratamico, P. *et al.* (eds) *Genomes of Foodborne and Waterborne Pathogens*, pp. 185–212. ASM Press, Washington DC.

Bytchenko, B. (1981) Microbiology of tetanus. In: Veronesi, R. (ed.) *Tetanus: Important new concepts*, pp. 28–39. Excerpta Medica, Amsterdam, Holland.

Call, J.E., *et al.* (1995) *In situ* characterization of *Clostridium botulinum* neurotoxin synthesis and export. *J. Appl. Bacteriol.*, **79**: 257–263.

Campbell, J.I., *et al.* (2009) Microbiologic characterization and antimicrobial susceptibility of *Clostridium tetani* isolated from wounds of patients with clinically diagnosed tetanus. *Am. J. Trop. Med. Hyg.*, **80**: 827–831.

Capogna, M., *et al.* (1997) Ca2+ or Sr2+ partially rescues synaptic transmission in hippocampal cultures treated with botulinum toxin A and C, but not tetanus toxin. *J. Neurosci.*, **17**: 7190–7202.

Carter, A.T., *et al.* (2009) Independent evolution of neurotoxin and flagellar genetic loci in proteolytic *Clostridium botulinum*. *BMC Genomics*, **10**: 115.

Carter, A.T., *et al.* (2014) Three classes of plasmid (47–63 kb) carry the type B neurotoxin gene cluster of group II *Clostridium botulinum*. *Genome Biol. Evol.*, **6**: 2076–2087.

Castor, C., *et al.* (2015) Cluster of two cases of botulism due to *Clostridium baratii* type F in France, November 2014. *Euro. Surveill.*, **20**: 1–3.

Cato, E.P., *et al.* (1986) Genus *Clostridium*. In: Sneath, P.H.A. *et al.* (eds) *Bergey's Manual of Systematic Bacteriology*, pp. 1141–1200. Williams and Wilkins, Baltimore, MD.

Chaudhry, R., *et al.* (1998) Outbreak of suspected *Clostridium butyricum* botulism in India. *Emerg. Infect. Dis.*, **4**: 506–507.

Chen, C., *et al.* (2008) Molecular basis for tetanus toxin coreceptor interactions. *Biochemistry*, **47**: 7179–7186.

Chen, C., *et al.* (2009) Gangliosides as high affinity receptors for tetanus neurotoxin. *J. Biol. Chem.*, **284**: 26569–26577.

Chen, Y.A., *et al.* (1999) SNARE complex formation is triggered by Ca2+ and drives membrane fusion. *Cell*, **97**: 165–174.

Chen, Y.A., *et al.* (2001) A discontinuous SNAP-25 C-terminal coil supports exocytosis. *J. Biol. Chem.*, **276**: 28503–28508.

Collins, M.D., *et al.* (1997) Phylogeny and taxonomy of the food-borne pathogen *Clostridium botulinum* and its neurotoxins. *J. Appl. Microbiol.*, **84**: 5–17.

Cordoba, J.J., *et al.* (1995) Studies on the genes encoding botulinum neurotoxin type A of *Clostridium botulinum* from a variety of sources. *Sys. Appl. Microbiol.*, **18**: 13–22.

Cornille, F., *et al.* (1995) Inhibition of neurotransmitter release by synthetic proline-rich peptides shows that the N-terminal domain of vesicle-associated membrane protein/synaptobrvin is critical for neuro-exocytosis. *J. Biol. Chem.*, **270**: 16826–16832.

Couesnon, A., *et al.* (2008) Receptor-mediated transcytosis of botulinum neurotoxin A through intestinal cell monolayers. *Cell Microbiol.*, **10**: 375–387.

Creti, R., *et al.* (1990) Occurence of *Clostridium botulinum* in the soil of the vicinity of Rome. *Curr. Microbiol.*, **20**: 317–321.

Deinhardt, K., *et al.* (2006) Tetanus toxin is internalized by a sequential clathrin-dependent mechanism initiated within lipid microdomains and independent of epsin1. *J. Cell Biol.*, **174**: 459–471.

Deinhardt, K., *et al.* (2006) Rab5 and Rab7 control endocytic sorting along the axonal retrograde transport pathway. *Neuron*, **52**: 293–305.

Diao, M.M., *et al.* (2014) Meta-analysis of D-values of proteolytic *Clostridium botulinum* and its surrogate strain *Clostridium sporogenes* PA 3679. *Int. J. Food Microbiol.*, **174**: 23–30.

Dineen, S.S., *et al.* (2003) Neurotoxin gene clusters in *Clostridium botulinum* type A strains: Sequence comparison and evolutionary implications. *Curr. Microbiol.*, **46**: 342–352.

Dineen, S.S., *et al.* (2004) Nucleotide sequence and transcriptional analysis of the type A2 neurotoxin gene cluster in *Clostridium botulinum*. *FEMS Microbiol. Lett.*, **235**: 9–16.

Dodds, K.L. (1993) *Clostridium botulinum* in the environment. In: Hauschild, A.H.W. *et al.* (eds) *Clostridium botulinum: Ecology and control in foods*, pp. 21–51. Marcel Dekker, Inc., New York.

Dong, M., *et al.* (2006) SV2 Is the Protein Receptor for Botulinum Neurotoxin A. *Science*, **312**: 592–596.

Dong, M., *et al.* (2007) Mechanism of botulinum neurotoxin B and G entry into hippocampal neurons. *J. Cell Biol.*, **179**: 1511–1522.

Dong, M., *et al.* (2008) Glycosylated SV2A and SV2B mediate the entry of botulinum neurotoxin E into neurons. *Mol. Biol. Cell.*, **19**: 5226–5237.

Dover, N., *et al.* (2009) Novel *Clostridium botulinum* toxin gene arrangement with subtype A5 and partial subtype B3 botulinum neurotoxin genes. *J. Clin. Microbiol.*, **47**: 2349–2350.

Dover, N., *et al.* (2013) *Clostridium botulinum* Strain Af84 Contains Three Neurotoxin Gene Clusters: Bont/A2, bont/F4 and bont/F5. *PLoS One*, **8**: e61205.

Dover, N., *et al.* (2014) Molecular characterization of a novel botulinum neurotoxin type H gene. *J. Infect. Dis.*, **209**: 192–202.

Eklund, M.W., *et al.* (1965) *Clostridium botulinum* type F from marine sediments. *Science*, **149**: 306.

Emsley, P., *et al.* (2000) The structures of the Hc fragment of tetanus toxin with carbohydrate subunit complexes provide insight into ganglioside binding. *J. Biol. Chem.*, **275**: 8889–8894.

Fach, P., *et al.* (2002) Detection by PCR-enzyme-linked immunosorbent assay of *Clostridium botulinum* in fish and environmental samples from a coastal area in Northern France. *Appl. Environ. Microbiol.*, **68**: 5870–5876.

Fenicia, L., *et al.* (1999) Intestinal toxemia botulism in two young people, caused by *Clostridium butyricum* Type E. *Clin. Infect. Dis.*, **29**: 381–387.

Fischer, A., *et al.* (2007) Crucial role of the disulfide bridge between botulinum neurotoxin light and heavy chains in protease translocation across membranes. *J. Biol. Chem.*, **282**: 29604–29611.

Fischer, A., *et al.* (2008) Botulinum neurotoxin devoid of receptor binding domain translocates active protease. *PLoS Pathog.*, **4**: e1000245.

Foran, P., *et al.* (1996) Botulinum neurotoxin C1 cleaves both syntaxin and SNAP-25 in intact and permeabilized chro-maffin cells: Correlation with its blockade of catecholamine release. *Biochemistry*, **35**: 2630–2636.

Fotinou, C., *et al.* (2001) The crystal structure of tetanus toxin Hc fragment complexed with a synthetic GT1b analogue suggests cross-linking between ganglioside receptors and the toxin. *J. Biol. Chem.*, **276**: 3274–3281.

Franciosa, G., *et al.* (2004) Differentiation of the gene clusters encoding botulinum neurotoxin type A complexes in *Clostridium botulinum* type A, Ab, and A(B) strains. *Appl. Environ. Microbiol.*, **70**: 7192–7199.

Franciosa, G., *et al.* (2006) A novel type A2 neurotoxin gene cluster in *Clostridium botulinum* strain Mascarpone. *FEMS Microbiol. Lett.*, **261**: 88–94.

Franciosa, G., *et al.* (2009) Evidence that plasmid-borne botulinum neurotoxin type B genes are widespread among *Clostridium botulinum* serotype B strains. *PLoS One*, **4**: e4829.

Fu, S.W., *et al.* (2008) An overview of type E botulism in China. *Biomed. Environ. Sci.*, **21**: 353–356.

Fu, Z., *et al.* (2006) Light chain of botulinum neurotoxin serotype A: Structural resolution of a catalytic intermediate. *Biochemistry*, **45**: 8903–8911.

Galloux, M., *et al.* (2008) Membrane interaction of botulinum neurotoxin A translocation (T) domain. The belt region is a regulatory loop for membrane interaction. *J. Biol. Chem.*, **283**: 27668–27676.

Gerona, R.R., *et al.* (2000) The C terminus of SNAP25 is essential for Ca(2+)-dependent binding of synaptotagmin to SNARE complexes. *J. Biol. Chem.*, **275**: 6328–6336.

Ghanem, F.M., *et al.* (1991) Identification of *Clostridium botulinum, Clostridium argentinense*, and related organisms by cellular fatty acid analysis. *J. Clin. Microbiol.*, **29**: 1114–1124.

Gil, C., *et al.* (2003) C-terminal fragment of tetanus toxin heavy chain activates Akt and MEK/ERK signalling pathways in a Trk receptor-dependent manner in cultured cortical neurons. *Biochem. J.*, **15**: 613–620.

Gill, D.M. (1982) Bacterial toxins: A table of lethal amounts. *Microbiol. Rev.*, **46**: 86–94.

Gimenez, D.F., *et al.* (1970) Another type of *Clostridium botulinum*. *Zentralbl. Bakteriol. Parasitenkd. Infektionskr. Hyg. Abt.*, **215**: 221–224.

Gonzalez-Escalona, N., *et al.* (2014) Whole-genome single-nucleotide-polymorphism analysis for discrimination of *Clostridium botulinum* group I strains. *Appl. Environ. Microbiol.*, **80**: 2125–2132.

Gupta, A., *et al.* (2005) Adult botulism type F in the United States, 1981–2002. *Neurology*, **65**: 1694–1700.

Gurtler, V., *et al.* (1991) Classification of medically important clostridia using restriction endonuclease site differences of PCR-amplified 16S rDNA. *J. Gen. Microbiol.*, **137**: 2673–2679.

Gutierrez, R., *et al.* (1997) A quantitative PCR-ELISA for the rapid enumeration of bacteria in refrigerated raw milk. *J. Appl. Microbiol.*, **83**: 518–523.

Hall, J.D., *et al.* (1985) Isolation of an organism resembling *Clostridium baratii* which produces type F botulinal toxin from an infant with botulism. *J. Clin. Microbiol.*, **21**: 654–655.

Hannett, G.E., *et al.* (2011) Biodiversity of *Clostridium botulinum* type E associated with a large outbreak of botulism in wildlife from Lake Erie and Lake Ontario. *Appl. Environ. Microbiol.*, **77**: 1061–1068.

Hardy, S.P., *et al.* (2013) Type C and C/D toxigenic *Clostridium botulinum* is not normally present in the intestine of healthy broilers. *Vet. Microbiol.*, **165**: 466–468.

Harvey, S.M., *et al.* (2002) Botulism due to *Clostridium baratii* type F toxin. *J. Clin. Microbiol.*, **40**: 2260–2262.

Hatheway, C.L. (1993) Bacteriology and pathology of neurotoxigenic Clostridia. In: DasGupta, B.R. (ed.) *Botulinum and Tetanus Neurotoxins*, pp. 491–502. Plenum Press, New York.

Hauschild, A.H.W. (1989) *Clostridium botulium*. In: Doyle, M.P. (ed.) *Foodborne Bacterial Pathogens*, pp. 111–189. Marcel Dekker, Inc., New York.

Hedeland, M., *et al.* (2011) Confirmation of botulism in birds and cattle by the mouse bioassay and Endopep-MS. *J. Med. Microbiol.*, **60**: 1299–1305.

Henderson, I., *et al.* (1996) Genetic characterization of the botulinum toxin complex of *Clostridium botulinum* strain NCTC2916. *FEMS Microbiol. Lett.*, **140**: 151–158.

Henkel, J.S., *et al.* (2009) Catalytic Properties of Botulinum Neurotoxin Subtypes A3 and A4. *Biochemistry*, **48**: 2522–2528.

Herreros, J., *et al.* (2001) Lipid rafts act as specialized domains for tetanus toxin binding and internalization into neurons. *Mol. Biol. Cell*, **12**: 2947–2960.

Hielm, S., *et al.* (1996) Detection of *Clostridium botulinum* in fish and envionmental samples using polymerase chain reaction. *Int. J. Food Microbiol.*, **31**: 357–365.

Hielm, S., *et al.* (1998) Prevalence of *Clostridium botulinum* in Finnish trout farms: Pulse-field gel electrophoresis typing reveals extensive genetic diversity among Type E isolates. *Appl. Environ. Microbiol.*, **64**: 4161–4167.

Hielm, S., *et al.* (1998) A high prevalence of *Clostridium botulinum* type E in Finnish freshwater and Baltic Sea sediment samples. *J. Appl. Microbiol.*, **84**: 133–137.

Hill, K.K., *et al.* (2007) Genetic diversity among botulinum neurotoxin-producing clostridial strains. *J. Bacteriol.*, **189**: 818–832.

Hill, K.K., *et al.* (2009) Recombination and insertion events involving the botulinum neurotoxin complex genes in *Clostridium botulinum* types A, B, E and F and *Clostridium butyricum* type E strains. *BMC Biol*, **7**: 66.

Hill, K.K., *et al.* (2013) Genetic diversity within *Clostridium botulinum* serotypes, botulinum neurotoxin gene clusters and toxin subtypes. *Curr. Top. Microbiol. Immunol.*, **364**: 1–20.

Hinderink, K., *et al.* (2009) Group I *Clostridium botulinum* strains show significant variation in growth at low and high temperatures. *J. Food Prot.*, **72**: 375–383.

Hippe, H., *et al.* (1992) The genus *Clostridium*-Nonmedical. In: Balows, A. *et al.* (eds) *The Prokaryotes*, pp. 1800–1866. Springer Verlag, New York.

Hosomi, K., *et al.* (2014) Complete nucleotide sequence of a plasmid containing the botulinum neurotoxin gene in *Clostridium botulinum* type B strain 111 isolated from an infant patient in Japan. *Mol. Genet. Genomics*, **289**: 1267–1274.

Humeau, Y., *et al.* (2000) How botulinum and tetanus neurotoxins block neurotransmitter release. *Biochimie*, **82**: 427–446.

Humeau, Y., *et al.* (2007) Fast changes in the functional status of release sites during short-term plasticity: Involvement of a frequency-dependent bypass of Rac at Aplysia synapses. *J. Physiol.*, **583**: 983–1004.

Hutson, R.A., *et al.* (1994) Nucleotide sequence of the gene coding for non-proteolytic *Clostridium botulinum* type B neurotoxin: Comparison with other Clostridial neurotoxins. *Cur. Microbiol.*, **28**: 101–110.

Hutson, R.A., *et al.* (1996) Genetic characterization of *Clostridium botulinum* type A containing silent type B neurotoxin gene sequences. *J. Biol. Chem.*, **271**: 10786–10792.

Hyytia, E., *et al.* (1998) Prevalence of *Clostridium botulinum* type E in Finnish fish and fishery products. *Epidemiol. Infect.*, **120**: 245–250.

Hyytia, E., *et al.* (1999) Characterisation of *Clostridium botulinum* groups I and II by randomly amplified polymorphic DNA analysis and repetitive element sequence-based PCR. *Int. J. Food Microbiol.*, **48**: 179–189.

Hyytia, E., *et al.* (1999) Biodiversity of *Clostridium botulinum* type E strains isolated from fish and fishery products. *Appl. Environ. Microbiol.*, **65**: 2057–2064.

Ihara, H., *et al.* (2003) Sequence of the gene for *Clostridium botulinum* type B neurotoxin associated with infant botulism, expression of the C-terminal half of heavy chain and its binding activity. *Biochim. Biophys. Acta*, **1625**: 19–26.

Jacobson, M.J., *et al.* (2008) Analysis of neurotoxin cluster genes in *Clostridium botulinum* strains producing botulinum neurotoxin serotype A subtypes. *Appl. Environ. Microbiol.*, **74**: 2778–2786.

Jin, Y., *et al.* (2009) Disruption of the epithelial barrier by botulinum haemagglutinin (HA) proteins – differences in cell tropism and the mechanism of action between HA proteins of types A or B, and HA proteins of type C. *Microbiology*, **155**: 35–45.

Johnson, E.A., *et al.* (2005) Characterization of *Clostridium botulinum* strains associated with an infant botulism case in the United Kingdom. *J. Clin. Microbiol.*, **43**: 2602–2607.

Johnson, J.L., *et al.* (1975) Taxonomy of the Clostridia: Ribosomal ribonucleic acid homologies among the species. *J. Gen. Microbiol.*, **88**: 229–244.

Kalb, S.R., *et al.* (2015) Functional Characterization of Botulinum Neurotoxin Serotype H as a Hybrid of Known Serotypes F and A (BoNT F/A). *Anal. Chem.*, **87**: 3911–3917.

Katitch, R.V. (1965) *Les maladies des animaux domestiques causées par les microbes anaérobies*. Vigot Frères, Paris, France.

Keller, J.E., *et al.* (2001) The role of the synaptic protein snap-25 in the potency of botulinum neurotoxin type A. *J. Biol. Chem.*, **276**: 13476–13482.

Keto-Timonen, R., *et al.* (2005) Efficient DNA fingerprint of *Clostridium botulinum* types A, B, E, and F by amplified fragment length polymorphism analysis. *Appl. Environ. Microbiol.*, **71**: 1148–1154.

Knock, G.G. (1952) Survey of soils for spores of *Clostridium botulinum* (Union of South Africa and South West Africa). *J. Sci. Food Agric.*, **3**: 86–90.

Koepke, R., *et al.* (2008) Global occurrence of infant botulism, 1976–2006. *Pediatrics*, **122**: e73–82.

Koriazova, L.K., *et al.* (2003) Translocation of botulinum neurotoxin light chain protease through the heavy chain channel. *Nat. Struct. Biol.*, **10**: 13–18.

Kozaki, S., *et al.* (1998) Characterization of *Clostridium botulinum* type B neurotoxin associated with infant botulism in Japan. *Infect. Immun.*, **66**: 4811–4816.

Kroken, A.R., *et al.* (2011) Novel ganglioside-mediated entry of botulinum neurotoxin serotype D into neurons. *J. Biol. Chem.*, **286**: 26828–26837.

Kull, S., *et al.* (2015) Isolation and functional characterization of the novel *Clostridium botulinum* neurotoxin A8 subtype. *PLoS One*, **10**: e0116381.

Kumaran, D., *et al.* (2009) Domain organization in *Clostridium botulinum* neurotoxin type E is unique: Its implication in faster translocation. *J. Mol. Biol.*, **386**: 233–245.

Lacy, D.B., *et al.* (1998) Crystal structure of botulinum neurotoxin type A and implications for toxicity. *Nature Struct. Biol.*, **5**: 898–902.

Lacy, D.B., *et al.* (1999) Sequence homology and structural analysis of the clostridial neurotoxins. *J. Mol. Biol.*, **291**: 1091–1104.

Lafuente, S., *et al.* (2012) Two simultaneous botulism outbreaks in Barcelona: *Clostridium baratii* and *Clostridium botulinum*. *Epidemiol. Infect.*, **19**: 1–3.

Lalli, G., *et al.* (2002) Analysis of retrograde transport in motor neurons reveals common endocytic carriers for tetanus toxin and neutrophin receptor p75[NTR]. *J. Cell Biol.*, **156**: 233–239.

Lalli, G., *et al.* (2003) The journey of tetanus and botulinum neurotoxins in neurons. *Trends Microbiol.*, **11**: 431–437.

Lawson, P.A., *et al.* (1993) Towards a phylogeny of the clostridia based on 16S rRNA sequences. *FEMS Microbiol. Lett.*, **113**: 87–92.

Li, Y., *et al.* (2001) Recombinant forms of tetanus toxin engineered for examining and exploiting neuronal trafficking pathways. *J. Biol. Chem.*, **276**: 31394–31401.

Lin, W.J., *et al.* (1995) Genome analysis of *Clostridium botulinum* type A by pulsed-field gel electrophoresis. *Appl. Environ. Microbiol.*, **61**: 4441–4447.

Lindberg, A., *et al.* (2010) Real-time PCR for *Clostridium botulinum* type C neurotoxin (BoNTC) gene, also covering a chimeric C/D sequence – application on outbreaks of botulism in poultry. *Vet. Microbiol.*, **146**: 118–123.

Lindstrom, M., *et al.* (2009) Comparative genomic hybridization analysis of two predominant Nordic group I (proteolytic) *Clostridium botulinum* type B clusters. *Appl. Environ. Microbiol.*, **75**: 2643–2651.

Lynch, K.L., *et al.* (2008) Synaptotagmin-1 utilizes membrane bending and SNARE binding to drive fusion pore expansion. *Mol. Biol. Cell*, **19**: 5093–5103.

Mahrhold, S., *et al.* (2006) The synaptic vesicle protein 2C mediates the uptake of botulinum neurotoxin A into phrenic nerves. *FEBS Lett.*, **580**: 2011–2014.

Maksymowych, A.B., *et al.* (1998) Binding and transcytosis of botulinum neurotoxin by polarized human carcinoma cells. *J. Biol. Chem.*, **273**: 21950–21957.

Maksymowych, A.B., *et al.* (2004) Structural features of the botulinum neurotoxin molecule that govern binding and transcytosis across polarized human intestinal epithelial cells. *J. Pharmacol. Exp. Ther.*, **210**: 633–641.

Manning, K.A., *et al.* (1990) Retrograde transneuronal transport properties of fragment C of tetanus toxin. *Neuroscience*, **34**: 251–263.

Marshall, K.M., *et al.* (2010) Conjugative Botulinum Neurotoxin-Encoding Plasmids in *Clostridium botulinum*. *PLoS One*, **5**.

Maskos, U., *et al.* (2002) Retrograde trans-synaptic transfer of green fluorescent protein allows the genetic mapping of neuronal circuits in transgenic mice. *Proc. Natl Acad. Sci. USA*, **99**: 10120–10125.

Matsumura, T., *et al.* (2008) The HA proteins of botulinum toxin disrupt intestinal epithelial intercellular junctions to increase toxin absorption. *Cell Microbiol.*, **10**: 355–364.

Mazuet, C., *et al.* (2012) Toxin detection in patients' sera by mass spectrometry during two outbreaks of type A botulism in France. *J. Clin. Microbiol.*, **50**: 4091–4094.

Mazuet, C., *et al.* (2015) An Atypical Outbreak of Food-Borne Botulism Due to *Clostridium botulinum* Types B and E from Ham. *J. Clin. Microbiol.*, **53**: 722–726.

McCroskey, L.M., *et al.* (1986) Characterization of an organism that produces type E botulinal toxin but which resembles *Clostridium butyricum* from the feces of an infant with type E botulism. *J. Clin. Microbiol.*, **23**: 201–202.

McCroskey, L.M., *et al.* (1991) Type F botulism due to neurotoxigenic *Clostridium baratii* from an unknown source in an adult. *J. Clin. Microbiol.*, **29**: 2618–2620.

Meng, X., *et al.* (1997) Characterization of a neurotoxigenic *Clostridium butyricum* strain isolated from the food implicated in an outbreak of food-borne type E botulism. *J. Clin. Microbiol.*, **35**: 2160–2162.

Meng, X., *et al.* (1999) Isolation and characterization of neurotoxigenic *Clostridium butyricum* from soil in China. *J. Med. Microbiol.*, **48**: 133–137.

Meunier, F.A., *et al.* (2002) Molecular mechanism of action of botulinal neurotoxins and the synaptic remodeling they induce in vivo at the skeletal neuromuscular junction. In: Massaro, J. (ed.) *Handbook of Neurotoxicology*, pp. 305–347. Humana Press, Totowa, NJ.

Meunier, F.A., *et al.* (2002) Botulinum neurotoxins: From paralysis to recovery of functional neuromuscular transmission. *J. Physiol.*, **96**: 105–113.

Moller, V., *et al.* (1960) Preliminary report on the isolation of an apparently new type of *Clostridium botulinum*. *Acta Pathol. Microbiol. Scand.*, **48**: 80.

Munro, P., *et al.* (2001) High sensitivity of mouse neuronal cells to tetanus toxin requires a GPI-anchored protein. *Biochem. Biophys. Res. Commun.*, **289**: 623–629.

Muraro, L., *et al.* (2009) The N-terminal half of the receptor domain of botulinum neurotoxin A binds to microdomains of the plasma membrane. *Biochem. Biophys. Res. Commun.*, **380**: 76–80.

Nakamura, K., *et al.* (2010) Characterization of the D/C mosaic neurotoxin produced by *Clostridium botulinum* associated with bovine botulism in Japan. *Vet. Microbiol.*, **140**: 147–154.

Nakamura, S., *et al.* (1979) Taxonomy of *Clostridium tetani* and related species. *J. Gen. Microbiol.*, **113**: 29–35.

Neill, S.D., *et al.* (1989) Type C botulism in cattle being fed ensiled poultry litter. *Vet. Rec.*, **124**: 558–560.

Nevas, M., *et al.* (2005) Diversity of proteolytic *Clostridium botulinum* strains, determined by a pulse-field gel electrophoresis approach. *Appl. Environ. Microbiol.*, **71**: 1311–1317.

Nishiki, T., *et al.* (1994) Identification of protein receptor for *Clostridium botulinum* type B neurotoxin in rat brain synaptosomes. *J. Biol. Chem.*, **269**: 10498–10503.

O'Connor, V., *et al.* (1997) Disruption of syntaxin-mediated protein interactions blocks neurotransmitter secretion. *Proc. Natl Acad. Sci. USA*, **94**: 12186–12191.

Oguma, K., *et al.* (1986) Biochemical classification of *Clostridium botulinum* type C and D strains and their nontoxigenic derivatives. *Appl. Environ. Microbiol.*, **51**: 256–260.

Oguma, K., *et al.* (1999) Structure and function of *Clostridium botulinum* progenitor toxin. *J. Toxicol.*, **18**: 17–34.

Otter, A., *et al.* (2006) Risk of botulism in cattle and sheep arising from contact with broiler litter. *Vet. Rec.*, **159**: 186–187.

Peck, M.W. (2006) *Clostridium botulinum* and the safety of minimally heated, chilled foods: An emerging issue? *J. Appl. Microbiol.*, **101**: 556–570.

Peck, M.W. (2009) Biology and genomic analysis of *Clostridium botulinum*. *Adv. Microb. Physiol.*, **55**: 183–265.

Peck, M.W., *et al.* (2011) *Clostridium botulinum* in the post-genomic era. *Food Microbiol.*, **28**: 183–191.

Peng, L., *et al.* (2011) Botulinum neurotoxin D uses synaptic vesicle protein SV2 and gangliosides as receptors. *PLoS Pathog.*, **7**: e1002008.

Popoff, M.R., *et al.* (1985) Experimental cecitis in gnotoxenic chickens monoassociated with *Clostridium butyricum* strains isolated from patients with neonatal necrotizing enterocolitis. *Infect. Immun.*, **47**: 697–703.

Popoff, M.R. (1990) Are anaerobes involved in neonatal necrotizing enterocolitis? In: Borriello, S.P. (ed.) *Clinical and Molecular Aspects of Anaerobes*, pp. 49–57. Wrighston Biomedical Publishing Ltd, Petersfield, Hampshire.

Popoff, M.R. (1995) Ecology of neurotoxigenic strains of Clostridia. *Curr. Top. Microbiol. Immunol.*, **195**: 1–29.

Popoff, M.R., *et al.* (1999) Structural and genomic features of clostridial neurotoxins. In: Alouf, J.E. and Freer, J.H. (eds) *The Comprehensive Sourcebook of Bacterial Protein Toxins*, pp. 174–201. Academic Press, London.

Popoff, M.R., *et al.* (2013) Botulism and Tetanus. In: Rosenberg, E. *et al.* (eds) *The Prokaryotes: Human Microbiology*, pp. 247–290. Springer-Verlag, Heidelberg, Berlin.

Poulain, B., *et al.* (2006) Attack of the nervous system by clostridial toxins: Physical findings, cellular and molecular actions. In: Alouf, J.E. and Popoff, M.R. (eds) *The Sourcebook of Bacterial Protein Toxins*, pp. 348–389. Elsevier, Academic Press, Amsterdam, UK.

Poulain, B., *et al.* (2008) How do the botulinum neurotoxins block neurotransmitter release: From botulism to the molecular mechanism of action. *Botulinum J.*, **1**: 14–87.

Qazi, O., *et al.* (2007) Identification and characterization of the surface-layer protein of *Clostridium tetani*. *FEMS Microbiol. Lett.*, **274**: 126–131.

Raphael, B.H., *et al.* (2012) Analysis of a unique *Clostridium botulinum* strain from the Southern hemisphere producing a novel type E botulinum neurotoxin subtype. *BMC Microbiol.*, **12**: 245.

Raphael, B.H., *et al.* (2014) *Clostridium botulinum* strains producing BoNT/F4 or BoNT/F5. *Appl. Environ. Microbiol.*, **80**: 3250–3257.

Raphael, B.H., *et al.* (2014) Distinguishing highly-related outbreak-associated *Clostridium botulinum* type A(B) strains. *BMC Microbiol.*, **14**: 192.

Ratts, R., *et al.* (2005) A conserved motif in transmembrane helix 1 of diphtheria toxin mediates catalytic domain delivery to the cytosol. *Proc. Natl Acad. Sci. USA*, **102**: 15635–15640.

Rethy, L., *et al.* (1997) Human lethal dose of tetanus toxin. *Lancet*, **350**: 1518.

Rossetto, O., *et al.* (2001) Tetanus and botulinum neurotoxins: Turning bad guys into good by research. *Toxicon*, **39**: 27–41.

Rummel, A., *et al.* (2003) Two carbohydrate binding sites in the H_{cc}-domain of tetanus neurotoxin are required for toxicity. *J. Mol. Biol.*, **326**: 835–847.

Rummel, A., *et al.* (2004) Synaptotagmins I and II act as nerve cell receptors for botulinum neurotoxin G. *J. Biol. Chem.*, **279**: 30865–30870.

Rummel, A., *et al.* (2004) The H_{cc}-domain of botulinum neurotoxins A and B exhibits a singular ganglioside binding site displaying serotype specific carbohydrate interaction. *Mol. Microbiol.*, **51**: 631–643.

Rummel, A., *et al.* (2007) Identification of the protein receptor binding site of botulinum neurotoxins B and G proves the double-receptor concept. *Proc. Natl Acad. Sci. USA*, **104**: 359–364.

Rummel, A., *et al.* (2009) Botulinum neurotoxins C, E and F bind gangliosides via a conserved binding site prior to stimulation-dependent uptake with botulinum neurotoxin F utilising the three isoforms of SV2 as second receptor. *J. Neurochem.*, **110**: 1942–1954.

Sakaba, T., *et al.* (2005) Distinct kinetic changes in neurotransmitter release after SNARE protein cleavage. *Science*, **309**: 491–494.

Sakaguchi, Y., *et al.* (2005) The genome sequence of *Clostridium botulinum* type C neurotoxin-converting phage and the molecular mechanisms of unstable lysogeny. *Proc. Natl Acad. Sci. USA*, **102**: 17472–17477.

Salem, N., *et al.* (1998) A v-SNARE participates in synaptic vesicle formation mediated by the AP3 adaptor complex. *Nat. Neurosci.*, **1**: 551–556.

Schiavo, G., *et al.* (2000) Neurotoxins affecting neuroexocytosis. *Physiol. Rev.*, **80**: 717–766.

Schuette, C.G., *et al.* (2004) Determinants of liposome fusion mediated by synaptic SNARE proteins. *Proc. Natl Acad. Sci. USA*, **101**: 2858–2863.

Sebaihia, M., *et al.* (2007) Genome sequence of a proteolytic (Group I) *Clostridium botulinum* strain Hall A and comparative analysis of the clostridial genomes. *Genome Res.*, **17**: 1082–1092.

Sharma, S.K., *et al.* (2003) Separation of the components of type A botulinum neurotoxin complex by electrophoresis. *Toxicon*, **41**: 321–331.

Skarin, H., *et al.* (2010) Molecular characterization and comparison of *Clostridium botulinum* type C avian strains. *Avian Pathol.*, **39**: 511–518.

Skarin, H., *et al.* (2011) *Clostridium botulinum* group III: A group with dual identity shaped by plasmids, phages and mobile elements. *BMC Genomics*, **12**: 185.

Smart, J.L., *et al.* (1987) Poultrry waste associated type C botulism in cattle. *Epidem. Inf.*, **98**: 73–79.

Smith, L.D.S. (1977) *Botulism. The Organism, Its Toxins, The Disease.* Charles C. Thomas Publisher, Springfield, Ill.

Smith, L.D. (1978) The occurence of *Clostridium botulinum* and *Clostridium tetani* in the soil of the United States. *Health Lab. Sci.,* **15**: 74–80.

Smith, L.D., *et al.* (1984) *Clostridium tetani.* In: Smith, L.D.S. (ed.) *The Pathogenic Anaerobic Bacteria,* 3rd edition. Charles C. Thomas, Publisher, Springfield, Ill.

Smith, L.D.S. (1992) The genus *Clostridium*-Medical. In: Balows, A. *et al.* (eds) *The Prokaryotes,* pp. 1867–1880. Springer Verlag, New York.

Smith, T.J., *et al.* (2005) Sequence variation within botulinum neurotoxin serotypes impacts antibody binding and neutralization. *Infect. Immun.,* **73**: 5450–5457.

Sonnabend, O., *et al.* (1981) Isolation of *Clostridium botulinum* types G and identification of botulinal toxin in humans: Report of five sudden unexpected deaths. *J. Infect. Dis.,* **143**: 22–27.

Sonnabend, W.F., *et al.* (1987) Isolation of *Clostridium botulinum* type G from Swiss soil specimens by using sequential steps in an identification scheme. *Appl. Environ. Microbiol.,* **53**: 1880–1884.

Stenmark, P., *et al.* (2008) Crystal structure of botulinum neurotoxin type A in complex with the cell surface co-receptor GT1b – insight into the toxin–neuron interaction. *PLoS Pathog.,* **4**: e1000129.

Stringer, S.C., *et al.* (2013) Genomic and physiological variability within Group II (non-proteolytic) *Clostridium botulinum. BMC Genomics,* **14**: 333.

Strotmeier, J., *et al.* (2010) Botulinum neurotoxin serotype D attacks neurons via two carbohydrate-binding sites in a ganglioside-dependent manner. *Biochem. J.,* **431**: 207–216.

Suen, J.C., *et al.* (1988) *Clostridium argentinense* sp. nov.: A genetically homogeneous group composed of all strains of *Clostridium botulinum* toxin type G and some nontoxigenic strains previously identified as *Clostridium subterminale* or *Clostridium hastiforme. Int. J. Syst. Bacteriol.,* **38**: 375–381.

Swaminathan, S., *et al.* (2000) Structural analysis of the catalytic and binding sites of *Clostridium botulinum* neurotoxin B. *Nature Struct. Biol.,* **7**: 693–699.

Swaminathan, S. (2011) Molecular structures and functional relationships in clostridial neurotoxins. *FEBS J.,* **278**: 4467–4485.

Tabita, K.S., *et al.* (1991) Distinction between *Clostridium botulinum* type A strains associated with food-borne botulism and those with infant botulism in Japan in intraintestinal toxin production in infant mice and some other properties. *FEMS Microbiol. Lett.,* **79**: 251–256.

Takeda, M., *et al.* (2005) Characterization of the neurotoxin produced by isolates associated with avian botulism. *Avian Dis.,* **49**: 376–381.

Tsukamoto, K., *et al.* (2008) Identification of the receptor-binding sites in the carboxyl-terminal half of the heavy chain of botulinum neurotoxin types C and D. *Microb. Pathog.,* **44**: 484–493.

Tucker, W.C., *et al.* (2004) Reconstitution of Ca2+-regulated membrane fusion by synaptotagmin and SNAREs. *Science,* **304**: 435–438.

Umland, T.C., *et al.* (1997) The structure of the receptor binding fragment H_c of tetanus neurotoxin. *Nature Struct. Biol.,* **4**: 788–792.

Vaidyanathan, V.V., *et al.* (1999) Proteolysis of SNAP-25 isoforms by botulinum neurotoxin types A, C, and E: Domains and amino acid residues controlling the formation of enzyme–substrate complexes and cleavage. *J. Neurochem.,* **72**: 327–337.

Van der Burgt, G.M., *et al.* (2007) Seven outbreaks of suspected botulism in sheep in the UK. *Vet. Rec.,* **161**: 28–30.

Van der Lugt, J.J., *et al.* (1995) Two outbreaks of type C and type D botulism in sheep and goats in South Africa. *J. S. Afr. Vet. Assoc.,* **66**: 77–82.

Van der Lugt, J.J., *et al.* (1996) Type C botulism in sheep associated with the feeding of poultry litter. *J. S. Afr. Vet. Assoc.,* **67**: 3–4.

Vidal, D., *et al.* (2013) Environmental factors influencing the prevalence of a *Clostridium botulinum* type C/D mosaic strain in nonpermanent Mediterranean wetlands. *Appl. Environ. Microbiol.,* **79**: 4264–4271.

Wang, D., *et al.* (2011) Syntaxin requirement for Ca2+-triggered exocytosis in neurons and endocrine cells demonstrated with an engineered neurotoxin. *Biochemistry,* **50**: 2711–2713.

Wang, X., *et al.* (2000) Genetic analysis of Type E botulism toxin-producing *Clostridium butyricum* strains. *Appl. Environ. Microbiol.*, **66**: 4992–4997.

Weedmark, K.A., *et al.* (2014) Whole genome sequencing of 175 *Clostridium botulinum* Type E strains reveals two novel toxin variants. *Appl. Environ. Microbiol.*, **80**: 6334–6345.

Wellhöner, H.H. (1989) Clostridial toxins and the central nervous system: Studies on *in situ* tissues. In: Simpson, L.L. (ed.) *Botulinum Neurotoxin and Tetanus Toxin*, pp. 231–253. Academic Press, San Diego.

Wilde, E., *et al.* (1989) *Clostridium tetanomorphum* sp. nov., nom rev. *Int. J. Syst. Bacteriol.*, **39**: 127–134.

Willems, A., *et al.* (1993) Sequence of the gene coding for the neurotoxin of *Clostridium botulinum* type A associated with infant botulism: Comparison with other clostridial neurotoxins. *Res. Microbiol.*, **144**: 547–556.

Williamson, L.C., *et al.* (1996) Clostridial neurotoxins and substrate proteolysis in intact neurons: Botulinum neurotoxin C acts on synaptosomal-associated protein of 25 kDa. *J. Biol. Chem.*, **271**: 7694–7699.

Woudstra, C., *et al.* (2012) Neurotoxin gene profiling of *Clostridium botulinum* types C and D native to different countries within Europe. *Appl. Environ. Microbiol.*, **78**: 3120–3127.

Wright, G.P. (1955) The neurotoxins of *Clostridium botulinum* and *Clostridium tetani*. *Pharmacol. Rev.*, **7**: 413–465.

Yeh, F.L., *et al.* (2011) SV2 mediates entry of tetanus neurotoxin into central neurons. *PLoS Pathog.*, **6**: e1001207.

Yowler, B.C., *et al.* (2004) Botulinum neurotoxin A changes conformation upon binding to ganglioside GT1b. *Biochemistry*, **43**: 9725–9731.

Zhang, Z., *et al.* (2013) Plasmid-borne type E neurotoxin gene clusters in *Clostridium botulinum* strains. *Appl. Environ. Microbiol.*, **79**: 3856–3859.

Clostridial Infections of the Gastrointestinal System

Diseases Produced by *Clostridium perfringens* Type A in Mammalian Species

Francisco A. Uzal

Introduction

Clostridium perfringens type A is frequently associated with enteric disease of poultry, ruminants, horses, pigs, dogs, and other species. However, while the role of this microorganism in avian necrotic enteritis is beyond doubt, with a few exceptions mentioned in this section, there is very little evidence supporting a role for *C. perfringens* type A in the pathogenesis of enteric disease of mammals. Type A strains producing NetF, a newly discovered toxin, seem to be strongly associated with canine hemorrhagic gastroenteritis (Chapter 9). A small percentage of *C. perfringens* type A strains producing enterotoxin (CPE) are responsible for highly prevalent food poisoning and antibiotic-associated diarrhea in humans. CPE-positive strains may also be associated with enteric disease in other mammalian species.

Yellow lamb disease

Introduction
Yellow lamb disease is a rare disease of sheep for which only a few references exist. The condition has been reported in the US and Europe, and anecdotal evidence indicates that a few cases may have been diagnosed in South America. Because *C. perfringens* type A is the most ubiquitous of all *C. perfringens* strains, and since it is found in the intestines of most clinically healthy mammals, diagnosis of yellow lamb disease is challenging; the mere isolation of this microorganism is of no diagnostic significance. Because of this, the occurrence of this disease may be underestimated.

Clostridial Diseases of Animals, First Edition. Francisco A. Uzal, J. Glenn Songer, John F. Prescott and Michel R. Popoff.
© 2016 John Wiley & Sons, Inc. Published 2016 by John Wiley & Sons, Inc.

Etiology

Yellow lamb disease has traditionally been associated with strains of *C. perfringens* type A that produce high levels of alpha toxin (CPA). Recently, however, an outbreak of what was thought to be yellow lamb disease was reported in lambs infected by a strain of *C. perfringens* type D that produced an unusually high amount of CPA. This toxin is a hemolytic lecithinase (phospholipase), which is consistent with the severe hemolysis and jaundice in yellow lamb disease. Because of the similarity in clinical signs and lesions, both type A and type D-associated yellow lamb disease are discussed in this section.

Epidemiology and clinical signs

Information on the epidemiology of yellow lamb disease is very scant. Factors predisposing to *C. perfringens* type D enterotoxemia (that is, sudden changes in diet to foods rich in carbohydrates) are also thought to predispose yellow lamb disease. Definitive evidence that this is the case is, however, lacking.

The most common clinical manifestations of yellow lamb disease are depression, anemia, icterus, and hemoglobinuria. Sudden death has occasionally been described. The cases of yellow lamb disease associated with *C. perfringens* type D were characterized by similar clinical signs plus abdominal pain, trembling, and tachycardia. Lethality in both forms of the disease has been reported to be close to 100%.

Gross changes

Necropsy findings in yellow lamb disease are not specific and may be compatible with several other diseases. The most frequently described gross findings include generalized icterus (Figure 8.1), red urine in the bladder, enlarged, pale,

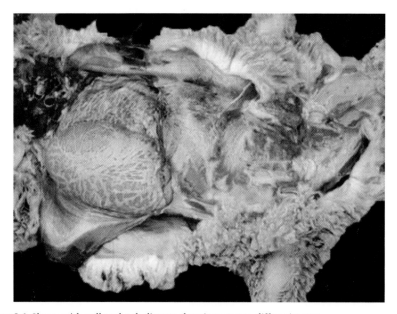

Figure 8.1 Sheep with yellow lamb disease showing severe, diffuse icterus.

and friable spleen, enlarged liver with an acinar pattern, and dark, swollen kidneys. Cases of type D-associated yellow lamb disease presented, in addition, serosanguineous fluid free in body cavities and severe pulmonary edema; these changes are presumably produced by epsilon toxin, the main action of which is to increase vascular permeability.

Microscopic changes

Microscopic changes include centrilobular necrosis of the liver (Figure 8.2), pigmentary (hemoglobinuric) nephrosis (Figures 8.3 and 8.4), splenic congestion, and pulmonary congestion and edema. The liver lesions are characterized by centrilobular to mid-zonal hepatocellular degeneration and necrosis, and bile stasis in bile canaliculi. The kidney lesions include multiple hemoglobin casts in the tubular lumen and the presence of numerous multifocal, eosinophilic, and granular to globular intracytoplasmic hyaline droplets that stain positively for hemoglobin, in the proximal and distal convoluted tubules (Figures 8.3 and 8.4). The lungs show diffuse proteinaceous alveolar and interstitial edema and fibrin in the alveoli. Most histological lesions are thought to be associated with acute intravascular hemolysis and anemia produced by CPA. These changes are not, by any means, specific to this condition, and a diagnosis of yellow lamb disease cannot be established on histological changes alone.

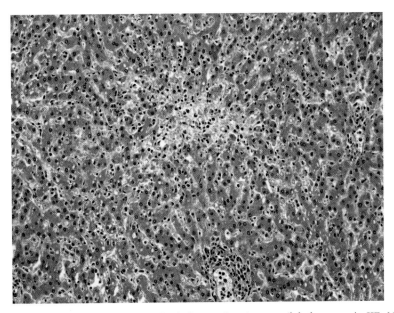

Figure 8.2 Liver of a lamb with yellow lamb disease showing centrilobular necrosis. HE, 100x.

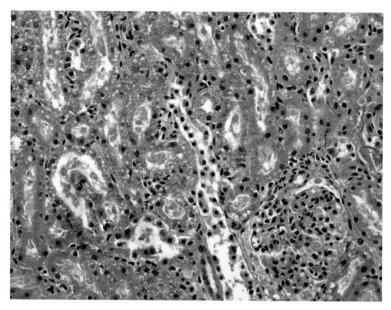

Figure 8.3 Kidney of a lamb with yellow lamb disease showing tubular degeneration and multiple protein (hemoglobin) droplets in the cytoplasm of tubular epithelial cells. HE, 400x. Courtesy of F. Giannitti.

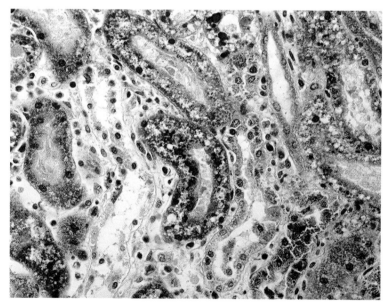

Figure 8.4 Kidney of a lamb with yellow lamb disease stained with Okajima stain to demonstrate hemoglobin (stained bright orange) in the cytoplasm of tubular epithelial cells. Okajima, 600x. Courtesy of F. Giannitti.

Diagnosis

Diagnostic criteria have not been clearly established for yellow lamb disease. It is, however, generally accepted that a presumptive diagnosis of yellow lamb disease can be established based on clinical, gross, and microscopic findings. This should be accompanied by ruling out other causes of intravascular hemolysis. Because *C. perfringens* type A and CPA are found with high prevalence in the intestines of healthy sheep, the mere detection of either or both of them cannot be considered diagnostic. A colony count of 10^4–10^7 CFU/g of *C. perfringens* type A in intestinal content has been considered diagnostic by some authors, although firm evidence to support this assertion is lacking; it can be considered suggestive, but nothing more. This is mostly because there is little information available about the number of type A organisms in healthy and sick animals, and a threshold for this count in sick animals has not been established. Similarly, CPA is usually present in the intestines of normal animals, but no information about the amount of this toxin present in healthy or diseased animals is available. To compound the problem, most of the ELISA techniques used currently to detect *C. perfringens* toxins are highly sensitive and can detect minimal concentrations of CPA.

Differential diagnosis includes other causes of hemolysis, such as chronic copper toxicosis, leptospirosis, hemoparasite infestations, and infectious necrotic hepatitis and bovine bacillary hemoglobinuria, caused by *Clostridium novyi* type B and *C. haemolyticum*, respectively. The hepatic lesions in the last two are almost pathognomonic of those diseases.

Prophylaxis, control, and treatment

There are no vaccines or vaccination protocols specifically designed to prevent yellow lamb disease, but many vaccines against the different types of *C. perfringens* used around the world serendipitously contain CPA toxoid, and it is possible that they afford at least some level of protection to animals against yellow lamb disease. This, however, has not been tested. No information is available in the literature about treatment and control of yellow lamb disease. It is possible, however, that at least some of the measures taken to control and treat cases of type D enterotoxemia might help with cases of yellow lamb disease.

Other enteric diseases produced by *Clostridium perfringens* type A in mammals

Introduction

In addition to CPA, some strains of *C. perfringens* type A can encode and/or produce several so-called non-typing toxins, including, but not limited to, enterotoxin (CPE), beta2 toxin (CPB2), and necrotic enteritis toxin B (NetB). As explained in Chapter 5, CPE is responsible for one of the most prevalent forms of human food poisoning and antibiotic-associated diarrhea, and NetB has been shown to be necessary for the development of avian necrotic enteritis. However, in contrast to the definitely established role of CPE and NetB in human and poultry enteric disease, respectively, the role of CPE in the pathogenesis of spontaneous animal disease has been less defined, as diagnostic criteria to establish CPE-mediated animal disease are not available. In addition, animals with diarrhea are very rarely tested for CPE in their feces or intestinal content, a criterion used to establish causality in humans. There are reports describing a possible association of CPE with gastrointestinal disease in several domestic and wild animal species including dogs, pigs, horses, goats, penguins, leopards, and tortoises. However, most of these reports are based on isolation of *cpe*-positive *C. perfringens* strains from the intestines of affected animals and, because CPE-positive type A strains may be found in the intestines of clinically healthy animals, isolation of these strains is not necessarily of diagnostic significance for CPE-associated disease in animals. The diagnostic utility of isolation of CPE-positive organisms is increased by a finding of numerous such organisms in feces or gut contents.

Hemorrhagic canine gastroenteritis (canine gastrointestinal hemorrhage syndrome)

Etiology

Hemorrhagic canine gastroenteritis is a sporadic, peracute, hemorrhagic disease of dogs which, in some cases, has been associated with *C. perfringens* type A, although the etiology has not been definitively established. Because CPE-positive *C. perfringens* type strains and/or CPE itself have been found in some dogs with this disease, it was thought that enterotoxigenic *C. perfringens* type A was responsible for hemorrhagic canine gastroenteritis. In other cases, however, no association with CPE has been demonstrated and a definitive role for this toxin in the pathogenesis has not been determined. Recent studies suggest that a novel toxin produced by some strains of *C. perfringens* type A, namely NetF, might be responsible for hemorrhagic canine gastroenteritis (Chapter 9). Because all the NetF-positive strains isolated so far are also *cpe* positive, it is possible that synergism between CPE and NetF occurs.

Clinical signs

Sudden death with dogs usually found in a pool of hemorrhagic diarrhea is characteristic of hemorrhagic canine gastroenteritis. In some cases, death may be peracute, occurring without diarrhea.

Gross and microscopic changes

Hemorrhagic enteritis and colitis, the latter usually being more severe than the changes in the small intestine, with occasional hemorrhagic gastritis, are characteristic gross findings of this condition. Histologically, there is full-thickness mucosal necrosis of the small intestine and colon and, occasionally, the stomach. The presence of large numbers of Gram-positive rods compatible with *C. perfringens*, lining the necrotic mucosal surface and/or mixed with the intestinal content, is also reported. It is not clear if this is a feature of the disease or the consequence of post-mortem proliferation of these organisms. No microorganisms have been described deep in intestinal tissue.

CPE-associated diarrhea in mammalian species

CPE has also been suspected to play a role in rare cases of diarrhea in horses, goats, and pigs. This assumption is based on the detection of CPE-positive *C. perfringens* strains and/or the detection of CPE in the intestinal content or feces of diarrheic animals. For instance, in one study CPE was detected in the feces of ~20% and 30%, respectively, of adult horses and foals with diarrhea, but not in the feces of healthy adult horses or foals. The clinical signs of CPE-associated diarrhea in these animal species are not specific and consist of acute, watery diarrhea. Gross and microscopic lesions in domestic animals with CPE-associated diarrhea have not been described in detail; necrotizing enteritis was described in one foal from which CPE-positive *C. perfringens* type A was isolated.

Diagnosis of CPE-associated disease

The detection of pre-formed CPE in the intestinal content and/or feces of animals with diarrhea is usually considered an indicator of CPE-associated disease. Isolation of *cpe*-positive *C. perfringens* from these specimens is also considered an indicator of this association. However, as explained previously, because the organism can be found in the intestine of healthy animals, this finding is not diagnostic.

Clostridium perfringens beta 2 toxin-associated gastrointestinal disease

Clostridium perfringens beta 2 toxin (CPB2)-producing *C. perfringens* type A strains have been associated with enteric disease in several animal species, including horses, pigs, sheep, and goats. However, very little scientific evidence is available to support the claim that CPB2 is responsible for enteric disease in any animal species. In most cases, this evidence is based solely on isolation of CPB2-positive *C. perfringens* from sick animals. However, *C. perfringens* type A carrying the *cpb2* gene is usually isolated with similar prevalence from the intestinal content or feces of healthy animals, which makes this diagnostic criterion doubtful. More importantly, Koch's postulates have not been fulfilled for CPB2, and the role of this toxin in the pathogenesis of enteric clostridial disease of animals remains, therefore, unconfirmed.

A special comment should be made, however, about the possible role of CPB2-positive *C. perfringens* type A in porcine clostridial enteritis. Because most type A strains isolated from pigs with enteric disease, but not from healthy pigs, carried the *cpb2* gene, it was suggested that in pigs, this toxin is associated with enteric disease. As with other animal species, however, Koch's postulates have not been fulfilled in pigs for CPB2. Clinical signs, gross and microscopic signs of CPB2-associated disease in pigs have not been described in detail. At least one study in horses reported finding beta2 toxin in association with intralesional bacterial rods in the gastrointestinal tract of horses with colitis. However, in the mentioned study, no normal horses were included as controls, and the association between beta2 toxin and the colonic inflammatory changes remains uncertain.

Bibliography

Bacciarini, L.N., *et al.* (2003) Immunohistochemical localization of *Clostridium perfringens* beta2-toxin in the gastrointestinal tract of horses. *Vet. Pathol.*, **40**: 376–381.

Bueschel, D., *et al.* (1998) Enterotoxigenic *Clostridium perfringens* type A necrotic enteritis in a foal. *J. Am. Vet. Med. Assoc.*, **213**: 1305–1307.

Bueschel, D., *et al.* (2003) Prevalence of cpb2, encoding beta2 toxin, in *Clostridium perfringens* field isolates: Correlation of genotype with phenotype. *Vet. Microbiol.*, **94**: 121–129.

Busch, K., *et al.* (2015) *Clostridium perfringens* enterotoxin and *Clostridium difficile* toxin A/B do not play a role in acute haemorrhagic diarrhoea syndrome in dogs. *Vet. Rec.*, **176**: 253.

Donaldson, M.T., *et al.* (1999) Prevalence of *Clostridium perfringens* enterotoxin and *Clostridium difficile* toxin A in feces of horses with diarrhea and colic. *J. Am. Vet. Med. Assoc.*, **215**: 358–361.

Giannitti, F., *et al.* (2014) Diagnostic Exercise: Hemolysis and Sudden Death in Lambs. *Vet. Pathol.*, **51**: 624–627.

Hazlett, M.J., *et al.* (2011) Beta 2 toxigenic *Clostridium perfringens* type A colitis in a three-day-old foal. *J. Vet. Diagn. Invest.*, **23**: 373–376.

Herholz, C., *et al.* (1999) Prevalence of beta$_2$-toxigenic *Clostridium perfringens* in horses with intestinal disorders. *J. Clin. Microbiol.*, **37**: 358–361.

Marks, S.L. (2003) Bacterial-associated diarrhea in the dog: A critical appraisal. *Vet. Clin. North Am. Small Anim. Pract.*, **33**: 1029–1060.

McClane, B.A. (1996) An overview of *Clostridium perfringens* enterotoxin. *Toxicon*, **34**: 1335–1343.

McGowan, G., *et al.* (1958) Lamb losses associated with *Clostridium perfringens* type A. *J. Am. Vet. Med. Assoc.*, **133**: 219–221.

Minamoto, Y., *et al.* (2014) Prevalence of *Clostridium perfringens*, *Clostridium perfringens* enterotoxin and dysbiosis in fecal samples of dogs with diarrhea. *Vet. Microbiol.*, **174**: 463–473.

Oda, M., *et al.* (2008) The relationship between the metabolism of sphingomyelin species and the hemolysis of sheep erythrocytes induced by *Clostridium perfringens* alpha-toxin. *J. Lipid Res.*, **49**: 1039–1047.

Silva, R.O., *et al.* (2013) Detection of toxins A/B and isolation of *Clostridium difficile* and *Clostridium perfringens* from dogs in Minas Gerais, Brazil. *Braz. J. Microbiol.*, **l44**: 133–137.

Silva, R.O., *et al.* (2015) *Clostridium perfringens*: A review of enteric diseases in dogs, cats and wild animals. *Anaerobe*, **33**: 14–17.

Uzal, F.A., *et al.* (2008) Ulcerative enterocolitis in two goats associated with enterotoxin- and beta2 toxin-positive *Clostridium perfringens* type D. *J. Vet. Diagn. Invest.*, **20**: 668–672.

Uzal, F.A., *et al.* (2008) Diagnosis of *Clostridium perfringens* intestinal infections in sheep and goats. *J. Vet. Diagn. Invest.*, **3**: 253–265.

9 NetF-Associated Necrotizing Enteritis of Foals and Canine Hemorrhagic Gastroenteritis

Iman Mehdizadeh Gohari, Valeria R. Parreira, and John F. Prescott

Introduction

Clostridium perfringens type A-associated diarrhea and enteric disease in dogs and foals is not well characterized, since the association of disease is complicated by the common presence of type A organisms in the bowel and feces of healthy animals. The recent description of a novel pore-forming toxin, NetF, which is strongly associated with these diseases, has shed light on the role of type A isolates in enteric disease of animals.

Etiology

There is a highly significant association between the presence of the toxin NetF and isolates of *C. perfringens* recovered from severe canine hemorrhagic gastro-enteritis as well as from necrotizing enterocolitis in foals aged 1–5 days. *C. perfringens* strains producing NetF are clonal (two clones), so that canine and equine strains cannot be distinguished.

The NetF toxin found in type A *C. perfringens* is a recently discovered toxin which is a member of the beta-pore-forming toxin leucocidin-hemolysin family, an important group of clostridial necrotizing toxins (Figure 9.1). The toxin was designated NetF for several reasons: it belongs to the same family of toxins as the relatively recently described NetB, associated with necrotic enteritis of chickens; it is associated with disease in foals (hence the "F"); and the strains could be considered to be "type F" if the current classification of *C. perfringens* as types A–E is to be expanded. *C. perfringens* strains producing NetF also produce another closely related toxin called NetE; both are encoded on the same large plasmid, whereas the enterotoxin (CPE) and often the beta2 toxin (CPB2) are encoded on

Clostridial Diseases of Animals, First Edition. Francisco A. Uzal, J. Glenn Songer,
John F. Prescott and Michel R. Popoff.
© 2016 John Wiley & Sons, Inc. Published 2016 by John Wiley & Sons, Inc.

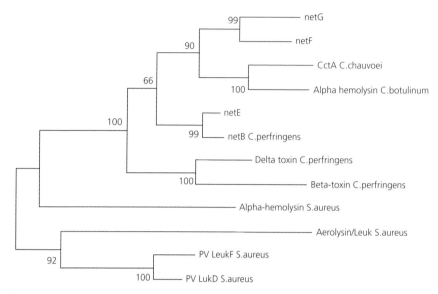

Figure 9.1 Phylogenetic analysis of representative members of the leukocidin/hemolysin superfamily. The tree is drawn to scale, with branch lengths in the same units as those of the evolutionary distances used to infer the phylogenetic tree. Toxins that were used include: alpha-hemolysin of *C. botulinum*, hemolysin II of *B. cereus*, alpha-hemolysin of *S. aureus*, putative CctA of *C. chauvoei*, and beta toxin of *C. perfringens*.

a separate large plasmid, sometimes in conjunction with another, similar toxin called NetG. Analysis of the upstream region of these *net* genes has shown the presence of potential VirR boxes in the promoter region of *netE* and *netG*, but not of *netF*. VirR is a critical regulator of virulence in *C. perfringens*. An equine ovarian cell line has been found to be most susceptible to NetF, with canine cell lines the next most susceptible cells. Unlike NetF, NetE and NetG do not seem to have toxic activity, but they are expressed *in vitro*. Interestingly, since all NetF-producing strains also encode CPE, there may be a synergistic pathogenic effect in the intestine of NetF and CPE, as has been described for beta toxin (CPB) and CPE in rabbits.

Epidemiology and clinical findings

Acute canine hemorrhagic gastroenteritis may occur in any breed and at any age, but small-breed dogs are over-represented, as are dogs aged 2–4 years. There is no apparent seasonal or gender predisposition, and rarely are there reports of recent dietary changes. Clinical signs commonly include a sudden onset of vomiting blood-stained material, followed by bloody diarrhea, although a small proportion of dogs may produce bloody but non-diarrheic feces. The feces have a characteristic foul odor. About 50% of dogs appear depressed and approximately 20% of dogs have painful abdomens on palpation. Ileus may be diagnosed radiographically in about half the cases, but most dogs do not appear dehydrated. Increased packed cell volume, hemoglobin concentration, and red blood cell count may reflect rapid fluid loss into the intestine.

Cases can vary from mild to severe, and many dogs respond well to symptomatic treatment (fluids, antidiarrheics, antiemetics, and antibiotics such as ampicillin). In a small proportion of cases, the disease may be fatal. In peracute cases, dogs that appeared healthy the previous evening may be found dead in the morning, surrounded by a pool of bloody feces, so that death may be attributed to some form of poisoning. The disease appears to be relatively common, although it occurs sporadically. However, information about the incidence and the full range of clinical and epidemiological features of NetF-associated acute hemorrhagic gastroenteritis is not available. This may be partly due to the fact that acute canine hemorrhagic gastroenteritis can have causes other than NetF-producing *C. perfringens*. The well-recognized association of this disease with small-breed dogs may speculatively be explained by the genetically associated predisposition to pancreatitis in small-, rather than in large-, breed dogs, since pancreatitis will disrupt pancreatic trypsin production. This speculation is based on analogy, since fatal type C *C. perfringens* enteritis in other species has commonly been associated with trypsin inhibition by foods such as sweet potatoes, or by trypsin inhibitory factors in colostrum, with the consequence that CPB toxin produced in the small intestine is not destroyed by the proteolytic action of trypsin but rather initiates intestinal necrosis and cascading clostridial disease. Although *netF* is highly associated with canine hemorrhagic gastroenteritis, the gene has been found in about 10% of *C. perfringens* isolates in dogs with undifferentiated diarrheal illness.

Enterocolitis in neonatal foals associated with type A *C. perfringens* is linked to high mortality but, because it has only recently been described, the clinical manifestations of NetF-positive type A *C. perfringens* remain to be fully described. Most foals with NetF-positive type A *C. perfringens*-associated enterocolitis are younger than six days of age, with no breed or gender predisposition. The disease may start as early as 12–24 hours of age, and foals may die within 24 hours of the onset of disease. Foals are usually diarrheic, dull and depressed, colicky, and dehydrated. Intestinal pain can be intense. Hematologically, there is either neutrophilia or neutropenia, with toxicity in white blood cells and increased fibrinogen. Metabolic acidosis and other electrolyte disturbances are common.

The strong association of this infection with neonatal foals supports a role for the trypsin-inhibitory action of colostrum in interfering with the breakdown of *C. perfringens* toxins as an important feature of its pathogenesis. Although *netF* is highly associated with type A *C. perfringens* necrotizing enteritis in foals, the gene is rare in *C. perfringens* isolates in foals or adult horses with undifferentiated diarrheal illness. Anecdotally, the disease can be endemic on some horse-breeding farms and is regionally distributed. It is likely that mares and fecally-contaminated environments are sources of the bacterium, which is acquired orally by the foal. *C. perfringens* can readily transiently multiply to large numbers in the stomach and intestines of young foals as part of the normal bacterial intestinal colonization process that occurs in neonates. Further work is required to describe the prevalence of these strains in healthy and diarrheic dogs and foals, and the epidemiology of infection.

Gross changes

The gross pathology of fatal cases of *netF*-positive *C. perfringens* canine hemorrhagic gastroenteritis is characterized by flaccidity, transmural congestion, and the presence of bloody content in the small intestine, with marked congestion and watery, red contents present both in the small intestine and in the colon. The serosal and mucosal surfaces of the entire gastrointestinal tract are often diffusely hemorrhagic. The stomach may contain a small amount of reddish-brown, foul-smelling liquid.

The gross pathology of fatal cases of *netF*-positive foal necrotizing enterocolitis is characterized by fibrinonecrotic enteritis (Figures 9.2 and 9.3) or by enterocolitis, in some cases with intestinal mural emphysema; necrohemorrhagic enteritis is less common. Disease is usually acute in onset but may develop into a severe chronic localized region of necrosis in a segment of the small intestine.

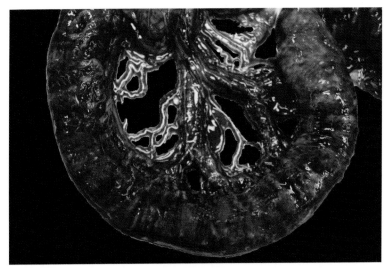

Figure 9.2 Jejunum of a 7-day-old foal showing thickening of the wall and serosal congestion associated with *netF*-positive type A *C. perfringens*. Courtesy of M. Spinato.

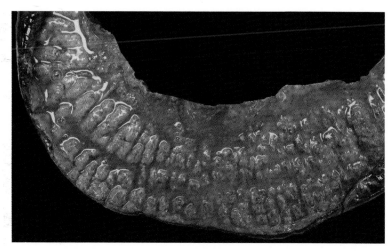

Figure 9.3 Jejunum of a 7-day-old foal showing diffuse necrotizing enteritis associated with *netF*-positive type A *C. perfringens*. Courtesy of M. Spinato.

Microscopic changes

In *netF*-associated canine hemorrhagic gastroenteritis, the villus epithelium in the small intestine and the superficial portion of the gastric glands show acute coagulative necrosis, which is separated from the underlying, more normal intestinal tissue by a band of mostly neutrophilic infiltration. The presence of large numbers of Gram-positive rods adhering to the necrotic intestinal mucosa is a prominent and striking characteristic feature of canine hemorrhagic gastroenteritis. The submucosal vessels are markedly congested.

Histopathological changes in the intestine in *netF*-associated foal necrotizing enterocolitis are similar to those observed in the canine disease, although focal mucosal ulceration may also be present in the large bowel.

Diagnosis

Diagnosis of *netF*-positive type A *C. perfringens* disease in dogs and foals depends on demonstration of the *netF* gene in isolates recovered from animals presenting with characteristic clinical or pathological features, or on the demonstration of this gene in feces by PCR. However, this finding should be interpreted cautiously, as NetF-positive strains of *C. perfringens* type A have been found in a small percentage of clinically healthy dogs. Ruling out other causes of enteric disease in dogs and horses lends additional support to a diagnosis of NetF-associated disease. The 100% correlation between the presence of *netF* and the *cpe* enterotoxin gene suggests that demonstration of CPE by ELISA testing of feces might be a rapid, indirect approach to diagnosis or to raising a suspicion of the presence of the disease.

Bibliography

Burrows, C.F. (1977) Canine hemorrhagic gastroenteritis. *J. Am. Anim. Hosp. Assoc.*, **13**: 451.

Diab, S.S., *et al.* (2011) Pathology of *Clostridium perfringens* Type C enterotoxemia in horses. *Vet. Pathol.*, **49**: 255.

Donahue, M., *et al.* (2002) Clostridial enterocolitis in horses. *Equine Dis. Quart.*, **10**: 4.

East, L.M., *et al.* (1998) Enterocolitis associated with *Clostridium perfringens* infection in neonatal foals: 54 cases (1988–1997). *J. Am. Vet. Med. Assoc.*, **212**: 1751.

Marks, S.L. (2010) *Clostridium perfringens-* and *Clostridium difficile-* associated diarrhea. In: Greene, C.E. (ed.) *Infectious Diseases of the Dog and Cat*, 4th edition, p. 393. Saunders Elsevier, St. Louis, MO.

Mehdizadeh, G.I., *et al.* (2015) A novel pore-forming toxin in type A *Clostridium perfringens* is associated with both fatal canine hemorrhagic gastroenteritis and fatal foal necrotizing enterocolitis. *PLoS One*, **10**: e0122684.

Schlegel, B.J., *et al.* (2012) *Clostridium perfringens* type A fatal acute hemorrhagic gastroenteritis in a dog. *Can. Vet. J.*, **53**: 549.

Silveira, R.O., *et al.* (2015) *Clostridium perfringens*: A review of enteric diseases in dogs, cats and wild animals. *Anaerobe*, **33**: 14.

Tillotson, K., *et al.* (2002) Population-based study of fecal shedding of *Clostridium perfringens* in broodmares and foals. *J. Am. Vet. Med. Assoc.*, **220**: 342.

Unterer, S., *et al.* (2014) Endoscopically visualized lesions, histologic findings, and bacterial invasion in the gastrointestinal mucosa of dogs with acute hemorrhagic diarrhea syndromes. *J. Vet. Intern. Med.*, **28**: 52.

10

Necrotic Enteritis of Poultry

Kerry K. Cooper and J. Glenn Songer

Introduction

Necrotic enteritis (NE) produced by *Clostridium perfringens* is the most severe clostridial enteric disease of poultry, and it is estimated that worldwide NE costs the poultry industry 2 billion dollars per year. The disease occurs in two forms: acute and chronic (subclinical). The acute form is associated with loss due to increased mortality rates at around 3–4 weeks of age, but it is the chronic or subclinical form that results in severe economic loss due to reduced weight gain and less efficient feed conversion. The subclinical form causes the greatest production loss, as it often goes undetected; reports estimate that as much as 40% of commercial broiler flocks are affected.

Epidemiology

Necrotic enteritis has been reported in a wide variety of avian species including chickens, turkeys, ostriches, quail, capercaillies, geese, bluebirds, lorikeets, and crows. NE has been reported in most countries around the world, with acute outbreaks occurring sporadically, and most commonly in broiler chickens aged 2–6 weeks. This is believed to be due to a window in the anti-clostridial immunity that occurs when maternal antibodies disappear at around 2 weeks of age, and lasts until the immune system reaches maturity at around 3–4 weeks of age. Acute outbreaks have also been reported in broilers up to 11 weeks of age, in 3–6-month-old commercial layers, and in 12–16-week-old replacement pullets. Only one outbreak of NE has been reported in 9-month-old chickens. Subclinical NE often goes unobserved, so it is difficult to get an exact sense of the epidemiology of this form of the disease.

Clostridial Diseases of Animals, First Edition. Francisco A. Uzal, J. Glenn Songer,
John F. Prescott and Michel R. Popoff.
© 2016 John Wiley & Sons, Inc. Published 2016 by John Wiley & Sons, Inc.

Etiology and pathogenesis

C. perfringens type A almost exclusively produces clostridial necrotic enteritis of poultry, although it is thought that type C may be involved on rare occasions. However, since most diagnoses of necrotic enteritis are based on gross, and occasionally microscopic, pathology alone, it is possible that type C is involved in at least some cases, but goes undetected.

The disease starts when *C. perfringens* multiplies anarchically in the intestine of chickens, producing toxins that cause necrosis. In fact, during initial disease development, a single *C. perfringens* clone arises to dominance in the bird's intestinal tract. After birds recover from the disease, whether naturally or via antimicrobial treatment, a diverse population of *C. perfringens* isolates returns. Furthermore, a high portion of NE isolates inhibits the growth of other *C. perfringens* strains, particularly compared to isolates from healthy birds. Recently, perfrin, a novel bacteriocin, was identified from an NE isolate, and is predominantly associated with NE isolates. This may be a critical virulence factor that allows the NE isolate to arise to dominance, fill open niches, multiply, and establish disease in the host. NE isolates adhere to extracellular matrix molecules, such as fibrinogen and collagen types III and IV, more efficiently than isolates from healthy birds. This suggests a role for some unknown attachment factor in initial colonization. Additionally, proteolytic enzymes affecting the basement membrane of the villous enterocytes help to establish the initial infection by these NE isolates. Overall, research is slowly deciphering the virulence factors needed to establish disease in the host.

For many years, alpha toxin (CPA, the only so-called "major" toxin produced by *C. perfringens* type A) has been considered the major virulence factor involved in necrotic enteritis, because crude preparations of this toxin obtained from *C. perfringens* type A cultures produced lesions typical of necrotic enteritis when injected into the intestine of conventional chickens. When these crude toxin preparations were neutralized with anti-CPA serum, no lesions were observed. In addition, CPA has been found in the feces and intestinal content of poultry with NE, and many NE isolates were found to produce higher levels of CPA *in vitro* than *C. perfringens* isolates from healthy birds. Thus, it was initially speculated that CPA was the major virulence factor responsible for NE. This was also supported by the fact that vaccination of chickens with recombinant CPA or CPA toxoids provides a degree of protection against NE.

Despite the evidence presented above, during the past few years, the role of CPA in the pathogenesis of NE has been questioned. Fulfillment of molecular Koch's postulates showed that a CPA null mutant produced lesions typical of NE. Based on that, researchers concluded that CPA was not critical for the pathogenesis of NE. However, additional work has found that CPA is still present in the intestinal tract of birds challenged with a CPA null mutant, as the type A normal flora in the bird's intestinal tract produces CPA in these circumstances. Additionally, spontaneously derived CPA mutants of NE strains lost the ability to produce disease; however, these mutants were never complemented for CPA production and then tested *in vivo*. Also, CPA vaccination research has shown that some anti-CPA antibodies bind to the cell wall of *C. perfringens* and prevent growth, thus potentially providing protection by binding directly to the bacteria rather than to the actual toxin. Therefore, additional work on the importance of CPA in the pathogenesis of NE is needed.

Recently, a toxin called necrotic enteritis toxin (NetB) was discovered and determined to have a critical role in the pathogenesis of NE. NetB shares 38% identity with *C. perfringens* beta toxin (CPB) and 31% with *Staphylococcus aureus* alpha hemolysin, both of which are pore-formers. NetB also forms heptameric pores; it also has enhanced activity in the presence of cholesterol and is toxic for chicken hepatocytes (LMH cells). Importantly, a *C. perfringens netB* null mutant strain did not produce NE lesions in chickens, and this mutant recovered full virulence when *netB* was restored. The *netB* gene is found on a large, conjugative plasmid within a 42 kb pathogenicity locus. It is regulated by the VirSR two-component signal transduction system, which is activated as a result of population density and regulates production of a number of other toxins in *C. perfringens*. Interestingly, IgY levels against both CPA and NetB are significantly higher in healthy chickens compared to birds with NE, which further supports the role of these two toxins in the pathogenesis of NE no matter how minor the effect may be on the disease.

Additional work does need to decipher the exact role of NetB in producing disease, because although some studies have found that 70–90% of NE isolates have *netB*, and very few *C. perfringens* isolates from normal chickens have this gene, others have found an almost equal distribution of *netB* between NE isolates and poultry normal flora isolates. Furthermore, the gene is very highly conserved, but less than 30% of *netB*-positive isolates from healthy birds actually produce the toxin, while over 90% of *netB*-positive isolates from NE cases produce the toxin. In addition, a study also reported a *netB*-negative NE isolate that produced disease in an experimental model. Furthermore, during studies with the *netB* mutant, the authors found a small number of NE lesions in birds challenged with the *netB* mutant, but concluded these were due to *netB*-negative normal flora strains. Conversely, other studies have found that *netB*-negative NE isolates do not produce disease, and all *netB*-positive isolates, regardless of the source, produce NE, but with significant differences in severity and incidence.

Beta2 toxin (CPB2) and *C. perfringens* enterotoxin (CPE), two toxins produced by some *C. perfringens* isolates, have also been suggested to play a role in poultry NE. However, there is no definitive evidence that either of these toxins plays a role in the pathogenesis of poultry NE. Both are uncommon finds in the genotyping process.

TpeL, a member of the large clostridial toxins (LCT), is present in strains that produce severe disease in experimental NE models. TpeL has been found in less than 10% of isolates from NE birds and is always associated with NetB; however, no isolates from healthy birds have been found to carry *tpeL*. Although there is no doubt of the role played by NetB in the pathogenesis of many cases of NE, further investigation is needed to determine the possible role of other toxins in some cases of this disease.

Several unknown virulence factors appear to have a potential role in the pathogenesis of NE, and additional approaches, such as comparative genomics, are helping to identify these factors. Comparative genomics of seven NE strains has revealed three highly conserved NE-associated loci including NELoc-1 (42 kb, encoding *netB*, two leukocidins, and 34 additional genes), NELoc-2 (11.2 kb), and NELoc-3 (5.6 kb). NELoc-1 and NELoc-3 are both located on large, distinct plasmids; in fact, *netB*-positive isolates have been found always to contain one to four large plasmids. Comparative genomic hybridization of 54 *C. perfringens* isolates from NE or healthy birds revealed 142 genomic regions variably present in poultry isolates with 49 significantly associated with NetB, while multilocus sequence typing (MLST) studies have identified two major NE clonal groups, and further correlated NetB with NE disease. Overall, this suggests type A strains acquire the plasmid carrying *netB*, and then through two different pathways acquire other virulence factors to emerge as NE strains.

Host response

Although little is known about the avian immune response to NE, some work has begun to shed light on the issue. Chicken immune microarrays demonstrated that both cell-mediated and humoral-mediated immune responses via MHC classes I and II were activated during NE. While toll-like receptor-2 (TLR-2) appears to be strongly involved in the immune response, several other toll-like receptors, such as TLR-4 and TLR-7, have a minor role in the immune response. A number of cytokines such as TNF-α, IL-8, IL-6, and IL-1β are all upregulated during NE. Mucin has a critical role in protecting the intestinal epithelium during infections. The presence of *C. perfringens* during NE results in the downregulation of both *MUC2* (widely expressed in goblet cells from the small and large intestines) and *MUC13* (the exact role is not known) genes in birds, and is suggested most likely to be the consequence of severe shedding of the jejunal mucosa during the disease. The presence of *C. perfringens* and the development of NE, as expected, also causes major intestinal microflora changes. In particular, various *Weissella* species and lactobacilli are suppressed by the presence of *C. perfringens* during disease development. Even though there is limited knowledge about the host's response to NE, we are beginning to gain a better understanding that will hopefully assist in the development of effective prevention methods.

Predisposing factors

A number of factors have been linked to increasing rates of NE in birds, particularly broiler chickens. The normal number of *C. perfringens* is negligible in the crop and steadily increases to the highest levels in the colon. Normal, healthy chickens typically have 10^2–10^4 colony-forming units (CFUs)/g of intestinal contents in the small intestine, while birds suffering from NE reach levels of 10^7–10^9 CFU/g, demonstrating that predisposing factors which allow high proliferation of *C. perfringens* are critical for disease development. A preceding or co-infection with *Eimeria* is known as a major precursor for NE in chickens. Damage caused by *Eimeria* results in the leakage of plasma proteins into the intestinal tract, which enhances *C. perfringens* growth and toxin production. High energy, high protein, and/or high non-starch-polysaccharide-containing diets induce higher rates of NE in birds. An increased level of animal protein such as fishmeal in feed has been a known predisposing factor for years, as animal protein is poorly digested, providing large amounts of cysteine, glycine, and proline to *C. perfringens* for growth and toxin production. Recently, inclusion of potato protein in the diet resulted in higher rates and more severe NE than either fishmeal or soybean diets. Additionally, potato protein contains higher trypsin inhibitor activity than fishmeal or soybean; trypsin destroys *C. perfringens* toxins, so inhibitors have been associated with a higher incidence of NE in birds. In addition to the physical damage and providing critical nutrients to *C. perfringens*, examination of the microbiota has revealed that fishmeal and *Eimeria* infection both cause a significant change in the alpha and/or beta diversity of the intestinal tract of broiler chickens which allows *C. perfringens* to colonize and expand in numbers. High non-starch polysaccharides, such as from wheat-, rye-, or barley-based diets, increase digesta viscosity, which slows intestinal movement, increases mucus production, and impairs oxygen transfer, allowing *C. perfringens* to grow. Additionally, the size of the feed particles can increase the incidence of NE, as finely ground feed provides more surface area for *C. perfringens* to metabolize the feed and proliferate faster.

Interestingly, the common feed contaminant *Fusarium* mycotoxin deoxynivalenol also has the potential to more than double the occurrence of subclinical NE, due to the intestinal epithelial damage the mycotoxin produces, which increases nutrient availability to *C. perfringens*. Aflatoxin B_1 also results in increased occurrence, severity, and mortality rates due to NE, which has been suggested to be due to suppression of the bird's immune system by the toxin. In addition to diet, higher stocking densities of broiler chickens increase the severity of the NE lesions. Although these predisposing factors can make birds more susceptible to disease, research has proven that a virulent *C. perfringens* NE isolate must be present under these conditions in order for disease to develop.

Clinical signs

Acute and subclinical forms of the disease have been described. Chickens with acute NE show a variety of clinical signs, which may include depression, reluctance to move, diarrhea, ruffled feathers, decreased appetite or anorexia, huddling, dribbling from the beak, and dehydration. The course of the acute disease is usually very short and most birds die within 1–2 hrs after the onset of clinical disease; finding birds dead without premonitory clinical signs is not uncommon. An early indicator of disease can be wet litter, although this can be coincident with, rather than prior to, disease development. Mortality rates due to acute NE can reach as high as 50%.

Chickens with the subclinical form of NE suffer a drop in production, but no other clinical signs are evident. The chronic damage to the intestinal mucosa results in reduced weight gain and higher feed conversion ratios due to decreased digestion. Clinical signs of NE in birds of other species are similar to those described in chickens, while subclinical disease has only been described in chickens.

Gross changes

Gross lesions in birds with acute NE are typically restricted to the small intestine, most frequently the jejunum and ileum, although lesions are occasionally observed in the duodenum and ceca (Figure 10.1). The reason for this small bowel predilection is unknown. A study suggested that cecal lesions only occur as a consequence of primary jejunal lesions releasing debris contaminated with *C. perfringens* into the ceca.

The affected area of the intestine is usually distended with gas, and contains a foul-smelling, dark brown, grey, or yellow-green fluid that contains fibrin mixed with sloughed-off mucosal cells and other components and digesta. The

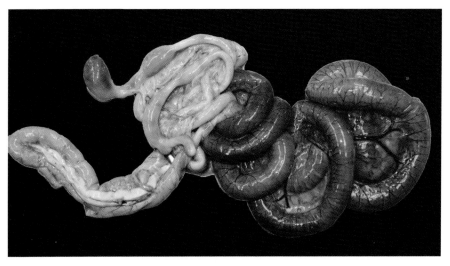

Figure 10.1 Serosal view of the intestinal tract of a chicken with acute necrotic enteritis, which demonstrates the predilection of the disease to develop in the small intestine, particularly the jejunum. Courtesy of F.A. Uzal.

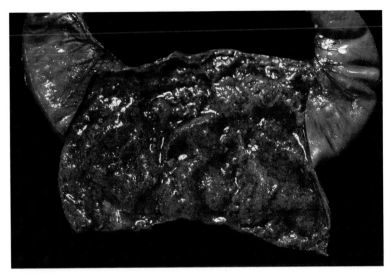

Figure 10.2 Mucosal view of the jejunum in a chicken with acute necrotic enteritis, which shows the thin intestinal wall, hyperemia, and diffuse mucosal necrosis typical of severe cases. Courtesy of F.A. Uzal.

intestinal wall is usually thin and quite friable. The mucosal surface presents multifocal to coalescent deep round or irregular mucosal ulcerations, which have peripheral hyperemia, and are typically covered by a yellow-green to yellow-brown pseudomembrane (Figure 10.2). These lesions can typically be seen from the serosa. Frank intestinal hemorrhage is not usually seen in field cases, although a few strands of blood can occasionally be seen in feces.

In subclinical NE, the lesions are similar to those described for acute cases and consist of small, multifocal mucosal ulcerations (usually 1–2 mm in diameter, but occasionally bigger; Figure 10.3). One exception is that in subclinical NE, the intestinal wall can be severely thickened by edema and/or granulation tissue.

Cholangiohepatitis may be seen occasionally in chickens with NE. It has been hypothesized that these hepatic lesions are associated with the intestinal damage that allows the increased numbers of *C. perfringens* in the intestinal tract to gain access to the portal bloodstream and biliary ducts. Grossly, the livers are enlarged, firm, and pale, with multifocal yellow necrotic foci. There is severe hepatic congestion, and occasionally the gall bladder and bile duct are distended with bile and have thickened walls.

Gross lesions of NE in turkeys are very similar to those in chickens, but can extend into the colon, and the duodenum is frequently more affected than in chickens. In outbreaks of NE in ostriches, gross lesions comprise diffuse, small intestinal fibrino-necrotic enteritis. The small intestine is dilated with gas and yellowish fibrino-hemorrhagic fluid.

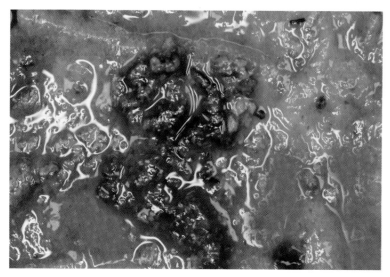

Figure 10.3 Mucosal view of the jejunum in a chicken with chronic necrotic enteritis, which shows multifocal ulceration. Courtesy of F.A. Uzal.

Microscopic changes

Recent studies of the early development of the disease have revealed that microscopic lesions of NE develop at the basement membrane of the enterocytes of the villi and progress throughout the lamina propria. Eventually, epithelial damage at the tips of the villus leads to necrosis throughout the villi. Commonly, microscopic lesions of NE involve extensive mucosal necrosis, while more severe disease can reach the submucosa, and the most severe forms may extend into the muscular layers. The progression of disease is marked by a clear line of demarcation between necrotic and viable tissue, characterized by large numbers of inflammatory cells at the edge of viable tissue (Figure 10.4), with heterophils dominant in acute infections and mononuclear cells in chronic disease. Research has shown that *C. perfringens* does not invade enterocytes and is only associated with the necrotic tissue. As disease progresses, the intestinal lumen fills with fibro-necrotic material, eventually forming a pseudomembrane composed of fibrin, bacilli, cell debris, and inflammatory cells. Outbreaks of NE in other avian species have nearly identical microscopic lesions to those described in chickens. When NE spreads beyond the intestinal tract, there can be multifocal coagulative necrosis in the liver and bile ducts, which is characterized by the presence of bacilli and fibrinous exudate.

During convalescence, the birds begin to regenerate the intestinal epithelial cells, typically starting in the crypts. This regeneration process results in an increase in cuboidal cells and a decrease in goblet and columnar epithelial cells, which overall leaves the intestinal tract with decreased villus height and increased villus width.

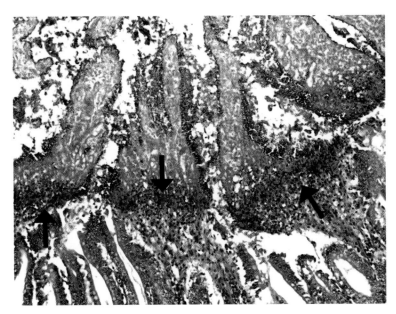

Figure 10.4 Microscopic view of the jejunum in a chicken with acute necrotic enteritis, showing the sharp line of demarcation between viable and necrotic tissue characterized by large numbers of inflammatory cells at the edge of the viable tissue (arrows). HE, 200x.

Prophylaxis

For decades, NE in poultry was controlled by the addition of antimicrobial growth promoters (AGPs) to the birds' feed or water. However, since 2006, the European Union has banned the use of AGPs in animal feed, which has resulted in an increase in the incidence of NE in poultry. North America, South America, and Asia still use AGPs, but with rising concerns about antibiotic resistance, many producers are slowly discontinuing their use due to the stigma. Therefore, there is a great need to develop alternative preventive methods to control NE in poultry; in fact, the major focus of research on NE over the last four to five years has been vaccination and other preventive methods. Current prevention methods include avoiding predisposing factors and the use of a few types of not very effective in-feed additives to reduce risk. The development of an effective vaccine is hampered by the fact that multiple doses are not practical in the poultry industry, and single 1-day-old chick vaccines have failed to prevent infection. Maternal vaccinations and the use of attenuated *Salmonella* vectors have shown some promise and are the most industrially feasible, but to date nothing has been completely effective against the disease.

The various preventive components that have been investigated recently include several different forms: various chemical and natural compounds, and biological control additives (prebiotics). Chemical compounds such as bismuth citrate, potassium diformate, and selenium, mixed with feed or, in the case of selenium, also delivered *in ovo,* have shown a decrease in the severity and mortality rates in experimentally produced NE. Natural compounds like plant-derived phytonutrients, essential oils, and organic acids from a variety of different sources have resulted in decreased disease severity, decreased numbers of *C. perfringens* and lower disease rates, while increasing body weight gain. The use of anti-clostridial bacteriocins and lysozyme added to feed or water resulted in decreased lesion scores and numbers of *C. perfringens,* while increasing body weight and improving feed conversion rates. Experiments with various prebiotics have also had relative success in controlling NE and improving feed conversion rates. Spores from several species of the genus *Bacillus,* a lytic *C. perfringens* bacteriophage, and several species of *Lactobacillus* have all reduced lesion scores and mortality, and improved feed efficiency and body weight during experimental NE. Unfortunately, to date nothing has proven to be as effective at preventing NE as AGPs.

The goal of vaccination is to provide protection for a 4–5 week window after maternal antibodies have waned at 2 weeks of age, and until the birds are fully raised at approximately 6–7 weeks of age. Protection is possible; it has been shown that previous *C. perfringens* infections induce protection against subsequent challenges. Numerous studies have looked into developing an effective vaccine against NE, but to date, no totally effective vaccine is commercially available. Recombinant CPA and attenuated *Salmonella* vectors expressing CPA provide partial protection against the disease, while *C. perfringens* type A and type C toxoid vaccines also significantly decreased the occurrence of the disease in experimental models. A maternal type A CPA toxoid vaccine increased antibodies against CPA in the hens that were transferred to the chicks, and resulted in an overall lower mortality rate during natural infection compared to chicks from unvaccinated control groups. Since the identification of NetB as a major virulence factor, it has been an obvious vaccine candidate; however, a recombinant NetB, NetB toxoid, and NetB genetic toxoid all only provided partial protection against experimental NE. *C. perfringens* and cell-free toxoids supplemented with recombinant NetB demonstrated significant protection against severe experimental NE challenge, while maternal vaccination with either a recombinant NetB or type A toxoid supplemented with recombinant NetB resulted in anti-NetB antibodies in the hens that were transferred to the progeny, but neither provided protection beyond 14 days of age.

Examination of serum from chickens recovered from NE revealed a number of different vaccine targets. Recombinant proteins of elongation factor Tu (EF-Tu) and pyruvate:ferredoxin oxidoreductase (PFO) in combination with CPA and NetB demonstrated significant but not complete protection against experimental NE challenge. Vaccination against recombinant endo-beta-N-acetylglucosamine (Naglu) resulted in significant protection but only against certain NE strains. However, recombinant phosphoglyceromutase (Pgm) did provide significant protection against all tested NE strains.

To date, only one vaccination study has reported complete protection against experimental challenge; supernatant fluid from eight different NE isolates was examined and the supernatant from one strain provided complete protection. It appears that in order to obtain complete protection, an effective vaccine needs the proper combination of *C. perfringens* immunogens. While there is an extreme need for an effective vaccine or preventative measure against NE, nothing to date reaches the protective levels of AGPs.

Diagnosis

There is no single, definitive diagnostic test or finding to diagnose NE in any avian species, but, rather, several criteria are required. First, a presumptive diagnosis can be made with a post-mortem finding in the intestinal tract of focal, multifocal, or diffuse necrotic lesions in the small intestine, and rarely in the proximal colon or cecum. Since these lesions are not pathognomonic of NE, histological examination and confirmation of the characteristic extensive mucosal necrosis with lining of the necrotic surface by Gram-positive rods can be used to further support the presumptive diagnosis, and can also rule out other diseases. In coccidiosis, numerous oocysts will be present in the intestinal villi and large schizonts found in the lamina propria. NE can be predisposed by coccidiosis, so that dual infections may be present. Ulcerative enteritis will exhibit ulcerations in the small intestine as well as focal crypt necrosis.

Isolation of *C. perfringens* is required for confirmation of NE. There are numerous conventional or selective media that can be used to isolate *C. perfringens* from the intestine, including, but not limited to, tryptose-sulfite cycloserine (TSC) agar and blood agar incubated anaerobically at 37 °C for 24 hours. Thioglycollate broth can be used, but solid media are preferred, since they will give semi-quantitative data on colony numbers. Colonies on blood agar will have the double zone of hemolysis characteristic of *C. perfringens* and on TSC agar usually have black colonies, especially after 48 hours of incubation. Unfortunately, *C. perfringens* type A is a common inhabitant of the intestinal tract of healthy birds, so that isolation of *C. perfringens* alone will not lead to a definitive diagnosis. PCR screening of *C. perfringens* isolates for the presence of *netB* will help support the presumptive NE diagnosis. More virulent *netB*-positive strains are likely also to possess the *tpeL* gene, and this can also be confirmed by PCR. It should be noted that not all isolates of *C. perfringens* from cases of NE will be positive for *netB*, even in isolates taken directly from the necrotic lesions. The reason for this discrepancy is unknown but may relate to co-infection with non-*netB*-positive strains, loss of the *netB* plasmids, or other reasons.

The development of direct PCR screening, DNA sequencing, and real-time PCR assays for *C. perfringens* NE isolates directly from the intestinal tract of birds without cultivation may significantly speed up the diagnostic process. Because of the common presence of *C. perfringens* as normal flora, the detection by ELISA of CPA in the intestinal tract is not reliable. Future developments might include ELISA detection of NetB or other NE-associated proteins, or identification of either of the two clonal types of *C. perfringens* associated with NE. Overall, the presence of characteristic necrotic lesions during gross examination that are confirmed by histopathology should lead to a presumptive diagnosis of NE, which can then be confirmed by the isolation of *netB* (and possibly *tpeL*)-positive *C. perfringens* strains to give a definitive diagnosis of necrotic enteritis.

Bibliography

Abildgaard, L., *et al.* (2010) *In vitro* production of necrotic enteritis toxin B, NetB, by *netB*-positive and *netB*-negative *Clostridium perfringens* originating from healthy and diseased broiler chickens. *Vet. Microbiol.*, **144**: 231–235.

Antonissen, G., *et al.* (2014) The mycotoxin deoxynivalenol predisposes for the development of *Clostridium perfringens*-induced necrotic enteritis in broiler chickens. *PLoS One*, **9**: e108775.

Barrios, M.A., *et al.* (2013) Comparison of 3 agar media in Fung double tubes and petri plates to detect and enumerate *Clostridium* spp. in broiler chicken intestines. *Poult. Sci.*, **92**: 1498–1504.

Cao, L., *et al.* (2012) Reduced lesions in chickens with *Clostridium perfringens*-induced necrotic enteritis by *Lactobacillus fermentum* 1.2029. *Poult. Sci.*, **91**: 3065–3071.

Cheung, J.K., *et al.* (2010) The VirSR two-component signal transduction system regulates NetB toxin production in *Clostridium perfringens*. *Infect. Immun.*, **78**: 3064–3072.

Cooper, K.K., *et al.* (2009a) Immunization with recombinant alpha toxin partially protects broiler chicks against experimental challenge with *Clostridium perfringens*. *Vet. Microbiol.*, **133**: 92–97.

Cooper, K.K., *et al.* (2009b) Necrotic enteritis in chickens: A paradigm of enteric infection by *Clostridium perfringens* type A. *Anaerobe*, **15**: 55–60.

Cooper, K.K., *et al.* (2010) Virulence for chickens of *Clostridium perfringens* isolated from poultry and other sources. *Anaerobe*, **16**: 289–292.

Cooper, K.K., *et al.* (2013) Diagnosing clostridial enteric disease in poultry. *J. Vet. Diagn. Invest.*, **25**: 314–327.

Coursodon, C.F., *et al.* (2010) *Clostridium perfringens* alpha toxin is produced in the intestines of broiler chicks inoculated with an alpha toxin mutant. *Anaerobe*, **16**: 614–617.

Coursodon, C.F., *et al.* (2012) TpeL-producing strains of *Clostridium perfringens* type A are highly virulent for broiler chicks. *Anaerobe*, **18**: 117–121.

Cravens, R.L., *et al.* (2013) The effects of necrotic enteritis, aflatoxin B$_1$, and virginiamycin on growth performance, necrotic enteritis lesion scores, and mortality in young broilers. *Poult. Sci.*, **92**: 1997–2004.

Crouch, C.F., *et al.* (2010) Safety and efficacy of a maternal vaccine for the passive protection of broiler chicks against necrotic enteritis. *Avian Pathol.*, **39**: 489–497.

Engberg, R.M., *et al.* (2012) The effect of *Artemisia annua* on broiler performance, on intestinal microbiota and on the course of a *Clostridium perfringens* infection applying a necrotic enteritis disease model. *Avian Pathol.*, **41**: 369–376.

Feng, Y., *et al.* (2010) Identification of changes in the composition of ileal bacterial microbiota of broiler chickens infected with *Clostridium perfringens*. *Vet. Microbiol.*, **140**: 116–121.

Femandes da Costa, S.P., *et al.* (2013) Protection against avian necrotic enteritis after immunization with NetB genetic or formaldehyde toxoids. *Vaccine*, **31**: 4003–4008.

Fernando, P.S., *et al.* (2011) Effect of diets containing potato protein or soya bean meal on the incidence of spontaneously-occurring subclinical necrotic enteritis and the physiological response in broiler chickens. *Br. Poult. Sci.*, **52**: 106–114.

Forder, R.E.A., *et al.* (2012) Quantitative analyses of genes associated with mucin synthesis of broiler chickens with induced necrotic enteritis. *Poult. Sci.*, **91**: 1335–1341.

Geier, M.S., *et al.* (2010) Comparison of alternatives to in-feed antimicrobials for the prevention of clinical necrotic enteritis. *J. Appl. Microbiol.*, **109**: 1329–1338.

Grilli, E., *et al.* (2009) Pediocin A improves growth performance of broilers challenged with *Clostridium perfringens*. *Poult. Sci.*, **88**: 2152–2158.

Henriksen, M., *et al.* (2009) Evaluation of PCR and DNA sequencing for direct detection of *Clostridium perfringens* in the intestinal tract of broilers. *Avian Dis.*, **53**: 441–448.

Hibberd, M.C., *et al.* (2011) Multilocus sequence typing subtypes of poultry *Clostridium perfringens* isolates demonstrate disease niche partitioning. *J. Clin. Microbiol.*, **49**: 1556–1567.

Jang, S.I., *et al.* (2012) Vaccination with *Clostridium perfringens* recombinant proteins in combination with Montanide™ ISA 71 VG adjuvant increases protection against experimental necrotic enteritis in commercial broiler chickens. *Vaccine*, **30**: 5401–5406.

Jayaraman, S., *et al.* (2013) *Bacillus subtilis* PB6 improves intestinal health of broiler chickens challenged with *Clostridium perfringens*-induced necrotic enteritis. *Poult. Sci.*, **92**: 370–374.

Jerzsele, A., *et al.* (2012) Efficacy of protected sodium butyrate, a protected blend of essential oils, their combination, and *Bacillus amyloliquefaciens* spore suspension against artificially induced necrotic enteritis in broilers. *Poult. Sci.*, **91**: 837–843.

Jiang, Y., *et al.* (2009) Immunization of broiler chickens against *Clostridium perfringens*-induced necrotic enteritis using purified recombinant immunogenic proteins. *Avian Dis.*, **53**: 409–415.

Keyburn, A.L., *et al.* (2010) Association between avian necrotic enteritis and *Clostridium perfringens* strains expressing NetB toxin. *Vet. Res.*, **41**: 21.

Keyburn, A.L., *et al.* (2013a) Maternal immunization with vaccines containing recombinant NetB toxin partially protects progeny chickens from necrotic enteritis. *Vet. Res.*, **44**: 108.

Keyburn, A.L., *et al.* (2013b) Vaccination with recombinant NetB toxin partially protects broiler chickens from necrotic enteritis. *Vet. Res.*, **44**: 54.

Knap, I., *et al.* (2010) *Bacillus licheniformis* prevents necrotic enteritis in broiler chickens. *Avian Dis.*, **54**: 931–935.

Kulkarni, R.R., *et al.* (2010) A live oral recombinant *Salmonella enterica* serovar Typhimurium vaccine expressing *Clostridium perfringens* antigens confers protection against necrotic enteritis in broiler chickens. *Clin. Vaccine Immunol.*, **17**: 205–214.

Lanckriet, A., *et al.* (2010) Variable protection after vaccination of broiler chickens against necrotic enteritis using supernatants of different *Clostridium perfringens* strains. *Vaccine*, **28**: 5920–5923.

Lee, K.W., *et al.* (2011) Identification and cloning of two immunogenic *Clostridium perfringens* proteins, elongation factor Tu (EF-Tu) and pyruvate:ferredoxin oxidoreductase (PFO) of *C. perfringens*. *Res. Vet. Sci.*, **91**: e80–e86.

Lee, K.W., *et al.* (2012) *Clostridium perfringens* alpha-toxin and NetB toxin antibodies and their possible role in protection against necrotic enteritis and gangrenous dermatitis in broiler chickens. *Avian Dis.*, **56**: 230–233.

Lee, S.H., *et al.* (2013) Dietary supplementation of young broiler chickens with *Capsicum* and turmeric oleoresins increases resistance to necrotic enteritis. *Br. J. Nutr.*, **110**: 840–847.

Lee, S.H., *et al.* (2014a) Effects of *in ovo* injection with selenium on immune and antioxidant responses during experimental necrotic enteritis in broiler chickens. *Poult. Sci.*, **93**: 1113–1121.

Lee, S.H., *et al.* (2014b) Immune and anti-oxidant effects of *in ovo* selenium proteinate on post-hatch experimental avian necrotic enteritis. *Vet. Parasitol.*, **206**: 115–122.

Lepp, D., *et al.* (2010) Identification of novel pathogenicity loci in *Clostridium perfringens* strains that cause avian necrotic enteritis. *PLoS One*, **5**: e10795.

Lepp, D., *et al.* (2013) Identification of accessory genome regions in poultry *Clostridium perfringens* isolates carrying the *netB* plasmid. *J. Bacteriol.*, **195**: 1152–1166.

Liu, D., *et al.* (2010) Exogenous lysozyme influences *Clostridium perfringens* colonization and intestinal barrier function in broiler chickens. *Avian Pathol.*, **39**: 17–24.

Lu, Y., *et al.* (2009) Expression profiles of genes in toll-like receptor-mediated signaling of broilers infected with *Clostridium perfringens*. *Clin. Vaccine Immunol.*, **16**: 1639–1647.

Martin, T.G., *et al.* (2009) Prevalence of *netB* among some clinical isolates of *Clostridium perfringens* from animals in the United States. *Vet. Microbiol.*, **136**: 202–205.

Martin, T.G., *et al.* (2010) The ability of disease and non-disease producing strains of *Clostridium perfringens* from chickens to adhere to extracellular matrix molecules and Caco-2 cells. *Anaerobe,* **16**: 533–539.

Mikkelsen, L.L., *et al.* (2009) Effect of potassium diformate on growth performance and gut microbiota in broiler chickens challenged with necrotic enteritis. *Br. Poult. Sci.,* **50**: 66–75.

Miller, R.W., *et al.* (2010) Bacteriophage therapy for control of necrotic enteritis of broiler chickens experimentally infected with *Clostridium perfringens. Avian Dis.,* **54**: 33–40.

Moran, E.T. (2014) Intestinal events and nutritional dynamics predispose *Clostridium perfringens* virulence in broilers. *Poult. Sci.,* **93**: 3028–3036.

Mot, D., *et al.* (2013) Day-of-hatch vaccination is not protective against necrotic enteritis in broiler chickens. *Avian Pathol.,* **42**: 179–184.

Mot, D., *et al.* (2014) Progress and problems in vaccination against necrotic enteritis in broiler chickens. *Avian Pathol.,* **43**: 290–300.

Palliyeguru, M.W.C.D., *et al.* (2010) Effect of dietary protein concentrates on the incidence of subclinical necrotic enteritis and growth performance of broiler chickens. *Poult. Sci.,* **89**: 34–43.

Palliyeguru, M.W.C.D., *et al.* (2011) Effect of trypsin inhibitor activity in soya bean on growth performance, protein digestibility and incidence of sub-clinical necrotic enteritis in broiler chicken flocks. *Br. Poult. Sci.,* **52**: 359–367.

Parreira, V.R., *et al.* (2012) Sequence of two plasmids from *Clostridium perfringens* chicken necrotic enteritis isolates and comparison with *C. perfringens* conjugative plasmids. *PLoS One,* **7**: e49753.

Saleh, N., *et al.* (2011) Clinicopathological and immunological studies on toxoids vaccine as a successful alternative in controlling clostridial infection in broilers. *Anaerobe,* **17**: 426–430.

Sarson, A.J., *et al.* (2009) Gene expression profiling within the spleen of *Clostridium perfringens*-challenged broiler fed antibiotic-medicated and non-medicated diets. *BMC Genomics,* **10**: 260.

Savva, C.G., *et al.* (2013) Molecular architecture and functional analysis of NetB, a pore-forming toxin from *Clostridium perfringens. J. Biol. Chem.,* **288**: 3512–3522.

Shojadoost, B., *et al.* (2012) The successful experimental induction of necrotic enteritis in chickens by *Clostridium perfringens*: A critical review. *Vet. Res.,* **43**: 74.

Skinner, J.T., *et al.* (2010) An economic analysis of the impact of subclinical (mild) necrotic enteritis in broiler chickens. *Avian Dis.,* **54**: 1237–1240.

Smyth, J.A., *et al.* (2010) Disease producing capability of *netB* positive isolates of *C. perfringens* recovered from normal chickens and a cow, and *netB* positive and negative isolates from chickens with necrotic enteritis. *Vet. Microbiol.,* **46**: 76–84.

Stanley, D., *et al.* (2012) Changes in the caecal microflora of chickens following *Clostridium perfringens* challenge to induce necrotic enteritis. *Vet. Microbiol.,* **159**: 155–162.

Stanley, D., *et al.* (2014) Differential responses of cecal microbiota to fishmeal, *Eimeria* and *Clostridium perfringens* in a necrotic enteritis challenge model in chickens. *PLoS One,* **9**: e104739.

Stringfellow, K., *et al.* (2009) Effect of bismuth citrate, lactose, and organic acid on necrotic enteritis in broilers. *Poult. Sci.,* **88**: 2280–2284.

Timbermont, L., *et al.* (2009a) Intra-species growth-inhibition by *Clostridium perfringens* is a possible virulence trait in necrotic enteritis in broilers. *Vet. Microbiol.,* **137**: 388–391.

Timbermont, L., *et al.* (2009b) Origin of *Clostridium perfringens* isolates determines the ability to induce necrotic enteritis in broilers. *Comp. Immunol. Microbiol. Infect. Dis.,* **32**: 503–512.

Timbermont, L., *et al.* (2010) Control of *Clostridium perfringens*-induced necrotic enteritis in broilers by target-released butyric acid, fatty acids and essential oils. *Avian Pathol.,* **39**: 117–121.

Timbermont, L., *et al.* (2011) Necrotic enteritis in broilers: An updated review on the pathogenesis. *Avian Pathol.,* **40**: 341–347.

Timbermont, L., *et al.* (2014) Perfin, a novel bacteriocin associated with *netB* positive *Clostridium perfringens* strains from broilers with necrotic enteritis. *Vet. Res.,* **45**: 40.

Tsiouris, V., *et al.* (2015) High stocking density as a predisposing factor for necrotic enteritis in broiler chicks. *Avian Pathol.*, **44**: 1–31.

Van Immerseel, F., *et al.* (2008) Rethinking our understanding of the pathogenesis of necrotic enteritis in chickens. *Trends Microbiol.*, **17**: 32–36.

Wu, S-B., *et al.* (2011) Real-time PCR assay for *Clostridium perfringens* in broiler chickens in a challenge model of necrotic enteritis. *Appl. Environ. Microbiol.*, **77**: 1135–1139.

Wu, S-B., *et al.* (2014) Two necrotic enteritis predisposing factors, dietary fishmeal and *Eimeria* infection, induce large changes in the caecal microbiota of broiler chickens. *Vet. Microbiol.*, **169**: 188–197.

Xu, S.Z., *et al.* (2015) Effects of dietary selenium on host response to necrotic enteritis in young broilers. *Res. Vet. Sci.*, **98**: 66–73.

Xu, S.Z., *et al.* (2015) Dietary sodium selenite affects host intestinal and systemic immune response and disease susceptibility to necrotic enteritis in commercial broilers. *Br. Poult. Sci.*, **56**: 103–112.

Yan, X-X., *et al.* (2013) Structural and functional analysis of the pore-forming toxin NetB from *Clostridium perfringens*. mBio 4: e00019.

Zhou, H., *et al.* (2009) Transcriptional profiling analysis of host response to *Clostridium perfringens* infection in broilers. *Poult. Sci.*, **88**: 1023–1032.

Infections by *Clostridium perfringens* Type B

Francisco A. Uzal and J. Glenn Songer

Introduction

Infections by *Clostridium perfringens* type B have been described in the Middle East, Europe, and South Africa. No cases of this infection have been reported from Australasia or the Americas, although anecdotal evidence suggests that infections by this microorganism have been occasionally diagnosed in North and South America. Disease has most frequently been reported in lambs, occasionally in calves, and very rarely in foals.

Etiology

C. perfringens type B isolates carry the genes encoding beta (CPB) and epsilon (ETX) toxins, but different strains can also encode several other non-typing toxins. It is assumed, however, that the two main virulence factors of type B strains are CPB and ETX. CPB is very sensitive to the action of proteases (for example, intestinal trypsin), while ETX needs one or more proteases to become fully activated; however, it seems likely that only one of these toxins is the main virulence factor in the pathogenesis of type B disease at a given time. Clinical signs and lesions are expected to be very different when ETX or CPB action predominates. This, however, has not been demonstrated and remains speculative.

Clostridial Diseases of Animals, First Edition. Francisco A. Uzal, J. Glenn Songer, John F. Prescott and Michel R. Popoff.
© 2016 John Wiley & Sons, Inc. Published 2016 by John Wiley & Sons, Inc.

Clinical signs

In young lambs (from birth to approximately 14 days of age), *C. perfringens* type B causes a condition known as "lamb dysentery", which is characterized clinically by acute abdominal pain, a distended abdomen, and hemorrhagic diarrhea. Older lambs may have a more chronic form of the disease, which in the UK is known as "pine," and is characterized by loss of condition, depression, and reluctance to suckle. Neurological signs including opisthotonus, blindness, and lack of coordination may be observed occasionally and are thought to be produced by the brain lesions caused by ETX. However, it is possible that at least some of these signs are associated with CPB.

In calves, the disease caused by *C. perfringens* type B is clinically similar to that described in lambs, with animals less than 10 days of age being mostly affected; a few cases have been reported in older animals. Although little information is available in this regard, it has been suggested that calves are more likely to recover than similarly affected lambs.

Rare cases of *C. perfringens* type B infection with hemorrhagic diarrhea have been described in foals within the first few days of life.

Gross changes

In lambs, intestinal gross lesions associated with infection by *C. perfringens* type B are essentially the same as those seen in *C. perfringens* type C necrotizing enteritis (Chapter 12), and are characterized by severe diffuse or multifocal to coalescing necrohemorrhagic or ulcerative enteritis. The ulcers are usually irregular, with well-defined margins, surrounded by a rim of hyperemia, and frequently covered by a fibrinous pseudomembrane. The intestinal contents usually have variable amounts of blood, from a few specks to almost pure blood. In more chronic cases in which the animals survive for a few days, little or no hemorrhage may be observed. In most cases, a small amount of clear or hemorrhagic fluid is present in the peritoneal cavity, but in cases with deeper mucosal ulcers and/or transmural inflammation, there may be intestinal perforations with fibrinous peritonitis that can lead to intestinal adhesions. Lesions characteristic of toxemia are usually present, including congested and edematous lungs, pale or congested, friable liver, enlarged and pulpy spleen, enlarged, edematous, and pale kidneys, hydropericardium, and epicardial and endocardial hemorrhages. Occasionally, focal symmetrical encephalomalacia indistinguishable grossly and histologically from that seen in the sub-acute and chronic forms of type D infection (Chapter 13) has been described in lambs with type B disease. Very rarely, gross lesions may be absent in peracute cases of type B infections.

With the exception of the central nervous system, the gross lesions in calves (Figure 11.1) and foals are essentially the same as those described for lambs.

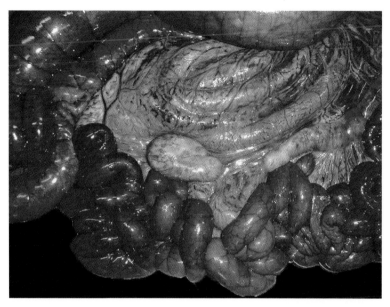

Figure 11.1 Diffuse hemorrhagic enteritis in a calf with *Clostridium perfringens* type B enterotoxemia. Courtesy of E. Paredes.

No gross changes have been described in the central nervous system of calves or foals with type B infection.

Microscopic changes

Histologically, the changes in the alimentary system of animals with type B disease are indistinguishable from those seen in animals with type C necrotic enteritis (Chapter 12). Briefly, there is multifocal to diffuse transmural hemorrhage of the small intestine, with mucosal coagulation necrosis that may extend to the muscularis and serosa. Thrombosis of mucosal blood vessels is an almost constant finding. A fibrin membrane may be seen over the necrotic mucosa and there are abundant, typically non-sporulated, large, Gram-positive rods in the lumen, the pseudomembrane, and the necrotic tissue. The inflammatory exudate is usually mild and mostly neutrophilic.

Lesions in the central nervous system have only been described occasionally in lambs and are similar to those seen in animals with type D disease (Chapter 13), including proteinaceous perivascular edema in acute cases and focal symmetrical necrosis in sub-acute and chronic cases.

Histological lesions in other organs are those associated with toxemia and include pulmonary congestion and edema, congested spleen, and hemorrhages of serous membranes.

Diagnosis

Clinical signs, gross and microscopic changes compatible with type B infection provide a reasonable presumptive diagnosis of this disease. A final diagnosis, however, relies on detection of both CPB and ETX in the intestinal content of affected animals, together with isolation of *C. perfringens* type B from the same specimen. Although small numbers of *C. perfringens* type B have rarely been isolated from intestinal contents of normal animals, isolation of large numbers of type B (especially in pure culture) from animals with compatible clinical signs and lesions is considered a very good diagnostic indicator of type B infection. As explained under type C disease (Chapter 12), failure to detect CPB does not preclude a diagnosis of type B disease, as this toxin is very sensitive to the action of trypsin and is destroyed rapidly in the intestine. Because of this, if CPB has been destroyed by intestinal proteases, a type B infection (alpha toxin [CPA], CPB, and ETX produced) may be misdiagnosed as type D (CPA and ETX toxins produced) if a diagnosis is based solely on toxin detection. This explains why a final diagnosis of type B infection should be based on toxin detection accompanied by clinical, pathological, and microbiological findings.

Prevention and treatment

Vaccines containing CPB and ETX toxoids should be used for the prevention of type B disease. Because most animals get sick at a very young age, vaccination of the dams a few weeks before parturition is essential to make sure an appropriate level of antibodies is present in the colostrum. This colostral immunity lasts for approximately 4 to 6 weeks, at which time a double vaccination, 4 to 6 weeks apart, should be applied. An annual booster is recommended.

Bibliography

Fernandez-Miyakawa, M.E. *et al.* (2007) Both epsilon-toxin and beta-toxin are important for the lethal properties of *Clostridium perfringens* type B isolates in the mouse intravenous injection model. *Infect. Immun.*, **75**: 1443–1452.

Gkiourtzidis, K., *et al.* (2001) PCR detection and prevalence of alpha-, beta-, beta 2-, epsilon-, iota- and enterotoxin genes in *Clostridium perfringens* isolated from lambs with clostridial dysentery. *Vet. Microbiol.*, **82**: 39–43.

Li, J. *et al.* (2013) Toxin plasmids of *Clostridium perfringens*. *Microbiol. Mol. Biol. Rev.*, **77**: 208–233.

Songer, J.G. (1996) Clostridial enteric diseases of domestic animals. *Clin. Microbiol. Rev.*, **9**: 216–234.

Stubbings, D.P. (1990) *Clostridium perfringens* enterotoxaemia in two young horses. *Vet. Rec.*, **127**: 431.

Uzal, F.A. (2004) Diagnosis of *Clostridium perfringens* intestinal infections in sheep and goats. *Anaerobe*, **10**: 135–143.

Uzal, F.A. *et al.* (2008) Diagnosis of *Clostridium perfringens* intestinal infections in sheep and goats. *J. Vet. Diagn. Invest.*, **20**: 253–265.

Uzal, F.A. *et al.* (2010) *Clostridium perfringens* toxins involved in mammalian veterinary diseases. *Open Toxin. J.*, **2**: 24–42.

Diseases Produced by *Clostridium perfringens* Type C

Santiago S. Diab

Diseases of mammalian species

Introduction

Intestinal infection by *C. perfringens* type C causes necrotizing enteritis or enterocolitis in domestic animals and humans. The disease occurs mostly in neonatal individuals of several animal species. In lambs, type C infection is referred to as hemorrhagic enteritis, while in adult sheep, the term "struck" is used because of the very sudden nature of death. The term necrotic enteritis is used for type C disease in goats, cattle, pigs, and horses. In humans, type C disease is also known as enteritis necroticans, pigbel, or darmbrand. The disease has been reproduced experimentally in pigs, sheep, calves, and goats, while rabbits, mice, and guinea pigs have been used in experimental models to study diverse aspects of the pathogenesis of type C disease (Table 12.1).

Etiology

C. perfringens type C has been associated with necrotizing enteritis in humans and domestic animals for many years. However, only in the last few years has the development of new research tools and the use of animal models (including pigs, guinea pigs, rabbits, mice, goats, and sheep) significantly expanded our understanding of the pathogenesis of type C infections. A detailed description of the toxins produced by *C. perfringens* is presented in Chapter 5. Briefly, all type C strains produce alpha (CPA) and beta (CPB) toxins. Additionally, certain strains of type C also produce other toxins, including, but not limited to, enterotoxin (CPE), beta2 toxin (CPB2), perfringolysin O (PFO), and the large clostridial toxin TpeL.

Clostridial Diseases of Animals, First Edition. Francisco A. Uzal, J. Glenn Songer, John F. Prescott and Michel R. Popoff.

Table 12.1 Most common spontaneous and experimental diseases associated with *C. perfringens* type C

Spontaneous	Sheep	Hemorrhagic enteritis in lambs; "struck" in adult sheep
	Pigs	Necrotizing enteritis (mostly in piglets)
	Cattle	Necrotizing enteritis (mostly in calves)
	Horses	Necrotizing enteritis (mostly in foals)
	Humans	Enteritis necroticans ("pigbel," "darmbrand")
Experimental	Rabbits[a]	Necrotizing enteritis (jejunum and ileum)
	Mice[b]	Depression, neurological disease, swollen abdomen, death. No significant damage to the intestine
	Pigs	Necrotizing enteritis (mainly jejunum and ileum; occasionally colon)
	Guinea Pigs	Necrotizing enteritis (mainly jejunum and ileum)
	Sheep	Necrotizing enteritis (mainly jejunum and ileum)
	Goats	Necrotizing enteritis (mainly jejunum and ileum)

Reprinted (slightly modified) with permission from Uzal *et al.* (2011) *Vet. Microbiol.*, 153: 37–43.
[a] Intestinal loop model.
[b] Intragastric and intraduodenal model.

Molecular Koch's postulates have been fulfilled for type C strains in several animal species, and it is now widely accepted that CPB plays a major role in the pathogenesis of *C. perfringens* type C disease and it is considered the most important virulence factor in type C infections. CPB is thermolabile and highly sensitive to proteases, including trypsin and pepsin, but it is resistant to low pH. It forms pores in the membranes of a variety of cultured cells, including endothelial cells of the intestinal mucosa of piglets and humans. These pores induce efflux of K^+ and influx of Ca^{++}, Na^+ and Cl^-; resulting in cellular swelling and lysis. Recent research suggests that during infection by type C, CPB initially affects the host intestine indirectly by causing intestinal endothelial cell damage and subsequent thrombosis with ischemic necrosis of the intestinal mucosa. This, however, has not been definitively proved and others believe that initial damage by CPB occurs in intestinal epithelial cells. Whatever the mechanism, the extensive mucosal necrosis allows CPB, as well as other toxins and/or enteric bacteria, to reach the circulation and produce lethal systemic effects, including neurological effects in both natural and experimental disease. Experimentally, CPB is capable of inducing neurological alterations in mice when administered intragastrically, intraduodenally, or intravenously in the absence of significant intestinal damage. Neurological alterations can also occur in natural hosts of type C disease. The pathogenesis of the neurological alterations in CPB-intoxicated animals has not yet been established.

Epidemiology

The epidemiology of type C disease in different animal species is poorly under-stood. Limited available data indicate that the prevalence of the disease varies among animal species, but the case fatality rate is usually high for all of them. In non-vaccinated swine populations, the incidence may be nearly 100%, while case fatality rates vary from 50 to 100%. Litters from non-immune sows are particularly at risk. Adequate herd immunity may significantly decrease the inci-dence of the disease. "Struck" of adult sheep occurs primarily in pastured, non-vaccinated animals; its prevalence may range from 5 to 15%. The prevalence of infections in foals is low, but the case fatality rate ranges from 80 to 100%.

C. *perfringens* type C disease is typically a condition of young animals but occurs occasionally in adults, as in ovine "struck." In swine, the disease can occur as early as 12 hours of age but is more commonly seen in 1- to 3-day-old piglets. Type C disease is rare in piglets older than 1 week. In foals, type C infec-tion occurs most commonly during the first week of life. Lambs, goats, and calves may develop type C disease as early as the second day of life.

Pathogenesis

C. *perfringens* type C is found in soil and in feces and the intestinal tracts of humans and other animals, and spores survive in the environment for long periods of time. However, this microorganism is not typically considered an important commensal in the intestinal tract of most animal species. Its presence is rare in the intestines of healthy horses, but it is commonly found in the feces of pigs on farms where the disease is endemic. *In vitro* studies have shown that type C strains may transfer the plasmid carrying the CPB-encoding gene to type A strains and, although not yet proven, it has been suggested that this might also happen *in vivo*.

Environmental contamination with feces from infected animals is an impor-tant source of infection. For instance, small numbers of C. *perfringens* type C may be detected in the feces of sows, exposing piglets to the microorganism shortly after birth. Although the main source of infection for piglets is sow feces, piglets may also be a source of infection for other piglets. *In vitro* studies have shown that a pH between 6.5 and 7.5 leads to high production of CPA, CPB, CPB2, and CPE toxins by C. *perfringens*. Therefore, gastrointestinal factors that increase the luminal pH in the stomach may increase intestinal colonization, growth, and toxin production by C. *perfringens*.

Dietary changes are also considered important predisposing factors for the disease. A sudden change in the diet and other factors may cause an imbalance of the normal intestinal flora, which favours overgrowth of C. *perfringens*. As noted previously, CPB is protease-labile and disease only occurs in situations where protease activity is very low or absent. In neonates, this occurs due to early failure to produce protective quantities of proteases and also because of the protease-inhibitor effect of colostrum. Human enteritis necroticans has often been associated with routine consumption of a protein-poor diet with occasional consumption of high-protein food rich in trypsin inhibitors and contaminated with type C. A classic scenario has been documented in the Highlands of Papua New Guinea over the past 60 years, although it seems likely that these cases have occurred there over a much longer period. The primary diet consisted of sweet potato, which contains a protease inhibitor, but is also low in protein, leading to a protease deficiency in the small intestine. Consumption of under-cooked meat from pigs slaughtered without careful attention to sanitation pro-vided the source of infection with *C. perfringens* type C. Under these conditions, production of CPB in the intestine was followed by fulminant disease. In Papua New Guinea, there remains a significant incidence of this disease, where it is known in the native dialect as "pigbel" (pig belly). Vaccination with a beta toxoid was quite effective in children, but that vaccine is no longer in production and the incidence has risen as a result.

On occasion, even when adequate levels of trypsin are present in the intestinal lumen, high levels of CPB may overpower the neutralizing effects of trypsin and cause disease, possibly explaining cases of type C disease in adult animals. The pres-ence of foods with high levels of trypsin inhibitors, such as sweet potato and soybeans, may predispose domestic animals to type C enteritis and enterotoxemia.

Concurrent infection with other pathogens can change the intestinal envi-ronment, creating circumstances that favor the proliferation of type C in the intestine. There is speculation that coinfection of pigs with transmissible gastro-enteritis virus, porcine epidemic diarrhea virus, rotavirus, or coccidia may predispose to type C disease. In calves, concurrent infections with rotavirus, *Cryptosporidium* spp., and *Salmonella* spp. have been described, but whether these really predispose to type C infection is not known. In horses, both *C. perfringens* type C and *C. difficile* have been identified in foals with hemorrhagic enteritis or enterocolitis.

Clinical signs

The clinical signs of necrotic enteritis are similar in the young of most species, although interspecies and individual variations occur. The disease is often peracute or acute, with occasional sub-acute and chronic presentations. In the peracute and acute forms, animals may be found dead or have rapidly progress-ing signs that include colic, lethargy, severe depression, and bloody diarrhea, although cases without diarrhea can occur. A slower progression of the disease results in sub-acute or chronic presentations, characterized by intermittent or persistent diarrhea that is usually not hemorrhagic, weight loss, progressive weakness, and dehydration. Many animals with the sub-acute and chronic forms will eventually die or, as frequently happens in pigs, be euthanized as "poor doers." Piglets may present with marked anal or perineal hyperemia and hemorrhage in both the acute and chronic forms (Figure 12.1).

In "struck" of adult sheep, animals can be found in a straining position that suggests acute abdominal pain, or may present with acute neurological signs or sudden death with no other clinical signs. Diarrhea is uncommon.

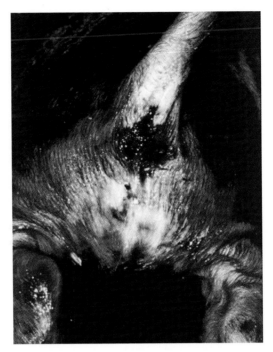

Figure 12.1 *Clostridium perfringens* type C necrotic enteritis in a piglet; observe perianal hemorrhage. Reprinted with permission from Songer *et al.* (2005) *J. Vet. Diagn. Invest.*, **17**: 528–536.

Type C disease is uncommon in adult goats and cattle, and therefore has been poorly documented, but generally resembles struck in sheep.

Gross changes

Lesions produced by *C. perfringens* type C are similar, regardless of animal species and the segment of the intestinal tract affected. They are most frequently observed in the small intestine, but can also be present occasionally in the cecum and colon and may be segmental or diffuse. In sheep and calves, the distal jejunum and ileum are most frequently affected. In piglets, lesions predominate in the jejunum, but are found occasionally in the cecum and spiral colon, with rare cases in which lesions are found in the large intestine only. In horses, lesions in the small intestine are accompanied by changes in the colon or cecum in approximately 40% of the cases and, as in pigs, only rarely do lesions present in the colon or cecum alone.

Affected portions of the intestinal tract can be externally dark red as a consequence of serosal congestion and/or hemorrhage accompanying severe mucosal and submucosal hemorrhage, and may occasionally be emphysematous (Figures 12.2 and 12.3).

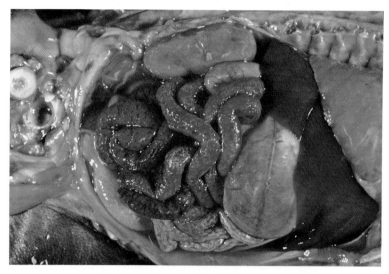

Figure 12.2 *Clostridium perfringens* type C necrotic enteritis in a piglet; observe dark red (hemorrhagic) and emphysematous small intestinal loops. Courtesy of M. Anderson.

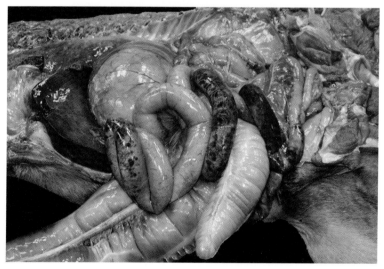

Figure 12.3 *Clostridium perfringens* type C necrotic enteritis in a foal. Transmural lesions extending through the jejunal wall are observed as patches of hemorrhage in the intestinal serosa. Reprinted with permission from Diab *et al.* (2012) *Vet. Pathol.*, **48**: 255–263.

In the acute disease, the small or large intestinal contents are fluid, frequently brown or red (bloody), and may contain fibrin clots and necrotic debris (Figures 12.4 and 12.5). In the sub-acute or chronic disease, particularly in piglets, the intestinal fluid may be mucoid and yellow or yellow-gray. The intestinal wall may be moderately to markedly thickened by gelatinous edema

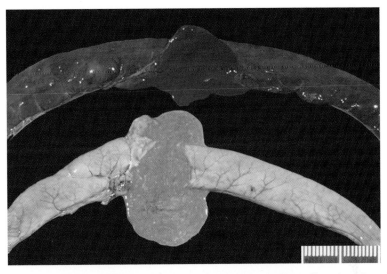

Figure 12.4 *Clostridium perfringens* type C necrotic enteritis in a foal. An affected portion of ileum (top) is diffusely dark red and contains frankly hemorrhagic fluid, whereas the unaffected duodenum (bottom) contains light brown, normal fluid. Reprinted with permission from Diab *et al.* (2012) *Vet. Pathol.*, **48**: 255–263.

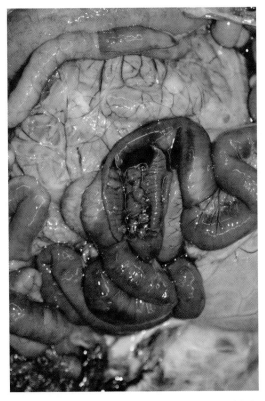

Figure 12.5 Experimental *Clostridium perfringens* type C necrotic enteritis in a goat. The lumen of the jejunum contains a small amount of hemorrhagic fluid and yellow, fibrinous exudate admixed with necrotic debris (pseudomembrane). Reprinted with permission from Garcia *et al.* (2012) *Vet. Microbiol.*, **157**: 412–419.

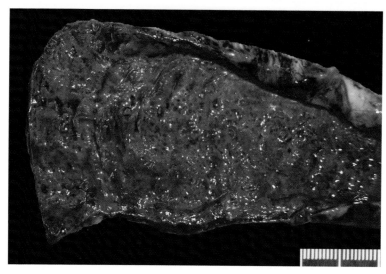

Figure 12.6 *Clostridium perfringens* type C necrotic enteritis in a foal. The mucosa of the small intestine is dull, orange/green and multifocally ulcerated. Reprinted with permission from Diab *et al.* (2012) *Vet. Pathol.*, **48**: 255–263.

or hemorrhage. The mucosa is often dark red due to hemorrhage and hyperemia or slightly brown or greenish (Figure 12.6); it may be multifocally ulcerated, and sometimes multifocally or diffusely covered by a tan, yellow, or slightly green pseudomembrane composed of cellular and inflammatory debris admixed with intestinal contents.

Extraintestinal lesions are usually the result of toxemia and/or septicemia. Typically, multifocal petechiae and ecchymoses of variable severity may be present in the intestinal serosa, mesentery, pericardium, endocardium, thoracic and visceral pleura, or diaphragm. A small amount of serous or hemorrhagic fluid with or without a few fibrin strands may be present in the abdominal and thoracic cavities and within the pericardial sac.

Microscopic changes

The characteristic microscopic lesion of natural disease in all species is severe necrotizing and hemorrhagic enteritis or colitis with mucosal or submucosal thrombosis. Necrosis of the epithelial lining and lamina propria usually begins at the villous tips and rapidly progresses to the deeper portions of the villi and into the crypts. The submucosa is often hyperemic and expanded by a combination of edema, hemorrhage, emphysema, and inflammatory cells, although inflammation is seldom a prominent feature (Figures 12.7 and 12.8). A mild to moderate number of neutrophils, lymphocytes, plasma cells, and histiocytes may be present in the lamina propria of the mucosa and in the submucosa. Lymphatic vessels in the submucosa may be greatly dilated and filled with fibrillar proteinaceous exudate and neutrophils. When lesions are transmural, inflammatory

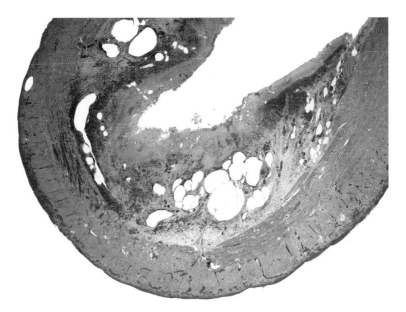

Figure 12.7 *Clostridium perfringens* type C necrotic enteritis in a foal. The mucosa of the small intestine is diffusely necrotic, and the submucosa is expanded by hemorrhage and emphysema; the hemorrhage extends into the muscular and serosal layers. HE, 200x. Reprinted with permission from Diab *et al.* (2012) *Vet. Pathol.,* **48**: 255–263.

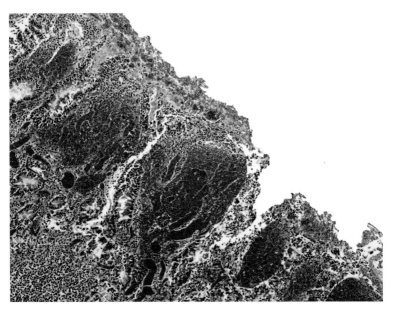

Figure 12.8 *Clostridium perfringens* type C necrotic enteritis in a calf. There is necrosis of the epithelium at the tip of the small intestinal villi and the mucosal surface is overlaid by a thin pseudomembrane containing abundant bacteria. Observe diffuse hemorrhage within the lamina propria. HE, 100x. Courtesy of F.A. Uzal.

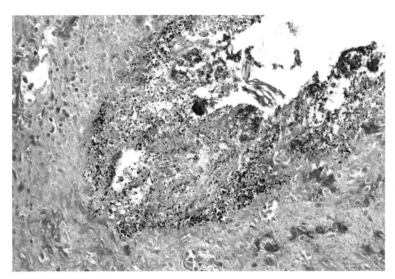

Figure 12.9 *Clostridium perfringens* type C necrotic enteritis in a foal. Abundant Gram-positive bacilli morphologically compatible with *Clostridium* spp. on the mucosal surface of the small intestine. Gram, 400x. Reprinted with permission from Diab *et al.* (2012) *Vet. Pathol.*, **48**: 255–263.

cells, edema, emphysema, and acute hemorrhage can be seen multifocally within the muscular and serosal intestinal layers. A variable number of large, thick, Gram-positive bacilli morphologically compatible with *Clostridium* spp. can be seen within the lumen or overlying the denuded intestinal mucosa (Figure 12.9).

Prophylaxis
Vaccination
C. perfringens vaccines for veterinary use are mostly prepared from semi-purified supernatants of cultures of *C. perfringens* types A, B, C, and D, or a combination of these types. Formalin inactivation of these supernatant fluids eliminates the toxicity but immunogenic activity is retained. Vaccines for type C stimulate most importantly the production of CPB antitoxin.

For prevention of type C disease in pigs, a first vaccination of the sow with type C toxoid at service or mid-gestation and a second vaccination 2 or 3 weeks before farrowing is recommended. Vaccine boosters should be given about 3 weeks before subsequent farrowing. Litters of non-immune sows can receive passive immunization with CPB antitoxin. Parenteral administration of anti-toxin should take place soon after farrowing, as the disease can affect piglets as young as a few hours.

Vaccination of sheep and goats against type C disease is usually concurrent with vaccination for the more prevalent type D enterotoxemia, and usually the same recommendations given for type D disease are followed (Chapter 13).

Vaccination of cattle against *C. perfringens* type C is rarely performed, probably because the disease is not frequently a problem in this species. When necessary, dry cows and heifers should be vaccinated twice 2 to 4 weeks apart and then receive yearly boosters 1 month before calving. Calves should be vaccinated with the same vaccine at approximately 8 and 12 weeks of age.

There are currently no vaccines against any type of *C. perfringens* or its toxins approved for horses, but foals may receive at least some protection from maternal antibodies when mares are immunized with a type C toxoid vaccine approved for other livestock species. It has been recommended that mares be vaccinated initially twice with type C toxoid (4 to 6 weeks apart), followed by an annual booster 2 to 3 weeks before parturition. Administration of type C antitoxin orally before approximately 6 hours of age may provide foals with passive immunity on farms where type C disease is a recurrent problem.

Other prophylactic measures

Avoiding carbohydrate and protein overload is important for *C. perfringens* disease prevention, regardless of the type. In lactating calves, environmental or management factors that may trigger ingestion of larger than normal volumes of milk or milk replacer should be avoided. Feeding more frequently with smaller volumes of milk per feeding has been used with variable success. To prevent induction of ileus, milk and milk replacer should be fed at or near body temperature. For grazing cattle, sheep, and goats, reducing the amount of carbohydrate in the diet and avoiding sudden dietary changes or alterations of the feeding routine are important for prevention of *C. perfringens*-associated disease.

In piglets, oral administration of antibiotics immediately after birth and for at least three days helps prevent the disease. The prophylactic use of antibiotics should be carefully evaluated, as *C. perfringens* may develop resistance.

In horses, preventive measures rely on correct peri-parturient management. These measures include reducing alfalfa or grain intake of peri-parturient mares, thorough cleaning and disinfection of stalls between foalings, minimizing foal exposure to fecal matter by washing the environment and the udder of the mare before the foal suckles for the first time, and administration of antibiotics for the first few days of the foal's life.

Treatment

Treatment options for a specific animal species are beyond the scope of this chapter. Treatment for type C enterotoxemia follows the principles of therapy for other acute diseases of the intestinal tract, including replacement of fluid and electrolytes, reduction of fluid secretion, promotion of mucosal repair, control of endotoxemia and sepsis, and reestablishment of normal flora. The usual fast course of the peracute and acute forms of the disease often precludes any therapeutic intervention and, even when treatment is established, the success rate is generally low. Animals that are raised individually or in small groups have a better chance of being found early in the course of the disease than those in large groups, which increases the possibility of successful treatment. If animals survive to the early acute stage of the disease, complications due to extensive intestinal mucosal damage and sepsis may arise after a few days. Treatment includes a combination of aggressive supportive therapy with intravenous fluids and electrolytes, variable use of antimicrobials, non-steroidal and steroidal anti-inflammatory drugs, hyperimmune plasma, toxin adsorbents, and administration of oral or parenteral specific type C antitoxin.

In recent years, the use of probiotics, plant extracts, essential oils, organic acids, bacteriophages, lysozymes, and antimicrobial peptides to treat *C. perfringens*-associated enteric disease has been investigated. Through different mechanisms, these substances aim to promote the growth and activity of harmless bacteria, increase the general gut health, and/or inhibit the growth of *C. perfringens* strains in the intestinal tract. However, variable and inconsistent results among these studies make it difficult to evaluate their real therapeutic value at this stage.

Necrotic enteritis of poultry

Necrotic enteritis is a disease of chickens first described in the 1930s in a Black Orpington chicken. However, it was only in the 1960s that researchers began to associate the genus *Clostridium* with the disease. In these early case descriptions, bacterial isolates obtained from intestinal samples of chickens with necrotic enteritis were suspected to be *C. perfringens* type C or F. Because of this doubtful implication of *C. perfringens* type C in these early reports, this toxinotype is still found in some of the more current literature as an uncommon cause of necrotic enteritis in chickens. However, research performed on clinical and experimental cases of necrotic enteritis of poultry in the last few decades has overwhelmingly shown that *C. perfringens* type A is the main etiologic agent for the disease, whereas the potential role of type C and CPB remains unclear. Details about necrotic enteritis caused by type A are provided in Chapter 10.

Bibliography

Allaart, J.G., *et al.* (2013) Predisposing factors and prevention of *Clostridium perfringens*-associated enteritis. *Comp. Immunol. Microbiol. Infect. Dis.*, **36**: 449–464.

Asha, N.J., *et al.* (2006) Comparative analysis of prevalence, risk factors, and molecular epidemiology of antibiotic-associated diarrhea due to *Clostridium difficile, Clostridium perfringens*, and *Staphylococcus aureus. J. Clin. Microbiol.*, **44**: 2785–2791.

Brown, C.C., *et al.* (2007) Diseases associated with enteric clostridial infections. In: Maxie, M.G. (ed.) *Jubb, Kennedy, and Palmer's Pathology of Domestic Animals*, 5th edition, pp. 214–221. Elsevier, Philadelphia.

Cooper, K.K., *et al.* (2013) Diagnosing clostridial enteric disease in poultry. *J. Vet. Diagn. Invest.*, **25**: 314–327.

Council of Europe (2004) *Clostridium perfringens* vaccine for veterinary use. In: *European Pharmacopoeia 5.0*, 5th edition, pp. 747–749. European Directorate for the Quality of Medicines and Healthcare.

Diab, S.S., *et al.* (2012) Pathology of *Clostridium perfringens* type C enterotoxemia in horses. *Vet. Pathol.*, **49**: 255–263.

Garcia, J.P., *et al.* (2013) The pathology of enterotoxemia by *Clostridium perfringens* type C in calves. *J. Vet. Diagn. Invest.*, **25**: 438–442.

Gardiner, M.R. (1967) Clostridial infections in poultry in Western Australia. *Aust. Vet. J.*, **43**: 359–360.

MacKay, R.J. (2001) *Update on equine therapeutics: Equine neonatal clostridiosis: Treatment and Prevention*. Compendium (www.vetlearn.com) 23.

Miclard, J., *et al*. (2009) *Clostridium perfringens* beta-toxin targets endothelial cells in necrotizing enteritis in piglets. *Vet. Microbiol.*, **137**: 320–325.

Miclard, J., *et al*. (2009) *Clostridium perfringens* beta-toxin binding to vascular endothelial cells in a human case of enteritis necroticans. *J. Med. Microbiol.*, **58**: 826–828.

Nairn, M.E., *et al*. (1967) Necrotic enteritis of broiler chickens in western Australia. *Aust. Vet. J.*, **43**: 49–54.

Paul, G.E., *et al*. (2009) Diseases caused by *Clostridium perfringens* toxins. In: Smith, B.P. (ed.), *Large Animal Internal Medicine*, 4th edition, pp. 870–874. Mosby, St. Louis, MO.

Pugh, D.G. (2002) Causes of diarrhea in older lambs and kids. In: Pugh, D.G. (ed.) *Sheep and Goat Medicine*, p. 84. Saunders, Philadelphia.

Quinn, P.J., *et al*. (2011) Enteropathogenic and enterotoxaemia producing clostridia. In: Quinn, P.J. *et al*. (eds) *Veterinary Microbiology and Microbial Disease*, 2nd edition, pp. 242–246. Wiley-Blackwell, Ames, IA.

Sayeed, S., *et al*. (2008) CPB is essential for the intestinal virulence of *Clostridium perfringens* type C disease isolate CN3685 in a rabbit ileal loop model. *Mol. Microbiol.*, **67**: 15–30.

Shane, S.M., *et al*. (1985) Etiology and pathogenesis of necrotic enteritis. *Vet. Res. Commun.*, **9**: 269–287.

Songer, J.G. (2012) Clostridiosis. In: Zimmerman, J.J. *et al*. (eds) *Diseases of Swine*, 10th edition, pp. 709–720. Wiley-Blackwell, Oxford, UK.

Songer, J.G., *et al*. (2005) Clostridial enteric infections in pigs. *J. Vet. Diagn. Invest.*, **17**: 528–536.

Tennant, S.M., *et al*. (2008) Influence of gastric acid on susceptibility to infection with ingested bacterial pathogens. *Infect. Immun.*, **76**: 639–645.

Tillotson, K., *et al*. (2002) Population-based study of fecal shedding of *Clostridium perfringens* in broodmares and foals. *J. Am. Vet. Med. Assoc.*, **2203**: 342–348.

Timbermont, L., *et al*. (2011) Necrotic enteritis in broilers: An updated review on the pathogenesis. *Avian Pathol.*, **40**: 341–347.

Titball, R.W. (2009) *Clostridium perfringens* vaccines. *Vaccine*, **27**: 44–47.

Uzal, F.A., *et al*. (2008) Diagnosis of *Clostridium perfringens* intestinal infections in sheep and goats. *J. Vet. Diagn. Invest.*, **203**: 253–265.

Uzal, F.A., *et al*. (2011) Recent progress in understanding the pathogenesis of *Clostridium perfringens* type C infections. *Vet. Microbiol.*, **153**: 37–43.

Uzal, F.A., *et al*. (2012) Animal models to study the pathogenesis of enterotoxigenic *Clostridium perfringens* infections. *Microbes Infect.*, **14**: 1009–1016.

Van Metre, D.C., *et al*. (2008) Infectious diseases of the gastrointestinal tract. *Clostridium perfringens* – Enterotoxemia. In: Divers, T.J. and Peek, S. (eds) *Rebhun's Diseases of Dairy Cattle*, 2nd edition, pp. 225–228. Saunders Elsevier, St. Louis, MO.

13 Diseases Produced by *Clostridium perfringens* Type D

Francisco A. Uzal, Federico Giannitti, John W. Finnie, and Jorge P. García

Introduction

Enterotoxemia caused by *Clostridium perfringens* type D, sometimes also called "overeating disease" or "pulpy kidney disease," is one of the most prevalent clostridial diseases of sheep and goats worldwide. The disease occurs rarely in cattle, and a few poorly characterized cases have been described in other species. Because the so-called focal symmetrical encephalomalacia (FSE) is one of the lesions that may be seen in the sub-acute and chronic forms of type D enterotoxemia of sheep, this term was used in the past and it is still occasionally used to refer to these forms of the disease. However, it is not recommended as a name for type D enterotoxemia, since this term refers only to the pattern of brain damage in those forms of type D disease. The name "pulpy kidney disease" should also be abandoned, as it refers to a likely post-mortem change and not to a lesion of this disease.

Type D enterotoxemia in sheep is a pure enterotoxemia, with no bacterial invasion of tissues, whereas in goats it may be a pure enterotoxemia, a localized enteric disease, or a combination of both. Although *C. perfringens* is acquired by the oral route and reaches the intestine, disease development in infected animals is dependent upon predisposing factors including individual intestinal environmental conditions that determine local toxin production. Therefore, type D enterotoxemia is considered a non-contagious disease, although it can occur in outbreaks under some specific circumstances. Because the disease is almost always fatal, it can result in significant economic losses for the livestock industry, particularly in unvaccinated flocks.

Clostridial Diseases of Animals, First Edition. Francisco A. Uzal, J. Glenn Songer, John F. Prescott and Michel R. Popoff.
© 2016 John Wiley & Sons, Inc. Published 2016 by John Wiley & Sons, Inc.

Etiology

C. perfringens type D produces two typing toxins, namely alpha (CPA) and epsilon (ETX), although most type D isolates may express several other toxins. However, the use of reverse genetic experiments *in vitro* and *in vivo* has demonstrated that ETX is the main virulence factor responsible for most and probably all clinical signs and lesions of *C. perfringens* type D disease in sheep and goats. ETX is the third most potent clostridial toxin, after botulinum and tetanus toxins. Because of its potency and potential as a biological weapon, this toxin was, until 2012, considered a class B select agent by the United States Department of Agriculture and the Center for Disease Control. A detailed description of all *C. perfringens* toxins is provided in Chapter 5. Whether there is host adaptation of type D strains to sheep, goats, and possibly cattle has not been determined, but if this is the case, it might explain the differences in the somewhat different nature of the disease among these species.

Epidemiology and pathogenesis

Type D enterotoxemia occurs in most areas of sheep and goat production in the world. The disease affects lambs and goat kids older than 2 weeks in particular, but it can also affect adult sheep and goats. Infrequent, poorly documented cases may have occurred in lambs younger than 2 weeks.

The most common predisposing factor for type D enterotoxemia in sheep and goats is sudden feeding of large amounts of grain or concentrate to unaccustomed animals; hence the synonym "overeating disease." Under field conditions, grazing of abundant, lush pasture has also been associated with cases of type D enterotoxemia, mostly in sheep. However, the mechanism by which these nutritional factors induce the disease is incompletely understood. Although the majority of *C. perfringens* type D cells ingested are destroyed in the pre-stomachs and abomasum, the few organisms that reach the intestine proliferate and produce toxins when the intestinal environment is favorable.

Traditionally, it was accepted that for type D enterotoxemia to occur, undigested starch in the small intestine was required. Starch would thus provide a suitable substrate for saccharolytic *C. perfringens*, allowing it to multiply and reach numbers that may approximate 10^9 organisms per gram of intestinal contents, with subsequent production of large amounts of ETX. Although this may be a predisposing factor, it has recently been demonstrated *in vitro* that the absence of glucose in a culture medium stimulates ETX production by *C. perfringens* type D. If this also occurs *in vivo*, it could be postulated that, while the presence of starch in the intestine stimulates the growth of *C. perfringens* type D, the absence of glucose stimulates ETX production. When ruminants have sudden and novel access to large amounts of starch-rich food, the ruminal microbiota requires several days or weeks to adapt, permitting substantial quantities of undigested starch to reach the intestine and providing a rich substrate for the proliferation of *C. perfringens* type D. Concomitantly, failure to digest starch would also result in a lack of glucose in the small intestine, stimulating ETX production.

ETX is produced in the exponential phase of bacterial growth and secreted from the bacterial cytosol as a relatively inactive prototoxin, which becomes fully activated in the extracellular environment by the removal of N- and C- terminal peptides by the action of proteolytic digestive enzymes, including trypsin and chymotrypsin, although *C. perfringens* lambda toxin can also activate this prototoxin. In the intestine, activated ETX seems to increase mucosal permeability, thus facilitating its own absorption into the bloodstream. Once absorbed, this toxin is distributed to several internal organs, including the brain, lungs, liver, heart, and kidneys. In target organs, the toxin binds a yet-unidentified receptor on the luminal surface of vascular endothelial cells, which can be experimentally and transiently prevented, via competitive inhibition, by prior injection of epsilon prototoxin. ETX-induced microvascular endothelial damage leads to increased vascular permeability and resulting severe vasogenic edema. The generalized edema in the brain produces raised intracranial pressure and marked neurologic disturbance and, in the lungs and perhaps other organs, hypoxic injury. Following blood–brain barrier breakdown, some of the toxin enters the brain and may have a direct and damaging effect on neurons.

In goats, the pathogenesis of the acute and sub-acute disease is believed to be similar to that in sheep, although intestinal lesions can also occur in the sub-acute form. Chronic disease in this species is confined to the colon and less commonly the small intestine, and is believed to be caused by local effects of ETX and perhaps other *C. perfringens* type D toxins. The disease in cattle seems to have a similar pathogenesis to that in sheep. The common occurrence of the disease in young, unvaccinated ruminants is related, at least in part, to the decline in maternally derived ETX-neutralizing antibodies.

Clinical signs

Sheep
Type D enterotoxemia in lambs is generally acute, with animals dying after a short period of mainly neurologic and respiratory signs, including convulsions, tachypnea, and bawling. Some animals may survive longer and show tachypnea, ptyalism, hyperesthesia, a wide-based stance, head pressing, blindness, opisthotonos, and terminal convulsions or coma. Sudden death, characterized by animals being found dead without premonitory clinical signs, may also occur. Sub-acute or chronic cases are most commonly seen in older sheep or younger but vaccinated animals, probably due to the presence of some anti-ETX antibodies from vaccination that afford some level of protection or exposure to small amounts of toxin absorbed from the intestine. These forms of type D enterotoxemia are characterized by neurologic clinical signs, including blindness, ataxia, head pressing, and paraparesis. Diarrhea may occasionally be observed, but this

is not a common clinical sign in ovine type D enterotoxemia. While *C. perfringens* type D ETX is usually incriminated in disease, a type D strain producing unusually high amounts of CPA was isolated from a lamb with hemolytic disease resembling "yellow lamb disease", a form of enterotoxemia characterized by acute intravascular hemolysis, typically associated with CPA produced by *C. perfringens* type A (Chapter 8). Hyperglycemia, largely from rapid mobilization of hepatic glycogen, and marked glycosuria can be found in all forms of the disease, albeit inconsistently, and are useful diagnostically when present. However, these biochemical changes do not occur consistently, and a diagnosis of type D enterotoxemia is not precluded by the absence of hyperglycemia or glycosuria.

Goats

Both kids and adult goats may be affected. As in sheep, acute, sub-acute, and chronic forms are recognized. The acute form of the disease is similar to that seen in lambs, and usually manifests as sudden death or acute neurologic and/or respiratory signs. It occurs more frequently in young, unvaccinated animals. The sub-acute form, which usually affects older goats, is characterized by diarrhea, which may be hemorrhagic, and severe abdominal discomfort, with or without neurologic or respiratory signs. Affected animals usually die within 2–4 days of the onset of clinical signs, but some may recover. The chronic form of the disease may persist for a few days or weeks and tends to occur in adult animals which have been vaccinated; animals may die or recover. This form of the disease presents as profuse, watery, and/or hemorrhagic diarrhea frequently containing mucus, abdominal discomfort, weakness, anorexia, weight loss, and agalactia in milking does. Hyperglycemia and glycosuria can occasionally occur in goats with any of the forms of type D disease.

Gross changes

Sheep

In the acute form of type D enterotoxemia in lambs, carcasses are usually well nourished. There may be evidence of diarrhea, although this is an unusual finding in sheep. Mild congestion and hemorrhage may sometimes be observed on the small intestinal mucosa, the small and large intestinal content may be moderately fluid, and the small intestine may be multifocally distended with gas, but no other gross changes are seen in the gastrointestinal tract. Pulmonary edema, with wide interlobar and interlobular septae (Figure 13.1) and a large amount of stable froth in the trachea and lower airways (Figure 13.2), is regularly found. Hydropericardium (Figure 13.3), hydrothorax, and ascites, with or without strands of fibrin, are characteristic, but not consistent, post-mortem findings in sheep. Due to their high protein concentration, these fluids tend to clot when the respective cavities are opened (Figure 13.3). Other gross changes include sub-endocardial and sub-epicardial hemorrhages, which are particularly marked in the left ventricle, serosal hemorrhages, and hepatic and splenic congestion.

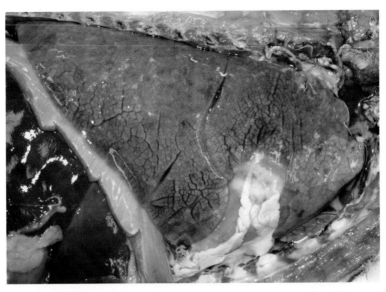

Figure 13.1 Pulmonary edema in a sheep with type D enterotoxemia. The interlobar and interlobular septae are diffusely expanded and filled by a clear fluid (edema). Reprinted with permission from Uzal *et al.* (2008) **20**: 253–265.

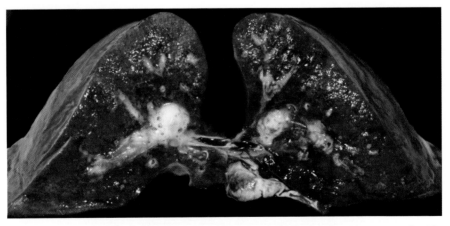

Figure 13.2 Pulmonary edema in a sheep with type D enterotoxemia. A large amount of stable froth is oozing mainly from the airways.

The so-called "pulpy kidney", characterized by softening of the renal parenchyma, is probably an accelerated autolytic process, but since it is not observed in freshly dead animals, it has scant diagnostic value.

Lambs and older sheep with sub-acute or chronic enterotoxemia may show gross brain lesions. These include herniation of the cerebellar vermis through the foramen magnum ("cerebellar coning") (Figure 13.4) and FSE (Figures 13.5 and 13.6). The former is highly suggestive of type D enterotoxemia, although it

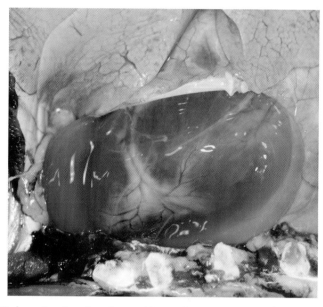

Figure 13.3 Hydropericardium in a sheep with type D enterotoxemia. There is abundant, clotted yellowish fluid in the pericardial sac.

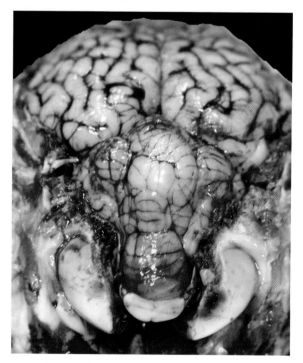

Figure 13.4 Herniation of the cerebellar vermis through the foramen magnum ("cerebellar coning") in a sheep with type D enterotoxemia. Courtesy of B. Barr.

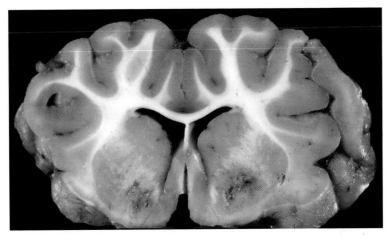

Figure 13.5 Focal symmetrical encephalomalacia in a sheep with type D enterotoxemia; both corpus striatum are affected. Courtesy of A. de Lahunta.

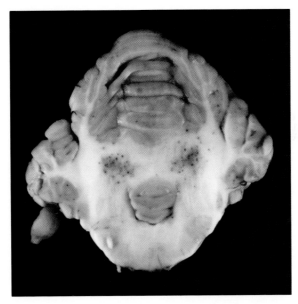

Figure 13.6 Focal symmetrical encephalomalacia affecting cerebellar peduncles of a sheep with type D enterotoxemia. Courtesy of J. Benavides and Moredun Research Institute.

can also occur as a consequence of other causes of increased intracranial pressure such as some encephalitides, and space-occupying hematomas and neoplasia, with their often substantial attendant edema. FSE is not frequently observed, but when present is considered pathognomonic of type D disease. Brain regions commonly damaged in FSE include the corpus striatum (Figure 13.5), the thalamus and cerebellar peduncles (Figure 13.6), with occasional lesions present in the substantia nigra, white matter of the frontal gyri, cerebral peduncles, and other regions. There seems to be a preference of ETX for the white matter of these areas. Gross lesions in acute type D enterotoxemia of adult sheep are similar to those in lambs.

Goats

Gross lesions in the acute form of type D enterotoxemia in goats are similar to those seen in sheep, but macroscopic brain lesions are rarely observed, with FSE only documented in one unconfirmed caprine case reported in the literature. In the sub-acute and chronic disease there is colitis, characterized by mild to severe mesocolonic edema, colonic distention, hyperemia (Figure 13.7), hemorrhage, and necrosis of the colonic mucosa, which may be covered by a fibrinous pseudomembrane (Figure 13.8). These lesions sometimes extend to the small intestine. The intestinal contents may contain mucus and/or fibrin and may be hemorrhagic. Hydropericardium, ascites, and pulmonary edema can be seen in the acute and sub-acute, but not chronic, forms of the disease in goats.

Other species

FSE has been described in one calf with experimental type D infection. Information on gross lesions produced by *C. perfringens* type D in other animal species is very scant.

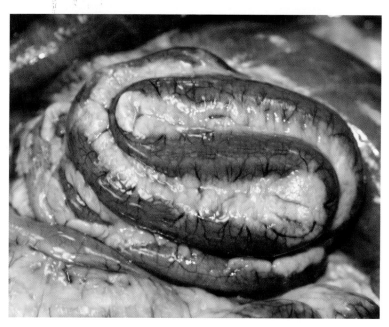

Figure 13.7 Colitis in a goat with type D enterotoxemia. The colonic serosa shows diffuse hyperemia, congestion, and edema.

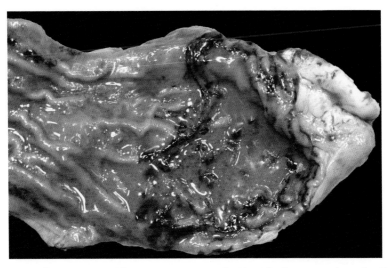

Figure 13.8 Colitis in a goat with type D enterotoxemia. The colonic mucosa shows focally extensive hemorrhage and an incipient pseudomembrane. Courtesy of L. Woods.

Microscopic changes

Sheep

The most consistent microscopic lesion of type D disease in sheep is perivascular proteinaceous edema, characterized by deposition of an albumin-rich fluid in the Virchow–Robins space around small- and medium-sized arterioles, venules, and capillaries (sometimes referred to as microangiopathy) in the brain (Figure 13.9). This leakage of plasma fluid and proteins following blood–brain barrier breakdown (vasogenic edema) is attended by upregulation of aquaporins-4 water channels in the astrocytic foot processes. Less frequently, protein hyaline droplets may also be seen around small vessels, sometimes being phagocytosed by macrophages. These lesions develop very soon after, or concurrently with, the onset of clinical signs. Since no other ovine disorder produces this lesion, it is regarded as diagnostic for type D enterotoxemia in this species, but although present in more than 90% of cases, it may occasionally be absent. Therefore, the absence of perivascular edema of the brain does not preclude a diagnosis of type D enterotoxemia in sheep.

In sub-acute and chronic cases, FSE may develop and is characterized by bilateral and approximately symmetrical foci of necrosis (malacia) in selectively vulnerable brain regions. These lesions are characterized by rarefaction of the neuropil with neuronal death, gliosis, myelin sheath swelling, swollen axons (spheroids), and the presence of vacuolated, lipid-laden macrophages (gitter cells) (Figures 13.10 and 13.11). These neuropathologic changes occur in a seemingly dose- and time-dependent manner.

Ultrastructurally, in the brain there is degeneration and necrosis of microvascular endothelium and astrocytic swelling. ETX-damaged endothelial cells

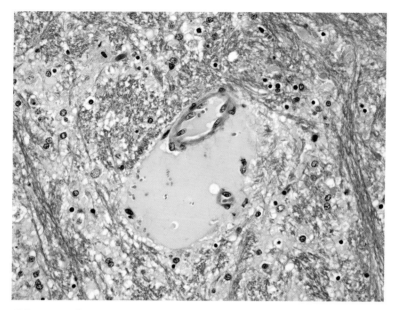

Figure 13.9 Perivascular proteinaceous edema (microangiopathy) in the brain of a sheep with type D enterotoxemia. Small arteries and capillaries are surrounded by abundant eosinophilic fluid in the Virchow–Robins space. HE, 200x.

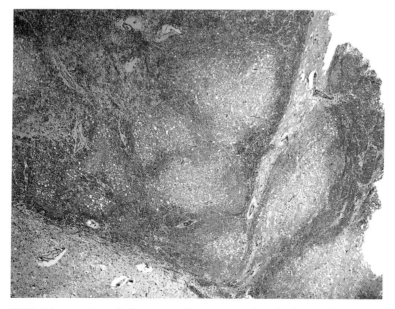

Figure 13.10 Sub-gross view of white matter (internal capsule) of a sheep with type D enterotoxemia showing multifocal necrosis, characterized by rarefaction of the neuropil. HE, 40x.

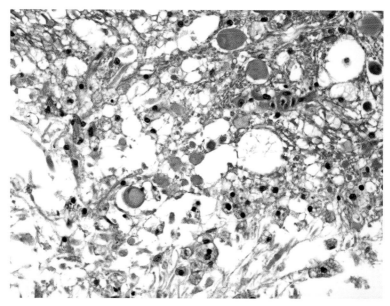

Figure 13.11 Higher magnification of Figure 13.10. The white matter shows severe dilation of myelin sheaths, neuronal death, gliosis, swollen axons (spheroids), and the presence of vacuolated macrophages (gitter cells). HE, 200x.

initially show swelling, luminal blebbing, loss of cytoplasmic organelles, and nuclear pyknosis; the cytoplasm eventually being reduced to an attenuated, electron-dense band (Figure 13.12). The astrocytic foot processes around blood vessels and the processes around neurons are most severely swollen and become detached from the adventitia of blood vessels by edema. In the neuropil surrounding microangiopathy, amyloid precursor protein (APP)-immunopositive damaged axons are found and, since this immunohistochemical technique is the most sensitive early marker of axonal injury, axons appear to be injured early in the disease process.

No significant microscopic lesions are typically found in the intestines of sheep with type D enterotoxemia. Because no histologic changes were observed in the kidneys of lambs experimentally inoculated with *C. perfringens* type D and necropsied immediately after death, it is assumed that changes previously described in the kidneys of sheep with enterotoxemia are a post-mortem phenomenon and should not be considered a diagnostic indicator of this disease.

Goats

In goats, perivascular edema similar to that described in sheep is very rarely observed in acute cases of type D enterotoxemia. In sub-acute and chronic cases, the predominant lesions are colonic and, less frequently, affect caudal segments of the small intestine. These lesions are characterized by suppurative and fibrino-necrotizing enteritis, colitis (Figure 13.13), or enterocolitis. FSE, presumably

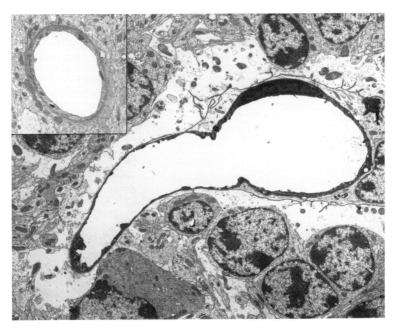

Figure 13.12 Transmission electron micrograph of the cerebellar granular layer of a sheep with type D enterotoxemia. The capillary endothelium exposed to ETX is markedly attenuated and electron dense, with nuclear pyknosis. Perivascular astrocytic foot processes are severely swollen. A normal capillary is shown in the inset. Uranyl acetate and lead citrate stain, 3750x.

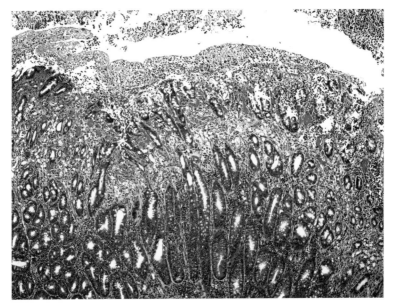

Figure 13.13 Colitis in a goat with type D enterotoxemia. The superficial colonic mucosa shows diffuse necrosis and suppurative effusion. HE, 100x.

attributed to type D enterotoxemia, has been described in only one report in a goat. The reasons for lesion differences between sheep and goats are unknown, but it is possible that enteric lesions are more severe in goats because the intestinal absorption of ETX into the bloodstream is slower in this species or because of possible but uninvestigated differences between sheep and goat strains. Although it was initially thought that serum antibodies provide only systemic but not local immune protection in the intestine, it has been demonstrated that circulating antibodies are effective in preventing the effects of ETX in the intestinal tract of goats.

Cattle

Documented cases of type D enterotoxemia in cattle are scant; the disease seems to occur very rarely in this species. Spontaneous disease with gross and microscopic brain lesions similar to those observed in sheep is occasionally seen; however, a direct causal relationship between these lesions and *C. perfringens* type D, or its ETX, has not been conclusively established in spontaneous cases. A disease with similar clinico-pathological features to ovine type D enterotoxemia has been experimentally produced in calves by intravenous administration of ETX, and was characterized by severe respiratory and neurologic signs that developed very rapidly after ETX exposure. Gross findings included severe pulmonary edema and hydropericardium, and microscopic changes were characterized by proteinaceous perivascular cerebral and pulmonary edema. A similar disease was also produced by intraduodenal inoculation of calves with *C. perfringens* type D; one of those animals developed lesions resembling FSE. Thus, while these studies confirmed that cattle are susceptible to *C. perfringens* type D infection and its ETX, the naturally occurring disease in this species seems to occur, albeit rarely.

Other species

Information on microscopic lesions in natural cases of *C. perfringens* type D in other animal species is very scant.

Diagnosis

Sheep

In sheep, a presumptive clinical diagnosis can be based on a history of access to heavy grain or concentrate feeding or abundant lush pasture, and clinical signs, especially in unvaccinated thriving lambs. Hyperglycemia and glycosuria, while neither pathognomonic nor consistent, can be diagnostically useful when present. Pulmonary edema, hydropericardium, and ascites, particularly if they are protein-rich, are suggestive but not specific of type D disease. Cerebellar vermis herniation at necropsy is highly suggestive of type D enterotoxemia. In recently dead animals, large numbers of Gram-positive rods can be found in smears of intestinal mucosa and this may support, but not confirm, a diagnosis of enterotoxemia. Isolation of *C. perfringens* type D from small or large intestinal content supports the diagnosis but it is also not confirmatory, since this microorganism can be found in a relatively small percentage of clinically normal animals. FSE, when present, is confirmatory, as is the histologic evidence of microvascular damage (microangiopathy) in selectively vulnerable brain regions, with perivascular deposition of a protein-rich edema fluid. Demonstration of ETX in intestinal content in animals with typical lesions is confirmatory. ETX is rarely found in bodily fluids other than intestinal content; the sample of choice for ETX diagnosis is the content of the small intestine, where this toxin is most frequently found in animals with type D enterotoxemia.

Goats

In goats, similar diagnostic criteria apply to acutely and sub-acutely affected animals, although perivascular edema in the brain is much less commonly found. In sub-acute and chronic cases, there is necrotizing colitis and, less frequently, enteritis. Cerebellar vermis herniation and FSE are more rarely found than in sheep, with FSE only documented in one unconfirmed case.

Cattle and other species

Diagnostic criteria have not been established in animal species other than sheep and goats, but they are probably similar to those reported for sheep.

Prophylaxis and treatment

Immunity in sheep is readily produced by vaccination, most vaccines being alum-adsorbed ETX toxoid. Two doses of vaccine, administered 4–6 weeks apart, are required to afford protective, approximately 1-year-duration, immunity in sheep. Lambs of vaccinated ewes and does should be first immunized at 4–6 weeks of age. An annual booster is recommended in this species.

For yet-unknown reasons, ETX toxoid antibody titers following immunization are lower and of shorter duration in goats, which therefore require, after the initial two-dose-vaccination, a booster every 3–4 months.

In order to afford colostral immunity to young lambs and goat kids, it is recommended that the annual booster in sheep and one of the boosters in goats be given to pregnant animals 2 to 4 weeks before parturition.

Although vaccination has substantially reduced its prevalence, the disease still occurs commonly. ETX antitoxin has been used experimentally to treat sheep and goats with type D enterotoxemia; however, there is no specific treatment currently available for this disease in livestock under field conditions. Nutritional management to avoid animals being exposed suddenly to large amounts of starch-rich feed is helpful in preventing cases of type D enterotoxemia in sheep and goats. No information is available about the prevention of the disease in cattle or other animal species.

Bibliography

Blackwell, T.E., *et al.* (1992) Clinical signs, treatment, and postmortem lesions in dairy goats with enterotoxemia: 13 cases (1979–1982). *J. Am. Vet. Med. Assoc.,* **200**: 214–217.

Buxton, D., *et al.* (1978) Pulpy kidney disease and its diagnosis by histological examination. *Vet. Rec.,* **102**: 241.

Dorca-Arévalo, J., *et al.* (2008) Binding of epsilon-toxin from *Clostridium perfringens* in the nervous system. *Vet. Microbiol.,* **131**: 14–25.

Fernández Miyakawa, M.E., *et al.* (2003) The early effects of *Clostridium perfringens* type D ETX in ligated intestinal loops of goats and sheep. *Vet. Res. Commun.,* **27**: 231–241.

Filho, E.J., *et al.* (2009) Clinicopathologic features of experimental *Clostridium perfringens* type D enterotoxemia in cattle. *Vet. Pathol.,* **46**: 1213–1220.

Finnie, J.W. (2003) Pathogenesis of brain damage produced in sheep by *Clostridium perfringens* type D ETX: A review. *Aust. Vet. J.,* **81**: 219–221.

García, J.P., *et al.* (2013) ETX is essential for the virulence of *Clostridium perfringens* type D infection in sheep, goats, and mice. *Infect. Immun.,* **81**: 2405–2414.

García, J.P., *et al.* (2015) Comparative neuropathology of ovine enterotoxemia produced by *Clostridium perfringens* type D wild-type strain CN1020 and its genetically modified derivatives. *Vet. Pathol.,* **52**: 465–475.

Giannitti, F., *et al.* (2014) Diagnostic exercise: Hemolysis and sudden death in lambs. *Vet. Pathol.,* **51**: 624–627.

Hughes, M.R., *et al.* (2007) Epsilon-toxin plasmids of *Clostridium perfringens* type D are conjugative. *J. Bacteriol.,* **189**: 7531–7538.

Knapp, O., *et al.* (2010) The aerolysin-like toxin family of cytolytic, pore-forming toxins. *Open Toxinol. J.,* **3**: 53–68.

Mantis, N.J. (2005) Vaccines against category B toxins. Staphylococcal, enterotoxin B, ETX and ricin. *Adv. Drug Deliv. Rev.,* **57**: 1424–1439.

Mete, A., *et al.* (2013) Brain lesions associated with *Clostridium perfringens* type D ETX in a Holstein heifer calf. *Vet. Pathol.,* **50**: 765–768.

Minami, J., *et al.* (1997) Lambda-toxin of *Clostridium perfringens* activates the precursor of epsilon-toxin by releasing its N- and C-terminal peptides. *Microbiol. Immunol.,* **41**: 527–535.

Miserez, R., *et al.* (1998) Detection of CPA- and epsilon-toxigenic *Clostridium perfringens* type D in sheep and goats using a DNA amplification technique (PCR). *Lett. Appl. Microbiol.,* **26**: 382–386.

Oliveira, D.M., *et al.* (2010) Focal symmetrical encephalomalacia in a goat. *J. Vet. Diagn. Invest.,* **22**: 793–796.

Petit, L., *et al.* (2001) *Clostridium perfringens* ETX induces a rapid change of cell membrane permeability to ions and forms channels in artificial lipid bilayers. *J. Biol. Chem.,* **276**: 15736–15740.

Soler-Jover, A., *et al.* (2004) Effect of ETX-GFP on MDCK cells and renal tubules in vivo. *J. Histochem. Cytochem.,* **52**: 931–942.

Songer, J.G. (1996) Clostridial enteric diseases of domestic animals. *Clin. Microbiol. Rev.,* **9**: 216–234.

Stiles, B.G., *et al.* (2013) *Clostridium perfringens* ETX: A malevolent molecule for animals and man? *Toxins,* **5**: 2138–2160.

Stubbings, D.P. (1990) *Clostridium perfringens* enterotoxaemia in two young horses. *Vet. Rec.,* **127**: 431.

Uzal, F.A., *et al.* (1996) Enterotoxaemia in goats. *Vet. Res. Commun.,* **20**: 481–492.

Uzal, F.A., *et al.* (1998) Experimental *Clostridium perfringens* type D enterotoxemia in goats. *Vet. Pathol.,* **35**: 132–140.

Uzal, F.A., *et al.* (2002) Effects of intravenous injection of *Clostridium perfringens* type D ETX in calves. *J. Comp. Pathol.,* **126**: 71–75.

Uzal, F.A., *et al.* (2004) Diagnosis of *Clostridium perfringens* intestinal infections in sheep and goats. *Anaerobe,* **10**: 135–143.

Uzal, F.A., *et al.* (2004) The pathology of peracute experimental *Clostridium perfringens* type D enterotoxemia in sheep. *J. Vet. Diagn. Invest.,* **16**: 403–411.

Uzal, F.A., *et al.* (2008) Ulcerative enterocolitis in two goats associated with enterotoxin- and beta2 toxin-positive *Clostridium perfringens* type D. *J. Vet. Diagn. Invest.,* **20**: 668–672.

Uzal, F.A., *et al.* (2008) Diagnosis of *Clostridium perfringens* intestinal infections in sheep and goats. *J. Vet. Diagn. Invest.,* **20**: 253–265.

Infections by *Clostridium perfringens* Type E

J. Glenn Songer

Introduction

Until the recent advent of PCR genotyping, *Clostridium perfringens* type E was relatively uncommonly reported as a cause of disease, with the first reports of enteric infection of domestic animals occurring in the late 1940s. However, in the past few years, an increasing number of cases of type E-associated disease have been reported in several domestic and wild animal species. Most of these reports were based, however, on isolation of *C. perfringens* type E from feces or intestinal content of animals with enteric disease, and the role of this microorganism in disease production remains mostly undetermined. Koch postulates have not been fulfilled for *C. perfringens* type E.

Etiology

Type E is probably the least commonly reported genotype of *C. perfringens*, but in specific conditions, it may be quite common. *C. perfringens* type E isolates are defined by their production of alpha (CPA) and iota (ITX) toxins. The role of ITX in disease of animals is poorly understood, although it is usually assumed that the pathogenesis of intestinal diseases produced by *C. perfringens* type E is mediated by ITX toxin. This toxin has been described in detail in Chapter 5. Briefly, ITX toxin is a guinea pig-dermonecrotic, mouse-lethal toxin which cross-reacts with the ITX-like toxin of *Clostridium spiroforme*. Antibodies against *C. spiroforme* or *C. perfringens* type E neutralize toxins from both species.

    C. perfringens genotype E isolates associated with hemorrhagic enteritis of neonatal calves produce CPA and ITX and, very frequently, carry sequences for the *cpe* gene, encoding *C. perfringens* enterotoxin (CPE), although they are usually

Clostridial Diseases of Animals, First Edition. Francisco A. Uzal, J. Glenn Songer,
John F. Prescott and Michel R. Popoff.
© 2016 John Wiley & Sons, Inc. Published 2016 by John Wiley & Sons, Inc.

unable to produce this toxin. These silent *cpe* sequences are highly conserved among type E isolates. In most cases, these silent sequences contain multiple nonsense and frameshift mutations and lack the initiation codon, promoters, and ribosome-binding site.

Pathogenesis

Little is known about the pathogenesis of type E infections. *In vitro* and *in vivo* models suggest that genotype E is well adapted to take advantage of changes caused by ITX on epithelial cell surfaces. In addition, type E produces metabolites that affect the growth of potential competitors. Enterocyte morphologic changes induced by ITX, associated with the specific increase of type E cell adhesion and the strong intra-specific growth inhibition of other strains, could be competitive traits that improve the fitness of type E isolates in the bovine gut. Further research is required to develop a clearer understanding of the interaction of ITX toxin with host tissues, as well as methods for prevention of these negative consequences.

Animal disease

The role of *C. perfringens* type E in animal disease is poorly understood, although this toxinotype has been associated with enteric disease in several animal species. Very little information is, therefore, currently available about clinical diseases produced by *C. perfringens* type E.

Historically, enterotoxemia of rabbits has been associated with *C. perfringens* type E. However, it is currently thought that most, if not all, of those cases are caused by *C. spiroforme*, with its similar toxin. The confusion in the diagnosis of infection by these two microorganisms probably originated when diagnoses of type E disease were established based on detection of what, at the time, was thought to be ITX in the intestine of affected animals. Since there is almost 100% cross-reactivity between ITX of *C. perfringens* type E and the toxin of *C. spiroforme*, it is likely that, on many occasions, infections by the latter were diagnosed as type E infections.

In a study of 27 rabbits with spontaneous diarrhea, all had a toxin in cecal contents that was neutralized by anti-ITX toxin antibodies. However, another four rabbits with clindamycin-associated colitis were positive for *C. spiroforme* by culture, and in all cases, the toxin in the intestinal content was neutralized by anti-ITX toxin antibodies.

In a study of calves up to 28 days of age, *C. perfringens* type E was found in the feces of 36.2% and 30.2% diarrheic and healthy animals, respectively. However, another study found that, at 50% of the total, type E was by far the most common genotype in diarrheic calves up to the age of about 2 months, with diarrhea, abomasitis, hemorrhagic enteritis, and sudden death, suggesting that type E may play a significant role as a pathogen of neonatal calves. In both cases, anaerobic cultures of abomasum yielded heavy growth of *C. perfringens* genotype E.

Type E disease has been reported in ostrich chick populations showing a high mortality rate associated with enteritis. In one study, about 10% of *C. perfringens* isolates were type E; isolates were often *netB* positive, whereas only about 10% of type A isolates recovered from the chicks had this gene.

C. perfringens type E has been detected in the intestine of normal reindeer, blackbuck, and collared peccary. Feces of Père David's deer in China yielded *C. perfringens* from 41 out of 155 samples. Fifteen isolates were type E, seven of which were *cpe* positive.

The sudden death of a neonatal goat was likely caused by type E; the only gross lesion was a thin intestinal wall, but microscopically large numbers of Gram-positive bacilli covered the epithelium of the small intestine. Lack of other pathogens in the face of heavy growth of type E suggests the latter as a pathogen in this case.

Type E is also thought to be an infrequent cause of enterotoxemia of lambs. However, descriptions of clinical disease, gross and microscopic lesions, and bacteriologic findings in sheep and goats are scant.

Diagnosis

There are currently no universally accepted diagnostic criteria for type E infections. While detection of ITX in the intestinal content and/or other bodily fluids was considered by several authors to be the gold standard for type E disease diagnosis, the cross-reaction with the toxin of *C. spiroforme* plus the lack of commercially available tests for the detection of these toxins, make this criterion of little practical use. Isolation of *C. perfringens* type E from the intestines of affected animals, while suggestive, is debatable as a diagnostic criterion because this microorganism can also be found in the intestines of some normal animals. Clinical and pathological findings are not specific to type E infection.

Bibliography

Billington, S.J., *et al.* (1998) *Clostridium perfringens* type E animal enteritis isolates with highly conserved, silent enterotoxin gene sequences. *Infect. Immun.*, **66**: 4531–4536.

Borriello, S.P., *et al.* (1983) Association of ITX-like toxin and *Clostridium spiroforme* with both spontaneous and antibiotic-associated diarrhea and colitis in rabbits. *J. Clin. Microbiol.*, **17**: 414–418.

Ermakova, M.P., *et al.* (1975) Morphologic changes in cultures of different tissues exposed to the toxins of *C. perfringens* types B, C, E and F. *Zh. Mikrobiol. Epidemiol. Immunobiol.*, **11**: 41–45.

Ferrarezi, M.C., *et al.* (2008) Genotyping of *Clostridium perfringens* isolated from calves with neonatal diarrhea. *Anaerobe*, **14**: 328–331.

Keokilwe, L., *et al.* (2015) Bacterial enteritis in ostrich chicks in the Western Cape Province, South Africa. *Poult. Sci.*, **94**: 1177–1183.

Kim, H.Y., *et al.* (2013) First isolation of *Clostridium perfringens* type E from a goat with diarrhea. *Anaerobe*, **22**: 141–143.

La Mont, J.T., *et al.* (1979) Role of clostridial toxin in the pathogenesis of clindamycin colitis in rabbits. *Gastroenterol.*, **76**: 356–361.

Miyamoto, K., *et al.* (2011) Identification of novel *Clostridium perfringens* type E strains that carry an ITX toxin plasmid with a functional enterotoxin gene. *PLoS One*, **6**: e20376.

Qiu, H., *et al.* (2014) Toxinotyping of *Clostridium perfringens* fecal isolates of reintroduced Père David's deer (*Elaphurus davidianus*) in China. *J. Wildl. Dis.*, **50**: 942–945.

Redondo, L.M., *et al.* (2013) Sudden death syndrome in adult cows associated with *Clostridium perfringens* type E. *Anaerobe*, **20**: 1–4.

Songer, J.G., *et al.* (1996) Clostridial enteric diseases of domestic animals. *Clin. Microbiol. Rev.*, **9**: 216–234.

Songer, J.G. (1998) Clostridial diseases of small ruminants. *Vet. Res.*, **29**: 219–232.

Songer, J.G., *et al.* (2004) *Clostridium perfringens* type E enteritis in calves: Two cases and a brief review of the literature. *Anaerobe*, **10**: 239–242.

Stiles, B.G., *et al.* (1986) *Clostridium perfringens* ITX toxin: Synergism between two proteins. *Toxicon*, **24**: 767–773.

Stiles, B.G., *et al.* (1986) Purification and characterization of *Clostridium perfringens* ITX toxin: Dependence on two nonlinked proteins for biological activity. *Infect. Immun.*, **54**: 683–688.

Uzal, F.A., *et al.* (2008) Diagnosis of *Clostridium perfringens* intestinal infections in sheep and goats. *J. Vet. Diagn. Invest.*, **20**: 253–265.

Uzal, F.A., *et al.* (2010) *Clostridium perfringens* toxins involved in mammalian veterinary diseases. *Open Toxinol. J.*, **2**: 24–42.

Wilkins, T., *et al.* (1985) Clostridial toxins active locally in the gastrointestinal tract. *Ciba Found. Symp.*, **112**: 230–241.

Diseases Produced by *Clostridium difficile*

Santiago S. Diab, Francisco A. Uzal, and J. Glenn Songer

Introduction

Clostridium difficile-associated disease (CDAD) affects numerous species, especially humans and animals with expanded large bowels (gerbils, guinea pigs, hamsters, horses, rabbits, swine, and others). *C. difficile* has been isolated from the gastrointestinal tract of a wide variety of other animal species in which it is not associated with disease, its role in disease is not known, or only single case reports have been published. These include bears, camels, cats, cattle, dogs, donkeys, ducks, elephants, geese, goats, sheep, non-human primates, ostriches, poultry, pet birds, and even reptiles.

In domesticated animals, CDAD is typically referred to as necrotizing enterotyphlocolitis and, with a few exceptions (notably pigs), is antibiotic-associated. In humans, the nature of the typical lesion gives rise to the common name of pseudomembranous colitis.

Etiology

C. difficile is a Gram-positive strict anaerobic rod, and its long-term survival, transmission, and, to an extent, the pathogenesis of its infections are mediated by the production of highly resistant spores, which are ubiquitous in the environment. *C. difficile* is well known for its widespread contamination of human and animal hospitals and other medical facilities, but can be found in surprisingly large numbers in any environment subject to fecal contamination. It is common in the large intestine and feces of domestic animals (particularly herbivores and swine) and, in consequence, can also be found in large numbers in

Clostridial Diseases of Animals, First Edition. Francisco A. Uzal, J. Glenn Songer,
John F. Prescott and Michel R. Popoff.
© 2016 John Wiley & Sons, Inc. Published 2016 by John Wiley & Sons, Inc.

manured soil. It is also common in meats and in vegetables that have been subjected to fecal contamination.

C. difficile is in cluster XIa ("Peptostreptococcaceae") (Chapter 1) and it appears morphologically as rods ~ 1.2 µm x 8 µm in size, occurring at times in short chains. Colonies are chartreuse under long-wave UV illumination. Solid media containing cefoxitin, cycloserine and fructose, often with taurocholate to initiate spore germination, are effective for isolation from feces and other contaminated environments. Spores are oval and subterminal. The vegetative forms of *C. difficile* do not survive for long periods of time in an aerobic environment; however, vegetative cells sporulate readily and the spores are highly resistant in air. The spores of *C. difficile* are resistant to most common disinfectants, making this microorganism a sturdy environmental contaminant.

The pathogenesis of *C. difficile* infections is mediated by toxins A (TcdA) and B (TcdB), both members of the family of large clostridial toxins (LCTs); a role for a separate, ADP-ribosylating toxin (CDTa) also seems likely (Chapter 6). The genes for these toxins (*tcdA, tcdB,* and *cdtA*) are located chromosomally.

General epidemiology and pathogenesis of *Clostridium difficile* infection

The epidemiology of *C. difficile* varies among animal species. Abundant ongoing research on humans, animals, and the human–animal interface, including the environment and food supply, will likely significantly expand the current knowledge on this subject. The most comprehensive epidemiological studies have been done on the human population, where the field continues to evolve as the incidence of *C. difficile* infection (CDI) continues to grow. CDI has become the most common cause of human healthcare-associated infection in Europe, Canada, and the United States, exceeding even methicillin-resistant *Staphylococcus aureus* infections.

In humans and pigs, but not in horses, the disease is age-dependent, affecting humans outside the neonatal period but contrarily piglets within the neonatal period, up to approximately 1 week of age. With the notable exception of piglets and neonatal foals, in most animals antibiotic administration is an important and critical risk factor. Hospitalization, a major risk factor for the human infection, is also important in horses. Hamsters and guinea pigs are often used as models for *C. difficile* infection in humans, since they readily develop *C. difficile* infection after colonization with spores and administration of antimicrobials. However, as in neonatal foals and piglets, disease may develop without prior antibiotic therapy.

Direct transmission of *C. difficile* from animals and food to people has not been clearly documented, but there is increasing evidence that this occurs. Some *C. difficile* ribotypes that are virulent for humans, including the emerging ribotype 078, have been found in the intestinal tract of multiple food animals and in or on retail food (including beef, pork, poultry, fish, and vegetables) in the USA,

Canada, and Europe. Colonization of the hamster intestinal tract by consumption of spore-contaminated food has been demonstrated experimentally, and exposure of humans through consumption of contaminated food may be more common than previously recognized. Thus, transmission may occur through direct contact with animals, from the environment, or by consumption of contaminated foods of animal or vegetable origin.

   C. difficile infection may be exogenous or endogenous. The exogenous route of infection is by far the most common and requires ingestion of *C. difficile* spores from a contaminated environment or from other animals. The fecal–oral route is the main source of exogenous infection, but *C. difficile* has also been found in air samples, air vents, and high horizontal surfaces from human hospitals and air samples from pig farms, suggesting that airborne transmission may also be possible. After ingestion, *C. difficile* spores resist the acidity of the stomach and germinate to the vegetative form in the small intestine and may subsequently colonize the large intestine. The endogenous form is less common and requires proliferation of endogenous *C. difficile* toxigenic strains carried in the intestinal tract of healthy animals, usually following destruction of the large bowel microflora by antibiotics that target anaerobic bacteria, resulting in bacterial multiplication, toxin production, and damage to the intestinal mucosa. This distinction between exogenous and endogenous infections is, however, somewhat artificial, as *C. difficile* is considered a ubiquitous opportunist that may be present in the environment and also in the intestinal tract of healthy animals. Differences in virulence between strains of *C. difficile* are well recognized (Chapter 6).

Animal diseases produced by *Clostridium difficile*

Enterocolitis of horses
Epidemiology
C. difficile infection in horses is not age-dependent and the disease may develop in foals as young as 2 days of age, as well as in older foals and adults. The exogenous fecal–oral route is the main form of transmission, although the endogenous form of infection is also possible. Potential sources of *C. difficile* spores include, but are not limited to, feces of foals and adult horses with and without diarrhea, soil from stud farms, small and large animal hospitals, and the stalls, floors, medical equipment, and footwear of medical personnel in large animal clinics. It is common for human medical personnel to carry the organism on their hands and, although this has not been demonstrated in veterinary medical personnel, it is safe to assume that they may also do so.

   The two main risk factors for the development of CDAD in horses are antibiotic therapy with broad-spectrum antibiotics and hospitalization. Although all antibiotics appear to be capable of predisposing to CDAD in horses, erythromycin, trimethoprim/sulfonamides, third-generation cephalosporins, clindamycin and gentamicin in combination with β-lactams, are most often associated with the disease. In neonatal foals, and occasionally in older foals and adult horses, the disease may occur without prior antibiotic administration or hospitalization. Interestingly, a single study shows that only 26% of horses with *C. difficile*-associated disease had a history of antibiotic therapy prior to the onset of diarrhea, suggesting that antibiotic therapy may not be a significant factor in certain geographic regions or environments.

In hospitalized horses, a potentially increased exposure to toxigenic *C. difficile* spores from a contaminated facility or contaminated medical instruments, the change to a hospital diet, pre- and post-surgical feed withdrawal, and antibiotic administration during hospitalization may all, alone or in combination, contribute to CDAD. Other, less clearly established risk factors, including stress, dietary changes, starvation, co-infections with other bacteria or parasites, colon impactions or torsions, transportation, surgical or medical treatment, and nasogastric intubation, have been proposed, but on the basis of anecdotal evidence rather than case-controlled reports.

The prevalence of *C. difficile* in the feces of healthy foals ranges between 0 and 3% in most studies. However, one research group found a 29% prevalence in healthy foals less than 14 days of age and a 44% prevalence in foals without diarrhea treated with antibiotics, suggesting that foals may be an important source of infection. The prevalence of *C. difficile* infection in the feces of healthy adult horses is also considered low, ranging from 0 to 10%. However, the cumulative prevalence obtained in a 1-year longitudinal study in healthy adult horses was higher, since 40% of the horses were *C. difficile* culture-positive at least once throughout the year. This suggests both that *C. difficile* shedding from healthy horses is transient and dynamic and that exposure to *C. difficile* may be more common than thought based on data obtained from horizontal prevalence studies. The reported prevalence of *C. difficile* in foals and adult horses with diarrhea and enterocolitis has varied greatly between authors, ranging from 5% to 63%, likely reflecting not only geographic and other differences, but also variations in diagnostic approaches.

Clinical signs

The clinical signs and severity of CDAD in horses are very variable. Diarrhea is the main clinical manifestation and may be accompanied by colic, abdominal distension, hyperemic mucous membranes, fever, prolonged capillary refill time, tachycardia, tachypnea, and dehydration. Adult horses with CDAD may have abdominal discomfort or fever without diarrhea and sometimes small intestinal ileus and gas distention may be the primary complaint. Neonatal foals may develop enterocolitis with mild abdominal discomfort and colic with pasty feces or watery diarrhea, but death may occur without prior clinical signs or after a short period of depression, watery or hemorrhagic diarrhea, and toxemia.

The clinical signs of CDAD are not specific, since other infectious enteropathogens such as *Salmonella* spp. or *Neorickettsia risticii* (equine ehrlichial colitis) may mimic CDAD. Type C or *netF*-associated type A *C. perfringens*-associated enterocolitis in foals may mimic CDAD, although both infections are more common in foals than in adult horses. The syndrome of duodenitis-proximal jejunitis of horses that is clinically characterized by abundant enterogastric reflux has been suggested to be associated with *C. difficile* infection. Although this association appears likely, definitive proof of causality is lacking.

Gross changes

The lesions in the intestinal tract of foals and adult horses with CDAD are characteristic but not specific for this condition. Other known causes of enterocolitis, such as *C. perfringens* type C, *Salmonella* spp., *Neorickettsia risticii*, non-steroidal anti-inflammatory drugs, or even colitis of undetermined origin (formerly known as "Colitis X") may cause similar or identical lesions. In naturally acquired CDAD, the distribution of the lesions in the intestinal tract is largely age-dependent, but occasional cases may present with a different distribution. Typically, foals under 1 month of age show lesions in the small intestine, whereas the colon and cecum may or may not be involved. In older foals and adult horses, the lesions are typically present in the colon and cecum, whereas the small intestine is usually spared. The serosal surface of affected small or large intestine may be normal or show grayish, bluish, or reddish discoloration as a consequence of severe mucosal and submucosal congestion or hemorrhage (Figure 15.1). The large intestine is often dilated by gas or fluid contents. In severe cases, the damage may extend through the intestinal wall, with multifocal patches of hemorrhage on the serosa. In foals, the intestinal content is often composed of

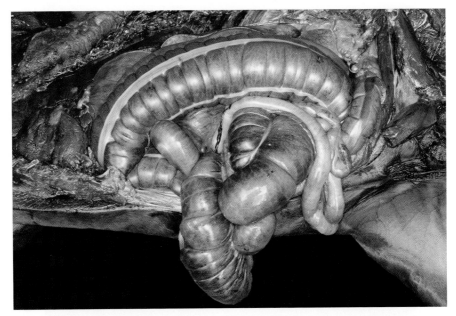

Figure 15.1 *Clostridium difficile*-associated disease; adult horse. The large colon and cecum show diffuse gray to bluish discoloration of the serosal surface due to mucosal and submucosal congestion and/or hemorrhage. Reproduced with permission from Diab *et al.* (2013) *Vet. Pathol.*, **50**: 1028–1036.

hemorrhagic fluid (Figure 15.2). In older horses, the large intestinal content may be similar to that in foals but also may consist of abundant green fluid or a mix of green fluid and roughage (Figure 15.3). The intestinal wall, especially in the large intestine, is frequently moderately to markedly thickened by clear, gelatinous edema (Figure 15.4). The mucosa of both the small and large intestines

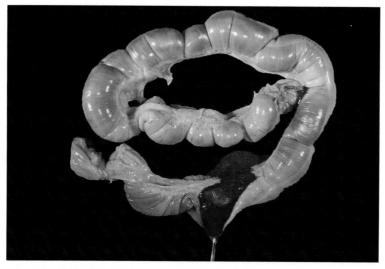

Figure 15.2 *Clostridium difficile*-associated disease; foal. Abundant red (hemorrhagic) fluid in the small colon. Reproduced with permission from Diab *et al.* (2013) *Vet. Pathol.*, **50**: 1028–1036.

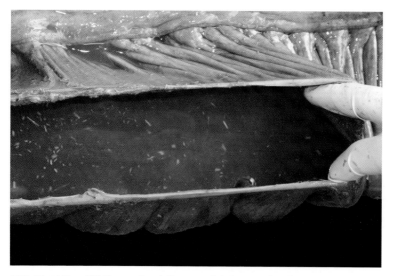

Figure 15.3 *Clostridium difficile*-associated disease; adult horse. Abundant green fluid in the colon. Reproduced with permission from Diab *et al.* (2013) *Vet. Microbiol.*, **167**: 42–49.

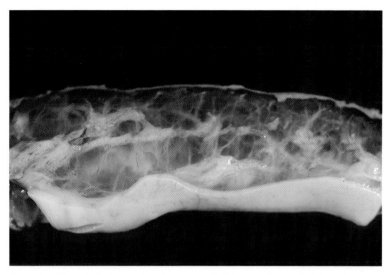

Figure 15.4 *Clostridium difficile*-associated disease; adult horse. The wall of the colon shows marked thickening by clear, gelatinous, submucosal edema. Reproduced with permission from Diab *et al.* (2013) *Vet. Pathol.*, **50**: 1028–1036.

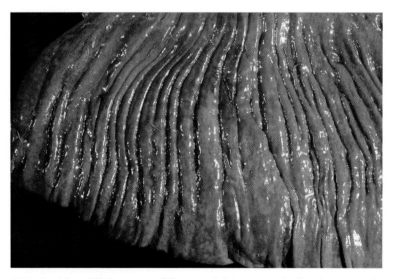

Figure 15.5 *Clostridium difficile*-associated disease; adult horse. Markedly edematous colon with dull, opaque, brownish to greenish discoloration of the mucosa. Reproduced with permission from Diab *et al.* (2013) *Vet. Microbiol.*, **167**: 42–49.

may appear dull, opaque, brownish or greenish (Figure 15.5) or, if hemorrhagic, diffusely bright or dark red. There is frequently multifocal or regional mucosal erosion or ulceration and the mucosa can be multifocally covered by a tan, yellow, or greenish pseudomembrane composed of cellular and inflammatory debris admixed with intestinal contents (Figure 15.6).

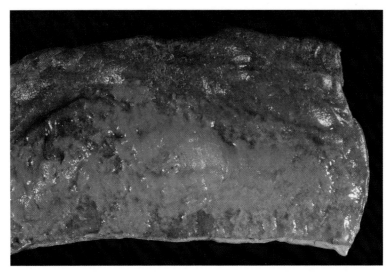

Figure 15.6 *Clostridium difficile*-associated disease; foal. Affected segment of small intestine shows multifocal to coalescing mucosal ulcers and a tan to light orange pseudomembrane. Reproduced with permission from Diab *et al.* (2013) *Vet. Microbiol.*, **167**: 42–49.

Extra intestinal lesions are usually the result of toxemia or septicemia. Typically, multifocal petechiae and ecchymoses of variable severity may be present in the intestinal serosa, mesentery, pericardium, endocardium, thoracic and visceral pleura, or diaphragm. A small amount of serous or hemorrhagic fluid, sometimes containing a few fibrin strands, may be present in the abdominal and thoracic cavities and within the pericardial sac. Pulmonary edema and hemorrhage as results of toxemia and septicemia are frequent; capillary thrombosis compatible with disseminated intravascular coagulation may be seen in the lung or other visceral organs.

Microscopic changes

The characteristic histological lesion of CDI infection in horses is severe, necrotizing, sometimes hemorrhagic, enteritis, colitis, and/or typhlitis with mucosal or submucosal thrombosis, very similar to the lesions of *C. perfringens* type C enterotoxemia (Figure 15.7). There is necrosis of the epithelial lining that usually begins in the more superficial mucosa and rapidly progresses to the deeper portions. The submucosa is often hyperemic and expanded by a combination of edema, hemorrhage, emphysema, and inflammatory cell infiltration, although inflammation is seldom a dominant feature in horses. A mild to moderate number of neutrophils, lymphocytes, plasma cells, and histiocytes may be present in the lamina propria of the mucosa and submucosa. The multifocal, superficial mucosal erosions from which fibrin and neutrophils exude ("volcano lesions") that are characteristic of the disease in pigs and humans are seen only sporadically in horses (Figure 15.8). Lymphatic vessels in the submucosa may be greatly

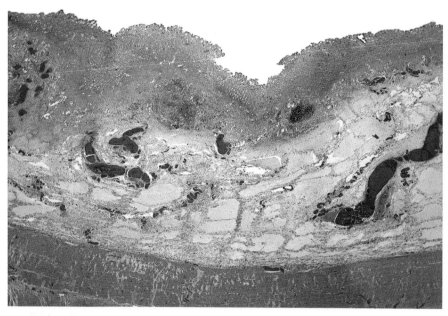

Figure 15.7 *Clostridium difficile*-associated disease; adult horse. Histology of the large colon shows diffuse necrosis of the mucosa, with total loss of the epithelial lining, marked submucosal edema and congestion. HE, 20x. Reproduced with permission from Diab *et al.* (2013) *Vet. Microbiol.*, **167**: 42–49.

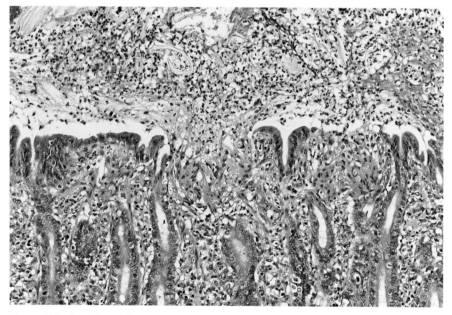

Figure 15.8 *Clostridium difficile*-associated disease; adult horse. Histology of the colon depicting a "volcano lesion" characterized by mucosal ulceration at the tip of the crypts from which fibrin and neutrophils exude. HE, 200x.

dilated and filled with fibrillar proteinaceous exudate and neutrophils. When lesions are transmural, inflammatory cells, edema, emphysema, and acute hemorrhage can be seen multifocally within the muscular and serosal layers. A variable number of large, thick, Gram-positive bacilli morphologically compatible with *Clostridium* spp. can be seen individually or in clusters within the lumen and overlying the denuded intestinal mucosa. The presence of large numbers of bacteria along with compatible intestinal lesions is suggestive of CDI, but their absence is not enough to rule out the disease.

Diagnosis

CDAD should be considered a differential diagnosis in horses with compatible clinical history, clinical signs, gross and/or microscopic findings, as described above. TcdA and/or TcdB detection in the intestinal contents or feces is considered the gold standard to confirm CDAD. Toxin detection can be achieved by several rapid, sensitive, and specific commercial ELISA tests or by a more sensitive and specific, but technically more demanding and expensive, cytotoxin assay to show the cytopathic effect of intestinal contents or fecal filtrates on cell lines. Isolation of *C. difficile* from intestinal contents, intestinal tissue, and/or feces demonstrates the presence of the organism in the intestinal tract and allows for a presumptive diagnosis of CDAD but, in the absence of toxin detection or with toxin-negative results, the disease cannot be confirmed. This is because approximately 5–15 % of clinically normal horses may carry *C. difficile* in their intestinal tracts and because some strains of *C. difficile* are not toxinogenic. Occasionally, TcdA and TcdB may be inactivated during sample transport or storage, thus yielding negative toxin detection test results. In these instances, positive *C. difficile* cultures help to establish a presumptive diagnosis of CDAD, with the caution noted above. Increasingly, DNA-based tests including quantitative PCR are used to diagnose CDI, often as part of "multiplex diarrhea panels"; as is the case with culture, these tests may overestimate the prevalence of infection since they do not distinguish between asymptomatic and symptomatic colonization. Toxin identification remains the gold standard. Diagnostic tests to rule out other common causes of diarrhea, such as *Salmonella, C. perfringens* type C, and *Neorickettsia risticii* are encouraged to rule out the possibility of co-infections.

The diagnostic issues noted above have contributed to difficulties in providing a comprehensive description of the clinical and pathological aspects of CDAD in horses.

Typhlocolitis of pigs

Epidemiology

C. difficile infection causes disease more commonly in neonatal piglets up to approximately 1 week of age, but the disease has also been described in postparturient sows with mastitis-metritis-agalactia treated with antibiotics. The prevalence of *C. difficile* is very high in the intestinal tract of neonatal piglets and decreases significantly with age. Piglets can test positive for *C. difficile* culture as soon as 1 hour after birth, and in some herds up to 100% of piglets can became positive by day 3. The prevalence then gradually decreases to less than 10% by around day 60. The prevalence in pigs at the nursery, grower-finisher group, breeding boars and sows, farrowing crates, air samples in pig farms, effluent from the farrowing barn, pig carcasses at a slaughter plant environment, and pork products is generally low, ranging between 3 and 9%, but in the case of pork products may be as high as 40%. The prevalence of *C. difficile* does not seem to vary between conventional and antimicrobial-free pigs at the farm and at slaughter.

C. *difficile* toxinotype V/ribotype 078, often associated with community-acquired *C. difficile* infection in humans, is the predominant ribotype found in pigs. Moreover, strains of *C. difficile* ribotype 078 found in neonatal piglets can be indistinguishable from human strains of ribotype 078. Several other ribotypes, such as 013, 014, 062, and 019 are found less frequently. Transmission of *C. difficile* from pigs, the pig farm environment, and retail meat to humans has not been demonstrated yet, but may be possible. Transmission from infected pig meat to hamsters has been demonstrated.

The source of infection for neonatal piglets is the sow and the contaminated environment in the farrowing wards, and transmission can be fecal–oral or even airborne. Experimental evidence indicates that transplacental vertical transmission of *C. difficile* from pregnant sows to piglets is unlikely. Morbidity and mortality are variable.

Clinical signs
Disease among neonatal pigs is usually mild and characterized by diarrhea. Dyspnea, mild abdominal distension, and scrotal edema with or without diarrhea are also clinical manifestations of the disease in piglets. Sudden death in piglets is uncommon, but may occur. One study documented the disease in sows after the use of antimicrobials to treat mastitis-metritis-agalactia. These sows developed diarrhea and respiratory distress, but had low mortality.

Gross changes
Mesocolonic edema is a characteristic, although not specific, gross lesion of *C. difficile* infection in piglets (Figures 15.9 and 15.10). The colon and cecum may be flaccid and dilated and contain watery or pasty yellowish to brown contents. Gross lesions in the mucosa of the colon and cecum may be subtle or marked and are characterized by multifocal to coalescing mucosal necrosis that can extend through the intestinal wall in the more severe cases. Enteric lesions may be accompanied by systemic manifestations, such as ascites, hydropericardium, pleural effusion, and scrotal edema, although these are not common. Adult sows that developed the disease after antibiotic treatment for mastitis-metritis-agalactia showed mesocolonic edema, hydrothorax, and ascites.

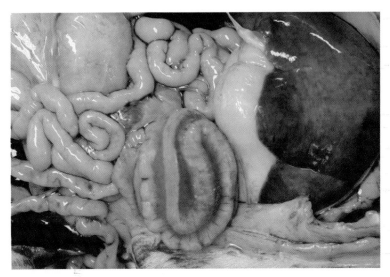

Figure 15.9 *Clostridium difficile*-associated disease; piglet. Marked mesocolonic edema, segmental dilation and yellow discoloration of the spiral colon. Courtesy of C.J. Perfumo.

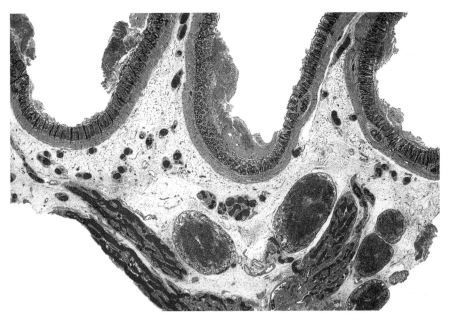

Figure 15.10 *Clostridium difficile*-associated disease; piglet. Histology of the spiral colon shows marked mesocolonic edema, congestion of mesocolonic vasculature, and multifocal mucosal necrosis with pseudomembrane formation. HE, 20x.

Microscopic changes

Suppurative, necrotizing, erosive/ulcerative colitis and typhlocolitis are characteristic of CDI in piglets (Figure 15.10). Often, "volcano lesions" are present, and are characterized by multifocal, superficial, mucosal erosions at the tip of the crypts; a fibrin and neutrophils exudate are present, although their absence does not rule out the disease. In severe cases, necrotizing intestinal lesions can be transmural, affecting all layers of the intestine. Postparturient sows with mastitis-metritis-agalactia treated with antibiotics showed fibrino-neutrophilic colitis and mesocolonic edema.

Diagnosis

A compatible clinical history and clinical signs along with the presence of mesocolonic edema and necrosuppurative typhlocolitis are suggestive of *C. difficile* disease in piglets. However, definitive diagnosis of *C. difficile* infection is often challenging because the prevalence of *C. difficile* in the intestinal tract of healthy piglets is relatively high and, although inconsistently, the two major *C. difficile* toxins, TcdA and TcdB, have been found in the intestinal tract of normal piglets. Therefore, the diagnosis must currently rely on a combination of gross and microscopic pathology, toxin detection, and demonstration of *C. difficile* by culture or DNA-based tests. Negative testing for other causes of diarrhea, such as colibacillosis, rotaviral enteritis, transmissible gastroenteritis, porcine epidemic diarrhea virus, and other clostridial enteritis should be part of the diagnostic work-up. As noted earlier, there are non-toxigenic strains of *C. difficile*, so that culture of the organism from the intestinal tract or feces without toxin detection has more value if the isolates are genotyped and found to have the gene encoding for at least one of the two major toxins. Detection of TcdA and/or TcdB in the intestinal contents or feces is of better diagnostic value than culture alone, for reasons described earlier.

C. difficile infection in other species

Epidemiology

Among laboratory animals, Syrian hamsters are the most susceptible to naturally acquired disease, although spontaneous or experimental *C. difficile* enteric disease also occurs in gerbils, guinea pigs, mice, rabbits, and rats. In particular, young SCID mice seem to be highly susceptible. All of these species are used as animal models of the disease in humans. Antibiotic therapy is a risk factor in gerbils, guinea pigs, and hamsters; hence, the disease may be a complication when antibiotic treatment to control other bacterial diseases, such as enteric helicobacteriosis in Mongolian gerbils, is applied. CDAD can also occur in the absence of antimicrobial treatment.

The role of *C. difficile* in enteric disease of dogs and cats is unclear but evidence indicates that this organism is not a common enteric pathogen. The existence of community-associated and hospital-associated colonization with toxigenic *C. difficile* has been demonstrated in dogs. The prevalence of *C. difficile* in the feces of healthy dogs and cats is variable, ranging approximately between 10 and 40%. However, the association between isolation of toxigenic *C. difficile* from feces and diarrhea in dogs is debatable. Causality has not been proven and the disease has not been reported to have been reproduced experimentally in healthy adult dogs. *C. difficile* ribotypes that can also be isolated from humans have been detected in dog and cat samples from animal shelters in Germany, suggesting that dogs and cats are a reservoir of potentially zoonotic strains of C. *difficile*. Alternatively, humans may be reservoirs of organisms for infection of small animals. There is a critical need to establish diagnostic criteria for the diagnosis of CDAD in dogs; this should include comparison of the sensitivity and specificity of toxin detection tests with those of agent detection.

The prevalence of *C. difficile* in domestic ruminants (cattle, sheep, and goats) has been studied mainly to investigate the potential for transmission of the disease from food animals to humans; however, to date, these animals seem quite resistant to *C. difficile*-associated disease despite some authors suggesting an association between *C. difficile* and diarrhea in calves. The prevalence of *C. difficile* in fecal samples of healthy cattle, ovine, and sheep is generally below 10%. This microorganism is frequently isolated from calves with diarrhea associated with multiple agents, including rota and coronaviruses, cryptosporidia and others, and the significance of this finding is, therefore, undetermined.

Clinical signs

Hamsters may display diarrhea, but often die so rapidly that signs are not observed. Mice (especially SCID mice) typically become diarrheic, lose weight, and become "poor-doers". Rabbits and other laboratory animals manifest severe diarrhea. Little and incomplete information is available on clinical disease of dogs and cats produced by *C. difficile*.

Gross lesions

The comparative distribution of lesions in different animal species is presented in Figure 15.11. With the exception of rabbits, in which the small intestine is primarily involved (Figure 15.12), lesions associated with naturally acquired *C. difficile*-associated disease in gerbils, guinea pigs, hamsters, mice, and rats occur mainly in the large intestine and variably affect the small intestine (Figure 15.13). Gross lesions vary in extent and severity, but may include a bloated abdomen, small or large intestine dilated with gas and tan or red fluid, serosal hemorrhage, mural edema, mucosal hyperemia, petechiation, ulceration, and a fibrinonecrotic pseudomembrane overlaying the mucosal surface.

Microscopic lesions

Histologically, in laboratory animals there is segmental or diffuse necrotizing enteritis, colitis, or typhlitis, with variable edema and leukocytic infiltration, and intestinal lumina may contain large numbers of Gram-positive bacilli morphologically compatible with *Clostridium* spp. In animals that survive the acute episode of

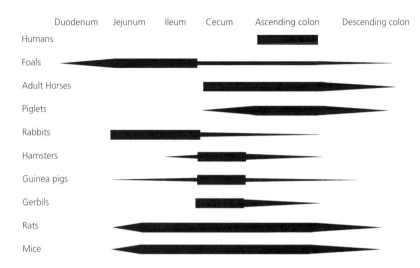

Figure 15.11 The comparative distribution of *C. difficile*-associated lesions in the intestinal tract of different animal species. Modified from Keel *et al.* (2006) *Vet. Pathol.*, **43**: 225–240.

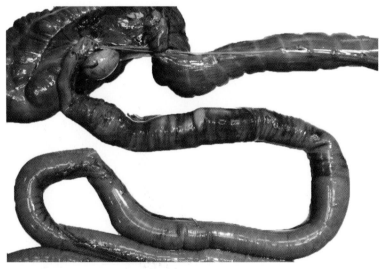

Figure 15.12 *Clostridium difficile*-associated disease; rabbit. Diffuse, severe, hemorrhagic ileitis with transmural necrotizing lesions. Courtesy of F. Giannitti.

disease, there may be hyperplasia of the intestinal mucosa. In hamsters, the cecum is most commonly involved and there is a sporadic, chronic form of the disease that is characterized by chronic typhlitis with mucosal hyperplasia and concurrent cholangiohepatitis, with amyloidosis of the liver, kidneys, and intestinal and cecal walls. Extra-intestinal lesions in mice include atrial thrombosis, pneumonia,

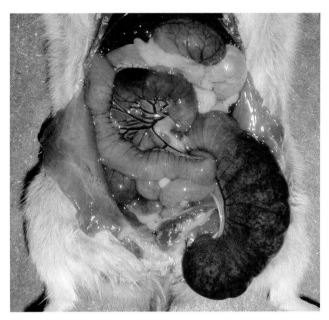

Figure 15.13 *Clostridium difficile*-associated disease; hamster. Diffuse, severe, necrotizing typhlitis is a characteristic lesion of CDAD in hamsters. Reproduced with permission from Keel *et al.* (2006) *Vet. Pathol.*, **43**: 225–240.

generalized lymphoid apoptosis, and renal tubular vacuolation. In rats, interstitial pneumonia and hepatitis have been recorded in experimental infections.

Diagnosis

As described above for horses and pigs, the diagnosis of *C. difficile*-associated disease in other animal species is also attained by a combination of compatible clinical history and signs, gross and microscopic pathology, TcdA and TcdB detection in the intestinal contents, and culture of the organism. Ruling out other enteropathogens, including *Clostridium spiroforme* in the cases of enterotoxemia of rabbits (Chapter 18), is always a good complement for the diagnosis of not only *C. difficile* disease but also other infectious causes of diarrhea and enteric disease.

Prophylaxis, control, and treatment

There is, generally speaking, no current effective means for prophylaxis of *C. difficile* infections. Although some literature suggests the use of antimicrobials to prevent the disease, there are few experimental data to support the effectiveness of this approach. Furthermore, antimicrobials are often associated with the development of the disease, for which prophylactic antimicrobial therapy is seldom practiced in most species. In special situations, such as outbreaks of CDAD in neonatal foals, metronidazole has been used prophylactically to prevent the disease in foals with certain exposure to *C. difficile*. In human medicine, metronidazole and vancomycin have been used, with clinical success rates of about 66%

and 78%, respectively, in the treatment of severe CDI, and the new macrolide drug fidaxomicin has clinical cure rates similar to those of vancomycin, but with less recurrence of infection.

There has been substantial research work on the use of non-toxigenic strains to block the establishment of a toxigenic strain. Human non-toxigenic strains have been tested extensively in hamsters and found to be highly effective in preventing and curing *C. difficile* infections. A similar study found that the effects of *C. difficile* were substantially ameliorated in piglets dosed at birth with a porcine non-toxigenic strain.

With *C. difficile*, as with most other enteric diseases of pigs, sanitation is a primary concern. Thorough cleaning in farrowing buildings is important. Without removal of all organic material, any further efforts at sanitation are unlikely to be successful. After cleaning, it is useful to disinfect with an effective product. In the case of *C. difficile*, the disinfectant of choice is Virkon, used at three times the recommended rate. It is important to maintain a sufficient contact time to allow the material to work; contact should be at least two hours and preferably four hours.

Experience suggests that it is not possible to completely control CDAD by environmental cleaning and disinfection. The onset of CDAD is often observed within the first 12 hours post-farrowing. In any case, action should be taken as soon as possible after observation of signs and the establishment of a diagnosis. In animals with high net worth or of emotional value, metronidazole is often the antimicrobial of choice. Vancomycin may be used in cases in which there is antimicrobial resistance to metronidazole. Because of the critical importance of vancomycin in human medicine, use of this drug should be avoided or used only as a last resort in definitely diagnosed CDAD of animals.

Additional supportive care includes intravenous administration of fluids and electrolytes, oral administration of di-tri-octahedral (DTO) smectite, a commercially available natural clay material that has been shown to neutralize *C. difficile* toxins *in vitro*. In swine, on the other hand, few antimicrobials are appropriate due to cost and the typical recommendation is tylosin. However, some strains of *C. difficile* carry a resistance element (for example, ErmX) that spreads rapidly under tylosin pressure, causing tylosin-resistant strains to dominate a population. Beta-lactam antimicrobials can also be useful at times, as well as rifamycin. A new macrolide antimicrobial, fidaxomicin, will be one of the possibilities for treatment of human CDAD.

Bibliography

Arroyo, L.G., *et al.* (2004) Experimental *Clostridium difficile* enterocolitis in foals. *J. Vet. Intern. Med.*, **18**: 734–738.

Cave, N.J., *et al.* (2002) Evaluation of a routine diagnostic fecal panel for dogs with diarrhea. *J. Am. Vet. Med. Assoc.*, **221**: 52–59.

Clooten, J.K., *et al.* (2003) Genotypic and phenotypic characterization of *Clostridium perfringens* and *Clostridium difficile* in diarrheic and healthy dogs. *J. Vet. Intern. Med.*, **17**: 123.

Clooten, J., *et al.* (2008) Prevalence and risk factors for *Clostridium difficile* colonization in dogs and cats hospitalized in an intensive care unit. *Vet. Microbiol.*, **129**: 209–214.

Czuprynski, C.J., *et al.* (1983) Pseudomembranous colitis in *Clostridium difficile*-monoassociated rats. *Infect. Immun.*, **39**: 1368–1376.

Debast, S.B., *et al.* (2009) *Clostridium difficile* PCR ribotype 078 toxinotype V found in diarrhoeal pigs identical to isolates from affected humans. *Environ. Microbiol.*, **11**: 505–511.

Diab, S.S., *et al.* (2012) Pathology of *Clostridium perfringens* type C enterotoxemia in horses. *Vet. Path.*, **49**: 255–263.

Diab, S.S., *et al.* (2013) *Clostridium difficile* infection in horses: A review. *Vet. Microbiol.*, **167**: 42–49.

Diab, S.S., *et al.* (2013) Pathology and diagnostic criteria of *Clostridium difficile* enteric infection in horses. *Vet. Path.* **50**: 1028–1036.

Fawley, W.N., *et al.* (2005) Molecular epidemiology of endemic *Clostridium difficile* infection and the significance of subtypes of the United Kingdom epidemic strain (PCR ribotype 1). *J. Clin. Microbiol.*, **43**: 2685–2696.

Goudarzi, M., *et al.* (2014) *Clostridium difficile* Infection: Epidemiology, pathogenesis, risk factors, and therapeutic options. *Scientifica* (Cairo): 916826.

Gould, L.H., *et al.* (2010) *Clostridium difficile* in food and domestic animals: A new foodborne pathogen? *Clin. Infect. Dis.*, **51**: 577–582.

Hassel, D.M., *et al.* (2009) Di-tri-octahedral smectite for the prevention of post-operative diarrhea in equids with surgical disease of the large intestine: Results of a randomized clinical trial. *Vet. J.*, **182**: 210–214.

Hensgens, M.P., *et al.* (2012) *Clostridium difficile* infection in the community: A zoonotic disease? *Clin. Microbiol. Infect.*, **18**: 635–645.

Honda, H., *et al.* (2014) The changing epidemiology of *Clostridium difficile* infection. *Curr. Opin. Gastroenterol.*, **30**: 54–62.

Hopman, N.E., *et al.* (2011) Acquisition of *Clostridium difficile* by piglets. *Vet. Microbiol.*, **149**: 186–192.

Keel, M.K., *et al.* (2006) The comparative pathology of *Clostridium difficile*-associated disease. *Vet. Path.*, **43**: 225–240.

Keessen, E.C., *et al.* (2011) Aerial dissemination of *Clostridium difficile* on a pig farm and its environment. *Environ. Res.*, **111**: 1027–1032.

Keessen, E.C., *et al.* (2011) *Clostridium difficile* infection in humans and animals, differences and similarities. *Vet. Microbiol.*, **153**: 205–217.

Kiss, D., *et al.* (2005) A new periparturient disease in Eastern Europe. *Clostridium difficile* causes postparturient sow losses. *Theriogenol.*, **63**: 17–23.

Knight, D.R., *et al.* (2013) Prevalence of gastrointestinal *Clostridium difficile* carriage in Australian sheep and lambs. *Appl. Environ. Microbiol.*, **79**: 5689–5692.

Marks, S.L., *et al.* (2011) Enteropathogenic bacteria in dogs and cats: Diagnosis, epidemiology, treatment, and control. *J. Vet. Intern. Med.*, **25**: 1195–1208.

Martirosian, G., *et al.* (1998) Dioctahedral smectite neutralization activity of *Clostridium difficile* and *Bacteroides fragilis* toxins in vitro. *Acta Microbiol. Polonica*, **47**: 177–183.

Metcalf, D.S., *et al.* (2010) *Clostridium difficile* in vegetables, Canada. *Lett. Appl. Microbiol.*, **51**: 600–602.

Metcalf, D., *et al.* (2011) *Clostridium difficile* in seafood and fish. *Anaerobe*, **17**: 85–86.

Nambiar, P.R., *et al.* (2006) Progressive proliferative and dysplastic typhlocolitis in aging Syrian hamsters naturally infected with *Helicobacter* spp.: A spontaneous model of inflammatory bowel disease. *Vet. Path.*, **43**: 2–14.

Norman, K.N., *et al.* (2009) Varied prevalence of *Clostridium difficile* in an integrated swine operation. *Anaerobe*, **15**: 256–260.

Percy, D.H., *et al.* (eds) (2007) *Pathology of Laboratory Rodents and Rabbits*, 3rd edition, Blackwell Publishing Ltd., Oxford, UK.

Perrin, J., *et al.* (1993) Intestinal carriage of *Clostridium difficile* in neonate dogs. *Zentralbl. Veterinarmed. B*, **40**: 222–226.

Rodriguez, C., *et al.* (2012) *Clostridium difficile* in young farm animals and slaughter animals in Belgium. *Anaerobe*, **18**: 621–625.

Rodriguez-Palacios, A., *et al.* (2007) *Clostridium difficile* in retail ground meat, Canada. *Emerg. Infect. Dis.*, **13**: 485–487.

Rodriguez-Palacios, A., *et al.* (2007) Natural and experimental infection of neonatal calves with *Clostridium difficile*. *Vet. Microbiol.*, **124**: 166–172.

Silva, R.O., *et al.* (2013) Detection of toxins A/B and isolation of *Clostridium difficile* and *Clostridium perfringens* from dogs in Minas Gerais, Brazil. *Braz. J. Microbiol.*, **44**: 133–137.

Songer, J.G., *et al.* (2005) Clostridial enteric infections in pigs. *J. Vet. Diagn. Invest.*, **17**: 528–536.

Songer, J.G., *et al.* (2006) *Clostridium difficile*: An important pathogen of food animals. *Anaerobe*, **12**: 1–4.

Songer, J.G. (2012) Clostridiosis. In: Zimmerman, J.J. *et al.* (eds) *Diseases of Swine*, pp. 709–722. Wiley Blackwell, Ames, IA.

Steele, J., *et al.* (2012) Systemic dissemination of *Clostridium difficile* toxins A and B is associated with severe, fatal disease in animal models. *J. Infect. Dis.*, **205**: 384–391.

Susick, E.K., *et al.* (2012) Longitudinal study comparing the dynamics of *Clostridium difficile* in conventional and antimicrobial free pigs at farm and slaughter. *Vet. Microbiol.*, **157**: 172–178.

Uzal, F.A., *et al.* (2012) *Clostridium perfringens* type C and *Clostridium difficile* co-infection in foals. *Vet. Microbiol.*, **156**: 395–402.

Weese, J.S., *et al.* (2001) The roles of *Clostridium difficile* and enterotoxigenic *Clostridium perfringens* in diarrhea in dogs. *J. Vet. Intern. Med.*, **15**: 374–378.

Weese, J.S., *et al.* (2006) *Clostridium difficile* associated diarrhoea in horses within the community: Predictors, clinical presentation and outcome. *Eq. Vet. J.*, **38**: 185–188.

Weese, J.S., *et al.* (2010) Longitudinal investigation of *Clostridium difficile* shedding in piglets. *Anaerobe*, **16**: 501–504.

Wetterwik, K.J., *et al.* (2013) *Clostridium difficile* in faeces from healthy dogs and dogs with diarrhea. *Acta Vet. Scand.*, **55**: 23.

Worsley, M.A. (1998) Infection control and prevention of *Clostridium difficile* infection. *J. Antimicrob. Chemother.*, **41**: 59–66.

Disease Caused by *Clostridium colinum*: Ulcerative Enteritis of Poultry and Other Avian Species

John F. Prescott

Introduction

Ulcerative enteritis produced by *Clostridium colinum* is an acute disease of game birds (grouse, quail, partridge, and pheasants), young chickens, and turkeys, and sometimes other birds including pigeons and American robins. It occurs worldwide. The disease was originally described in quail and therefore at one time it was called quail disease. Disease caused by this bacterium has only been described in birds.

Etiology

Ulcerative enteritis is caused by *C. colinum*, a close relative of *Clostridium piliforme* (Figure 1.1), a Gram-positive anaerobe that forms colonies on routine solid medium incubated at 37 °C in 48 hours. Optimal growth is obtained on tryptose-phosphate agar with 0.2% glucose, 0.5% yeast extract, and 8% horse plasma, but the organism grows well on other rich media conventionally used for anaerobes, such as Columbia or Brucella blood agar. Virtually nothing is known about the basis of virulence of this organism; its genome has not been characterized and the basis of its remarkable virulence is unknown.

Epidemiology

Disease is most frequent in young birds of all types aged 4–12 weeks, but may occur, albeit uncommonly, in adults. An outbreak may last three weeks, peaking 5–14 days after initial infection. Chickens are often predisposed to infection by prior infection with coccidia, or by immunosuppressive infections such as infectious bursal disease or infectious anemia.

Clostridial Diseases of Animals, First Edition. Francisco A. Uzal, J. Glenn Songer, John F. Prescott and Michel R. Popoff.
© 2016 John Wiley & Sons, Inc. Published 2016 by John Wiley & Sons, Inc.

The infection is transmitted by ingestion of fecally contaminated water or feed, or is acquired directly from infected birds. It is likely that the spores persist for months or years in contaminated environments that are not disinfected, and still persist, to some degree, in environments that are disinfected. Birds recovered from infection may remain carriers, and are likely an important source of infection, but little is known about the persistence of infection and fecal shedding.

Clinical signs

Clinically, ulcerative enteritis is characterized by the development of diarrhea, which is initially watery but may become hemorrhagic. Affected birds are dull and depressed, become huddled and exhibit feather ruffling. Birds may become emaciated. Mortality varies from 2–10% in chickens to 100% in highly susceptible species such as quail. The latter may just be found dead without clinically apparent illness being observed.

Gross changes

In quail, acute lesions are characterized by marked hemorrhagic enteritis mainly of the duodenum, with punctate multifocal hemorrhages often visible through the serosa. Over time, the punctate hemorrhages develop into ulcers, both in the duodenum and throughout the intestinal tract, including the cecum, although lesions are most common in the small intestine. Early hemorrhagic and ulcerative lesions are characteristically surrounded by a pale yellow halo, and expand and coalesce to form large fibrinous and necrotic plaques (Figure 16.1). The ulcers

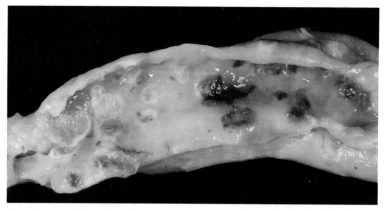

Figure 16.1 Jejunum of a quail with ulcerative enteritis. Numerous multifocal hemorrhagic ulcers are present. In the left side of the picture, the less hemorrhagic ulcers have a characteristic pale yellow halo around the necrotic ulcerated tissue. Courtesy of Gabriel Senties-Cue.

may perforate through the serosa to produce peritonitis. More chronic lesions typically include large, transmural, white focal areas of necrosis (Figure 16.2). The watery intestinal content is bloody in acute cases. Liver lesions are a hallmark of ulcerative enteritis. They vary considerably, from multifocal hemorrhagic or white on the liver surface to large, yellow, irregular multifocal to coalescing areas of necrosis present both on the liver surface and throughout the parenchyma (Figure 16.3). The spleen is usually enlarged and may also show multifocal areas of hemorrhage or necrosis.

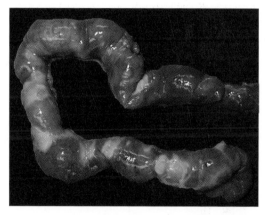

Figure 16.2 Jejunum of a quail with ulcerative enteritis. Multifocal transmural necrosis is typical of the more chronic disease. Courtesy of F.A. Uzal.

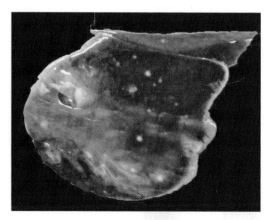

Figure 16.3 Liver of a quail with ulcerative enteritis. Multifocal areas of variably sized pale necrosis are visible on the liver surface. As the disease progresses, large, colorfully yellow areas of necrosis can be found throughout the parenchyma. Courtesy of Tahseen Abdul-Aziz.

Microscopic changes

Microscopic lesions include multifocal or coalescing areas of mucosal necrosis and ulceration in the intestine, which are covered by a pseudomembrane (Figure 16.4) and that commonly extend into the submucosa and muscularis. The ulcerated areas are surrounded by coagulative necrosis and a border of inflammatory cells (Figure 16.5). Mucosal and submucosal vascular congestion and frank hemorrhage are common. Large clumps of bacteria are commonly found in focal necrotic areas both in the intestinal lesions (Figure 16.6) and in the liver lesions. Large, transmural necrotic foci are common in more chronic cases. The liver lesions consist of multifocal, random areas of coagulation necrosis (Figure 16.7) in which abundant Gram-positive bacilli, single or in clusters, may be seen.

Diagnosis

Diagnosis of ulcerative enteritis by *C. colinum* is presumptively based on gross and microscopic changes (ulcerative enteritis and necrotizing hepatitis), and confirmed by isolation of *C. colinum* from the liver, spleen, and/or intestinal lesions. Gross lesions of ulcerative enteritis have similarities to those of necrotic

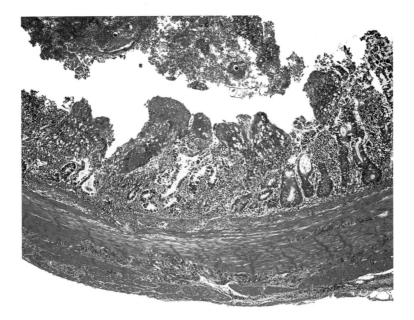

Figure 16.4 Jejunum of a quail with ulcerative enteritis. Extensive ulceration of the mucosa, which has sloughed its necrotic surface, forming a pseudomembrane. HE, 100x. Courtesy of F.A. Uzal.

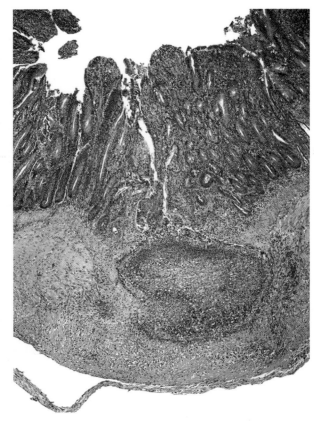

Figure 16.5 Jejunum of a quail with ulcerative enteritis. A large focal area of inflammation and necrosis is present in the mucosa and extends into the submucosa and muscularis; this lesion will develop into the transmural necrosis shown in Figure 16.2. HE, 100x. Courtesy of F.A. Uzal.

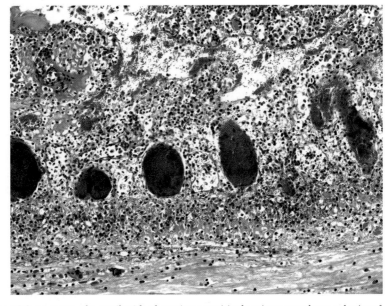

Figure 16.6 Jejunum of a quail with ulcerative enteritis showing many large colonies of bacteria. HE, 200x. Courtesy of F.A. Uzal.

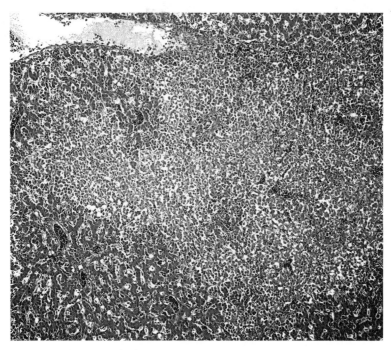

Figure 16.7 Liver of a quail with ulcerative enteritis. Hepatic lesion showing a large area of coagulative necrosis, with minimal inflammatory response. HE, 200x. Courtesy of F.A. Uzal.

enteritis caused by *C. perfringens*, especially as ulcerative enteritis lesions mature. They differ in the hemorrhagic nature of the initial ulcers, in the pale yellow halo surrounding the early lesions, in the large transmural necrotic intestinal lesions of the chronic lesions, and in the solid nature of the necrotic lesions in the liver. Liver lesions in necrotic enteritis are generally uncommon. Gross intestinal lesions in ulcerative enteritis are also similar to those observed in coccidiosis, which may be present concurrently. Microscopic lesions of ulcerative enteritis also have similarities to necrotic enteritis caused by *C. perfringens*; they differ, however, in that, in ulcerative enteritis, the bacterial microcolonies are focal in nature whereas in necrotic enteritis, extensive palisades of bacteria line the edges of the necrotic intestinal mucosa.

The liver and spleen may be fruitful diagnostic sources of *C. colinum* uncontaminated with intestinal bacteria such as *C. perfringens* and *E. coli*. Bacterial rods sized about 3–4 μm long and 1 μm wide with subterminal spores are found in smears of the liver, spleen, and intestine. They are far more likely to stain Gram-negative than *C. perfringens*, which differs also from *C. colinum* in that *C. perfringens* often fails to form spores. *C. colinum* can be isolated on pre-reduced enriched blood agar media such as Columbia or Brucella agar incubated anaerobically. The organism forms flat, 2–3 mm, non-hemolytic, round, gray colonies with irregular flowing margins after 48 hours of incubation at 37 °C. The isolated bacteria commonly show subterminal enlargements, but these are not usually obvious spores. Identification can be made by MALDI-TOF or by specific 16S rRNA sequence-based PCR.

Bibliography

Bano, L., *et al.* (2008) Development of a polymerase chain reaction assay for specific identification of *Clostridium colinum*. *Avian Path.*, **37**: 179–181.

Berkhoff, G.A., *et al.* (1974) Etiology and pathogenesis of ulcerative enteritis ("Quail disease"). Isolation of the causative anaerobe. *Avian. Dis.*, **18**: 186–204.

Cooper, K.K., *et al.* (2013) Diagnosing clostridial enteric diseases in poultry. *J. Vet. Diagn. Invest.*, **25**: 314–327.

Ononiwu, J.C., *et al.* (1978) Ulcerative enteritis caused by *Clostridium colinum* in chickens. *Can. Vet. J.*, **19**: 226–229.

Perelman, B., *et al.* (1991) An unusual *Clostridium colinum* infection in broiler chickens. *Avian Path.*, **20**: 475–480.

Pizarro, M., *et al.* (2005) Ulcerative enteritis (quail disease) in lories. *Avian Dis.*, **49**: 606–608.

Songer, J.G. and Uzal, F.A. (2013) Ulcerative Enteritis. In: Swayne, D.E. *et al.* (eds) *Diseases of Poultry*, 13th edition, pp. 944–949. Wiley-Blackwell, Danvers, MA.

17 Clostridial Abomasitis

John F. Prescott, Paula I. Menzies, and Russell S. Fraser

Introduction

Clostridial abomasitis is not an uncommon problem encountered mostly in young farmed pre-ruminants (calves, lambs, goat kids, and others), and it is associated with several clostridial species. The etiology is usually multiple, including, amongst others, *Sarcina* spp. (which are really true species of *Clostridium*, Chapter 1). This and the generally sporadic and multifactorial nature of clostridial abomasitis complicate understanding of the disease and consequently its effective diagnosis, treatment, and control. This chapter discusses what is currently known about clostridial abomasitis. Further research is required to understand this often frustrating and demoralizing disease process.

Braxy (*Clostridium septicum*)

Introduction
Braxy (also known as "bradsot") is the name used to describe abomasitis of sheep and other ruminants caused by *Clostridium septicum*.

Etiology
Braxy is caused by *C. septicum*, a species sometimes associated with other enteric infections as well as wounds of animals. It is not known whether the strains of *C. septicum* involved in braxy have any features uniquely associated with abomasitis, since no genetic characterization has been done. The organism causes severe localized abomasal infection and toxemia, and may disseminate through the bloodstream to other tissues. The toxins produced by this microorganism are described in Chapter 4.

Clostridial Diseases of Animals, First Edition. Francisco A. Uzal, J. Glenn Songer, John F. Prescott and Michel R. Popoff.
© 2016 John Wiley & Sons, Inc. Published 2016 by John Wiley & Sons, Inc.

Epidemiology

Braxy, first described in Scandinavian countries, is a disease that most commonly affects lambs post-weaning up to approximately 1 year of age. The disease is associated with grazing on cold or frozen pastures. Braxy is well recognized in more northerly countries, but it has been described in most sheep-rearing countries. The disease has also been described in calves. Speculatively, sheep may alter their grazing behavior in the winter when grasses are of poorer quality, which may increase ingestion of woody forages and soil containing spores of *C. septicum*. These elements may damage the abomasal mucosa, thus providing a port of entry for *C. septicum*. Freezing may make those high-lignin-containing plants more readily consumed. Experimentally, abomasal damage caused by an infusion of acetic acid through a cannula resulted in death due to *C. septicum* infection around the cannula site. This supports the importance of local trauma in the pathogenesis of the disease. In enzootic areas, losses can reach 8% of sheep at risk, with mortality being as high as 50% of affected sheep.

Clinical signs

Clinically, there is sudden onset of illness, complete anorexia, depression, and abdominal discomfort with moderate bloating. Fever may reach 42 °C. Affected animals become recumbent and die within 12–36 hours of the onset of disease. There may be bloody discharge from the nose of comatose animals.

Gross changes

Characteristically, the abomasal wall is markedly edematous and congested. Congestion may be focal but is commonly diffuse. Focal mucosal necrosis is usual; because of the rapid progression of disease, these lesions rarely become extensive. Gas bubbles that extend from the submucosa are commonly seen on the mucosal surface (Figure 17.1). The blood-tinged abomasal content smells foul.

Microscopic changes

Microscopically, there is marked necrosis, ulceration, edema, and congestion of the mucosa and submucosa. There is heavy neutrophilic infiltration around necrotic areas and throughout the lamina propria and submucosa (Figure 17.2). Large numbers of Gram-positive rods, sporulated or not, are present in clumps or chains in the necrotic areas. Thrombosis may be present in severely inflamed areas of the mucosa and submucosa.

Diagnosis

Diagnosis is based on clinical signs, gross and microscopic changes, and on identification of *C. septicum* by anaerobic culture, PCR, immunohistochemistry, and/or a fluorescent antibody technique. *C. septicum* grows within 24–36 hours on blood agar incubated anaerobically at 37 °C as a swarming colony, and characteristically forms long filaments. It can, however, be a post-mortem contaminant,

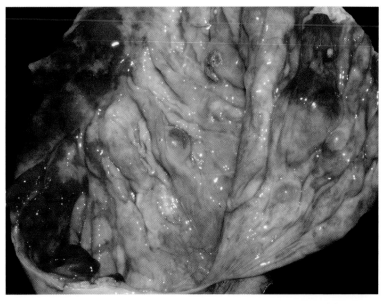

Figure 17.1 Abomasum of a sheep with braxy. The abomasum shows generalized edema and patches of marked congestion. Large gas bubbles are visible under the mucosa. Several multifocal ulcers are also present. Courtesy of the Department of Pathobiology, University of Guelph.

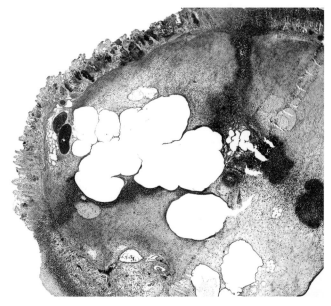

Figure 17.2 Abomasum of a lamb with braxy. There is marked mucosal necrosis, edema, emphysema, and congestion of the mucosa and submucosa. A rim of heavy neutrophilic infiltration surrounds necrotic areas. HE, 40x. Courtesy of F.A. Uzal.

since the organism invades readily from the intestine after death, and it is therefore important to use material collected from freshly dead animals for identification results to be significant. Isolation (or detection by other means) of *C. septicum* from tissues of animals in the advanced stage of post-mortem decomposition is not considered diagnostically significant. Identification of isolated microorganisms can be performed by conventional biochemical methods, by PCR, and/or by MALDI-TOF. PCR can also be performed directly on tissues.

Immunohistochemistry can be used to identify *C. septicum* in tissue sections, and fluorescent antibody staining can detect organisms directly in smears.

Prophylaxis and control

Disease at the flock level is usually sporadic, but can be prevented effectively in animals at risk by routine annual immunization with commercially available clostridial bacterin–toxoid vaccines containing *C. septicum* (Chapter 20). In countries where the disease is endemic, sheep management practices such as feeding hay before putting animals onto frozen pasture have been found to be useful. Prevention of the sporadic disease seen in calves should take the approaches recommended under other agents of clostridial abomasitis described below.

Treatment

Because of the rapid nature of the disease, treatment with antibiotics such as penicillin G is usually ineffective.

Other agents of clostridial abomasitis

Introduction

Clostridial abomasitis of calves, lambs, and goat kids in which *C. septicum* is not the causative agent is a well-recognized but not well-understood disease. It has been attributed to several different *Clostridium* spp. as well as to *Sarcina* spp. (which are true *Clostridium* spp., Chapter 1). It is possible that the disease may be caused concurrently by more than one clostridial species, taking advantage of host or environmental predisposition that is likely multifactorial. Although often sporadic, outbreaks associated with significant levels of morbidity and mortality may occur in animals at risk and be difficult to control. The full clinical and pathologic manifestations of clostridial abomasitis in calves, lambs, and goat kids have not been fully characterized. The condition may present as acute diffuse abomasitis, the most widely recognized presentation, but also as severe abomasal bloat or deep to perforating abomasal ulcers. Severe clostridial enteritis may occur with or without abomasitis in the same outbreak. A working assumption is that predisposition to the disease and its pathogenesis is similar in young calves, lambs, and goat kids, and the etiologic agents may vary with the circumstances, but final evidence for this is lacking.

Etiology

Several agents have most commonly been associated with clostridial abomasitis, including *Clostridium perfringens* type A, *Clostridium sordellii*, and *Sarcina* spp., or combinations of these agents. Other clostridia such as *Clostridium fallax* have been generally less consistently isolated.

Numerous questions remain about both the etiology of clostridia-associated abomasal bloat and abomasitis in young pre-ruminants, including its microbiology. Microbiologic issues yet to be resolved include the impact of dietary components (milk replacer, stored colostrum, different carbohydrates and proteins in both milk replacer and solid "starter" feed, and the effect of feed texture in solid starter) on bacterial growth and fermentation. Additionally, the cleanliness and effectiveness of the cleaning protocols of milk-feeding equipment may play a role. Clostridia including *Sarcina* are notable gas producers. Nothing is known about the interaction of the agents listed above in the abomasum, for example the possible role of quorum signaling by *Sarcina* on growth or expression of virulence determinants of other clostridia, or the role of *Sarcina* in providing an anaerobic environment in which other clostridia can establish and flourish.

Current understanding of the microbiology of abomasal disease and abomasitis in young farmed pre-ruminants is shown in Figure 17.3. The current knowledge of the etiology of clostridial abomasitis varies in different species.

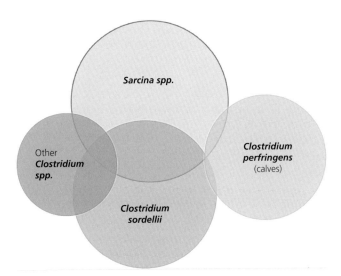

Figure 17.3 Venn diagram of current understanding of the microbiological complexities of abomasal bloat and abomasitis in young calves, lambs, and goat kids. It helps to see the circles as dynamic and changing, depending in part on the environmental and host predisposing factors. The figure also indicates our current inadequate understanding of the pathogenesis (and control) of the problem(s).

Calves

C. perfringens type A is commonly isolated in large numbers from the abomasum in fatal cases of abomasitis in young calves. In the single experimental study that has reproduced the disease, inoculation of *C. perfringens* type A into the rumen of healthy calves resulted in anorexia, bloat, depression, diarrhea, and, in some cases, death. Necropsy showed variable degrees of abomasitis that included petechial and/or ecchymotic hemorrhages and ulcers of variable size and depth, including those that were almost perforating. Microscopically, lesions in experimental calves were similar to those described in the naturally occurring infection, except that they lacked the emphysema that is sometimes described in the latter. The experimental reproduction of a disease resembling the naturally occurring condition is convincing evidence that *C. perfringens* type A can cause abomasitis in calves. Isolates have been inconsistently positive for the *cpb2* gene and a complete genome sequence of a type A isolate from a case of bovine clostridial abomasitis failed to reveal any novel toxin genes. The conclusion from a subsequent study by Schlegel and others (2012) was that no virulence "signature" has been identified in the *C. perfringens* strains associated with abomasitis, so that the involvement of *C. perfringens* is apparently not strain specific. Therefore, host or environmental predisposing factors are likely critical to the development of disease.

Other bacterial agents that have been associated with abomasitis in calves include *C. sordellii* and *Sarcina* spp. These are discussed below under lambs, in part since they appear to be more commonly associated with abomasal disease in those animals.

Lambs

Clostridial abomasal disease in lambs varies from bloat attributed to *Sarcina* spp., to severe abomasitis and emphysema associated with *C. sordellii*. In some cases, there may be both bloat and abomasitis with emphysema, and either or both agents (and others such as *C. fallax*) may be present.

Vatn and others (2000) have described the association of *Sarcina* spp. with fatal abomasal bloat, hemorrhage, and ulcers in young lambs. They also reported that bezoars comprised of wool and plant fiber were often present in the abomasum of lambs with *Sarcina* spp.-associated abomasal disease. In these lambs, *Sarcina*-like bacteria were visible as packets of Gram-positive cocci on mucosal smears, and immersed in the mucous in histological sections of abomasum. In some cases, large numbers of rods were seen, which were likely *Clostridium* spp. In the study by Vatn and others (2000) mentioned above, *Sarcina* observed on smears or histologically was associated with about 80% of cases of abomasal bloat, ulcers, and hemorrhage, *C. fallax* with about 40%, and *C. sordellii* with 20%. *Sarcina*-like bacteria were less commonly seen in lambs with more extensive hemorrhage and ulcers. *C. perfringens* type A was present in similar proportions in the abomasum of affected animals and in healthy controls, in contrast to *C. fallax* and *C. sordellii*, which were not found in healthy animals. With a few exceptions, the *Sarcina* spp. involved in abomasal disease have not usually been isolated or speciated. One of these exceptions is *Sarcina ventriculi*, which has been isolated from the abomasum of lambs with bloat. This particular species of Sarcina is a vigorous gas producer and has the remarkable ability to multiply over a broad range of acidity, even down to pH 1. This suggests adaptation to the stomach environment.

Goat kids
The only description of abomasal bloat and abomasitis in goat kids was that of an epizootic of abomasal bloat that killed 200 kids. This was attributed to the large numbers of *Sarcina*-like organisms observed on histological sections of the abomasum.

Epidemiology and clinical signs
Calves
Acute clostridial abomasitis occurs sporadically in pre-ruminant calves, ranging in age from 2 days to about 3 weeks. Calves affected may be of beef breeds suckling on their mothers on pasture, or dairy calves reared without their mothers and being fed pooled stored colostrum or milk replacer. Clostridial abomasitis has also been observed in 3–4-month-old beef calves, in which the disease was attributed to an increase in the consumption of coarse roughage as the amount of milk consumption diminished.

Proposed predisposing factors include: dietary changes, especially the introduction of coarse roughage (unlikely in milk-fed calves); pica, secondary to chronic enteritis and/or mineral deficiencies; abomasal trichobezoars and trichophytobezoars; undefined environmental or physical "stress"; vitamin E deficiency; lactic acidosis; mycotic infection; and low immune status attributed to copper deficiency. It is possible that the trypsin-inhibitory action of colostrum might prevent degradation of at least some clostridial exotoxins in *Clostridium*-contaminated colostrum. If milk replacer has a high soybean protein component, the trypsin-inhibitory effects of soybeans might have a similar effect.

It seems likely that, at least in dairy calves reared away from their mothers, dietary factors including overfeeding (for example with automated feeders) or heavy feeding at infrequent intervals, feeding of cold or partially thawed colostrum, and/or feeding of bacterially contaminated colostrum or milk replacer are important contributors to the disease. Factors contributing to disease in suckling beef cattle are less obvious, since those listed for dairy calves are not present.

Clinically, the disease is usually acute or peracute. Calves present with severe abdominal pain, bloat, depression, and diarrhea. Affected calves may also be found moribund or dead. Clinical pathology may show metabolic acidosis and other electrolyte abnormalities. Hematology may be normal or show moderate neutrophilia with left shift. Perforation of ulcers may lead to peritonitis, which may culminate in death.

Lambs

Abomasal disease with bloat, hemorrhage, and ulcers as major gross changes is a well-recognized problem in pre-ruminant lambs aged 2–5 weeks. Abomasitis in older (4–10 week) suckling or weaned lambs, and ewes, associated with *C. sordellii* frequently leads to sudden death.

Epidemiologically, abomasal bloat in 2–5-week-old lambs has occurred around the time that they are turned out to pasture. In a Norwegian study of abomasal disease in lambs on pasture by Lutnæs and Simensen (1982/1983), the incidence varied from less than 0.5% in more than half the flocks surveyed, to over 5% in nearly 20% of flocks. Since lambs are usually born in the spring, age may be more important than management. The highest incidence of bloat was noted in flocks with built-up litter and higher access to silage. Silage was thought to give litter a wet consistency, so that lambs were more likely to consume feces when nibbling straw. Substitution of litter by wooden slats or perforated metal floors decreased the incidence of abdominal bloat.

Lambs reared on liquid milk replacer are at risk of bloat; disease tends to be seen in the more robust feeders and the fastest-growing lambs. Abomasal bloat in lambs and goat kids has been associated with infrequent, high-volume feeding of warm milk replacer either by bottle or by lamb bar. This encourages the rapid consumption of milk, resulting in large volumes of milk in the abomasum and possible rapid growth of bacteria. To lower this risk, ad lib feeding of cool (20 °C) milk replacer is encouraged to reduce the possibility of gorging.

Anecdotally, an increased prevalence (15%) of fatal abomasal disease was observed in nursing lambs on a cement yard, with free access to a pelleted high-protein ration, along with insufficient energy in the ewes' ration which resulted in poor milk production. Vitamin E deficiency may also have been a possible contributor to the high incidence of lamb death due to clostridial abomasitis in this flock.

Clinically, lambs present with acute onset of severe abdominal pain, abdominal tympany (bloat), and marked depression with anorexia. Affected lambs may also be found moribund or dead. Diarrhea is not usually noted. Affected lambs may be naturally or artificially reared. Lambs often have trichophytobezoars present in the abomasum.

Sudden death due to abomasitis in 4–10-week-old suckling or weaned lambs and ewes attributed to *C. sordellii* has been associated with well-managed flocks at pasture, with high milk production by the ewes of affected lambs and with free access to creep feed. A management change such as access to new pasture often preceded the onset of illness by a few days. Disease is usually sporadic.

Goat kids

Abomasal disease with bloat, hemorrhage, and ulcers has been recognized in pre-ruminant goat kids fed artificial milk replacer or solid supplements. In these kids, disease was attributed to bacterial contamination of the feeding equipment and infrequent, high-volume feeding of warm milk replacer, as noted for lambs.

Most often, kids presented as sudden death cases, but some animals also had bloat, depression, and recumbency shortly after feeding. Diarrhea has not usually been noted.

Gross changes
Calves
Grossly, there is abomasal dilatation and variable abomasitis, characterized by congestion, hemorrhage, edema, extensive mucosal necrosis, and ulceration (Figures 17.4 and 17.5). Lesions may be diffuse or focal. Gas bubbles may be present, especially in the abomasal folds. The abomasal contents commonly contain red-brown ("coffee ground") clotted material (Figure 17.5). In one description of severe sporadic disease in dairy calves fed colostrum or milk replacer, abomasal folds were blackened and the mucosa and submucosa presented hemorrhage, necrosis, and emphysema in the form of ~1 cm gas bubbles.

The small intestine may be segmentally or diffusely reddened, and sometimes contains reddish fluid or is distended with gas. The cecum and parts of the colon can be similarly affected.

Lambs
Gross pathology is often similar to that generally described in calves, with the addition that a small proportion of affected animals may show mesenteric volvulus and abomasal perforation or rupture. These lesions have been attributed to a combination of rolling because of pain and mucosal ulceration. Some lambs

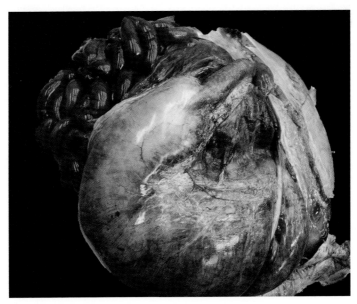

Figure 17.4 Serosal view of the abomasum of a calf with abomasitis showing marked gaseous distension, congestion, and hemorrhage. Courtesy of T. Van Dreumel.

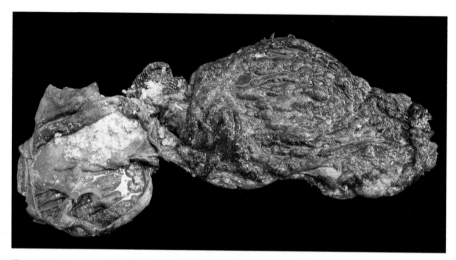

Figure 17.5 Mucosa of the abomasum of a calf with abomasitis showing edematous, hemorrhagic, and emphysematous folds. The abomasal content was foul smelling. Courtesy of T. Van Dreumel.

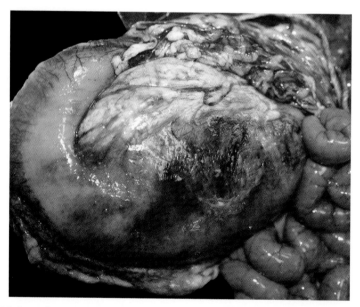

Figure 17.6 Serosal view of the abomasum of a lamb with abomasitis showing severe bloat, congestion, and hemorrhage.

show little abomasal gas but more marked ulcers or severe petechial hemorrhages (Figures 17.6 and 17.7). In 2–5-week-old lambs affected by abomasal bloat associated with *Sarcina* spp., there may be no other gross changes in the abomasal wall apart from mucosal ulcers.

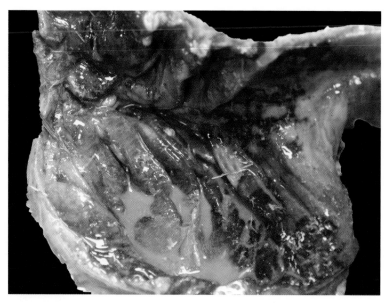

Figure 17.7 Abomasal mucosa of a lamb with abomasitis showing markedly edematous and congested folds, with multifocal hemorrhage and ulceration.

In lambs and older sheep in the United Kingdom with abomasitis attributed to *C. sordellii*, a partially distended and displaced abomasum was consistently present, as was gross thickening (up to 1 cm) of the abomasal wall due to a combination of edema and emphysema. Serosal surfaces were pale gray and glistening, with obvious subserosal emphysema and edema. Areas of erosion and intense congestion were present on the abomasal folds, but congestion was less marked between the folds.

Microscopic changes

Calves

The abomasal mucosa is hemorrhagic and edematous, with necrosis of surface epithelial cells. Mucosal ulcerations may extend into the submucosa, and are surrounded by intense infiltration of neutrophils and macrophages. The submucosa is edematous, and tissues are congested and may show thrombi in the lymphatics. Congestion can, in some cases, be severe. Gas bubbles may be evident in the submucosa as large, clear spaces (Figure 17.8). Scattered large numbers of Gram-positive rods consistent with *Clostridium* can be found in the mucosa and submucosa (Figure 17.9). Organisms consistent with *Sarcina* spp. may sometimes be found in necrotic material adhering to the damaged mucosa.

Lambs

Histologically, only moderate epithelial damage and submucosal edema may be present in 2–5-week-old lambs dead with bloat; these changes can be attributed to the physical effects of bloat. In some lambs, however, there may be severe

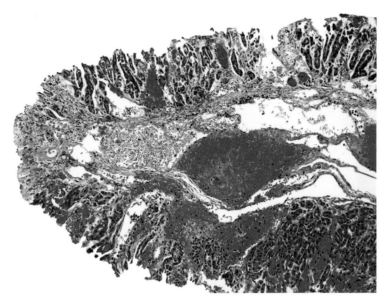

Figure 17.8 Abomasum of a calf with abomasitis. There is marked mucosal necrosis, mucosal and submucosal hemorrhage, edema, and emphysema. HE, 40x. Courtesy of F.A. Uzal.

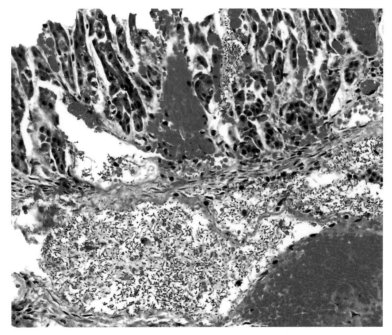

Figure 17.9 Higher magnification of Figure 17.8, showing large clusters of Gram-positive rods with typical *C. perfringens* morphology in the mucosa and submucosa of the abomasum. HE, 400x. Courtesy of F.A. Uzal.

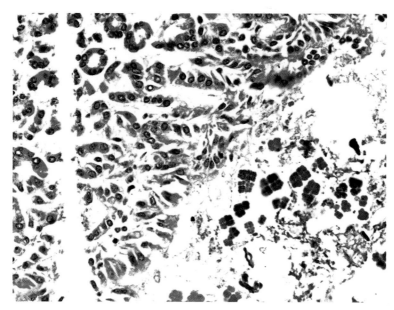

Figure 17.10 Abomasum of a lamb with abomasal bloat, showing bacterial clusters typical of *Sarcina* spp. on the mucosal surface. HE, 400x. Courtesy of the Department of Pathobiology, University of Guelph.

mucosal ulceration with marked mucosal and submucosal edema, neutrophil infiltration, congestion, hemorrhage, and emphysema. *Sarcina* spp. may be observed in the mucus covering the mucosal surface (Figure 17.10) and surrounded by neutrophils on the surface of mucosal ulcers. Gram-positive rods may also be observed in large numbers.

Diagnosis

Diagnosis is made on the basis of clinical presentation, gross and microscopic pathology, and microbiology, including anaerobic culture, examination of Gram-stained mucosal smears, fluorescent antibody technique, and immunohistochemistry. Identification of isolated colonies can be made by colonial and microscopic characteristics, followed by conventional biochemical techniques, MALDI-TOF, or PCR. The fluorescent antibody technique and immunohistochemistry allow identification of the clostridial species involved, on mucosal smears and tissue sections, respectively. In the case of *Sarcina*-associated disease, packets of *Sarcina*-like microorganisms may be found on Gram-stained mucosal smears or in tissue sections.

Prophylaxis

A *C. perfringens* type A toxoid vaccine is available in the United States for the control of abomasal tympany, ulcers, and hemorrhage of calves. Its safety has been demonstrated in pregnant cows but there are no published details on the efficacy of cow immunization in preventing clostridial abomasitis in their calves. The vaccine can also be used in calves from about 4 weeks of age. Multivalent clostridial vaccines used to immunize pregnant ewes in order to prevent early clostridial disease in their lambs contain *C. sordellii*, but there are no studies of their efficacy in preventing abomasal disease in lambs. No vaccines have been described for the prevention of *Sarcina*-associated abomasal bloat.

Control

Control of these sporadically occurring and multifactorial diseases requires identification of the numerous possible predisposing factors and of the relevant causative bacteria. Table 17.1 identifies possible predisposing factors that may need to be identified and corrected. There is no one-size-fits-all solution, and further research and detailed case studies are required to understand abomasal bloat and abomasitis in pre-ruminants.

Control of bacterial contamination of feeding equipment and of the environment likely is important. Feeding equipment for milk replacer consists of nipples, bottles, and buckets which should be cleaned with hot water and sanitized

Table 17.1 Factors that may predispose to abomasal bloat and abomasitis in young calves, lambs, and goat kids, and that may need to be investigated and corrected in order to control disease. Predisposing factors may be multiple and additive

Category	Possible factors in each category
Overfeeding	Limit feeding milk replacer infrequently so that animals gorge; restricting feed to ewes to promote excess creep feeding by lambs; overfeeding milk replacer; access to rich pasture.
Feed components	Pooled colostrum may have trypsin-inhibitory factors; soybean protein may have trypsin-inhibitory factors; protein content; readily fermented carbohydrates in milk replacer or starter ration; texture of starter ration; other.
Hygiene	Contamination of pooled colostrum; contamination of milk replacer; dirty and fecally contaminated environment; infrequent or ineffective cleaning protocols of milk-feeding equipment; contamination of milk-feeding equipment.
Immunosuppression or mineral deficiencies	Vitamin E deficiency; copper deficiency; iron deficiency.
Hair balls	Abomasal irritant or evidence of the need for hay.
Hunger	Gorging on food; eating straw contaminated by feces; formation of trichophytobezoars.
Antibody status	Implementation and maintenance of a clostridial vaccination program may be helpful. This includes a primary series, usually at 12 and 16 weeks of age, and annual vaccination suggested as being most effective 2–4 weeks prior to parturition. This will optimize colostral antibody production and passive transfer of protective antibodies to the nursing offspring.

after each use. Ad lib feeding systems should have plastic tubes and non-return valves to deliver the milk. These also need to be cleaned and sanitized daily to prevent bacterial growth. The environment of the nursing lamb or kid should be kept clean. This includes restricting access to manure piles located in yards, and bedding well with clean straw in pens.

Abomasal bloat in artificially ad lib or twice-daily fed lambs has been markedly reduced by the addition of 0.10% (v/w) formalin (37% formaldehyde) to 20% solids milk replacer, without affecting growth. This reduces contamination of the milk held at room temperature and also reduces fermentation in the abomasum. "Acidified" milk replacers containing citric or other organic acids are recommended to prevent bacterial growth after reconstitution. At this point, there is no evidence that they reduce the risk of clostridial abomasitis.

The factors predisposing to *C. perfringens*-associated abomasitis in beef calves at pasture with their dams are not understood, so that effective control measures remain unclear, including the unproven value of immunization of cows with type A toxoid vaccine to provide colostral immunity.

Treatment

Affected animals may respond to medical treatment including general nursing, antimicrobial drug treatment, and correction of electrolyte imbalances. Calves are more likely to be found dead or to be unresponsive to treatment because of the acuteness and severity of the disease. Treatment, including limitation of feeding, should be undertaken immediately when abomasal disease is suspected. Surgical resection of ulcerated or perforated areas in the abomasum may help in some cases.

Bibliography

DeBey, B.M., *et al.* (1996) Abomasal bloat associated with *Sarcina*-like bacteria in goat kids. *J. Am. Vet. Med. Assoc.*, **209**: 1468–1469.

Gorill, A.O., *et al.* (1975) Effects of formalin added to milk replacers on growth, feed intake, digestion and incidence of abomasal bloat in lambs. *Can. J. Anim. Sci.*, **55**: 557–563.

Lewis, C.J. and Naylor, R.D. (1998) Sudden death in sheep associated with *Clostridium sordellii*. *Vet. Rec.*, **142**: 417–421.

Lutnæs, B. and Simensen, E. (1982/1983) An epidemiological study of abomasal bloat in young lambs. *Prevent. Vet. Med.*, **1**: 335–345.

Nowell, V.J., *et al.* (2012) Genome sequencing and analysis of a Type A *Clostridium perfringens* isolate from a case of bovine clostridial abomasitis. *PLoS One*, **7**: e32271.

Roder, B.L., *et al.* (1988) Experimental induction of abomasal tympany, abomastitis, and abomasal ulceration by intrarumial inoculation of *Clostridium perfringens* type A in neonatal calves. *Am. J. Vet. Res.*, **49**: 201–207.

Roeder, B.L., *et al.* (1987) Isolation of *Clostridium perfringens* from neonatal calves with ruminal and abomasal tympany, abomasitis, and abomasal ulceration. *J. Am. Vet. Med. Assoc.*, **190**: 1550–1555.

Saunders, G. (1986) Diagnosing braxy in calves and lambs. *Vet. Med.*, **81**: 1050–1052.

Schlegel, B.J., *et al.* (2012) Toxin-associated and other genes in *Clostridium perfringens* type A isolates from bovine clostridial abomasitis (BCA) and jejunal hemorrhage syndrome (JHS). *Can. J. Vet. Res.*, **76**: 248–254.

Smith, L. (1975) *Clostridium perfringens*. In: Hitchner, S.B., *et al.* (eds) *The Pathogenic Anaerobic Bacteria*, p. 115. C.C. Thomas, Springfield, Ill.

Songer, J.G. (1996) Clostridial enteric diseases of domestic animals. *Clin. Microbiol. Rev.*, **9**: 216–234.

Songer, J.G. and Miskimmins, D.W. (2005) Clostridial abomasitis in calves: Case report and review of the literature. *Anaerobe*, **11**: 290–294.

Van Kruiningen, H.J., *et al.* (2009) Clostridial abomasitis in Connecticut dairy calves. *Can. Vet. J.*, **50**: 857–860.

Vatn, S. *et al.* (2000) *Sarcina*-like bacteria, *Clostridium fallax* and *Clostridium sordellii* in lambs with abomasal bloat, haemorrhage and ulcers. *J. Comp. Pathol.*, **122**: 193–200.

18

Diseases Produced by *Clostridium spiroforme*

J. Glenn Songer and Francisco A. Uzal

Introduction

Several clostridial species, including *Clostridium perfringens, Clostridium difficile,* and *Clostridium spiroforme,* affect the intestinal tract of rabbits. This chapter describes enteric disease produced by *C. spiroforme*, which is considered the most prevalent clostridial pathogen responsible for rabbit enteric disease, particularly in young animals. This microorganism also causes enteric disease in hares.

Etiology

C. spiroforme is a helically coiled, anaerobic, Gram-positive, spore-forming bacillus, which consists of an aggregation of individual semicircular cells joined end to end (Figure 18.1). It belongs phylogenetically in cluster XVIII of the low G+C Gram-positive bacteria and is not a genuine member of the genus *Clostridium* (Chapter 1). This microorganism is isolated frequently from the cecal contents of rabbits with spontaneous diarrhea in numbers as high as 10^6 spores per gram of content. *C. spiroforme* may also be related to clindamycin-associated colitis in rabbits, although at a lower concentration. The presence of *C. spiroforme* toxin (CST) is a consistent finding in the cecal content of diarrheic but not of healthy rabbits, and CST has been proposed as being responsible for diarrhea, enterocolitis, and death in rabbits infected with this organism.

CST is a binary toxin which, like other clostridial binary toxins such as *C. botulinum* C2 toxin, *C. difficile* transferase, *C. perfringens* iota toxin, as well as the *Bacillus* binary toxins, including *Bacillus anthracis* toxins, consists of two independent proteins, one being the binding component which mediates the internalization into the cell of the intracellularly active component and the other

Clostridial Diseases of Animals, First Edition. Francisco A. Uzal, J. Glenn Songer, John F. Prescott and Michel R. Popoff.
© 2016 John Wiley & Sons, Inc. Published 2016 by John Wiley & Sons, Inc.

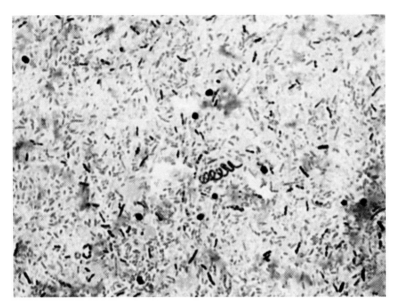

Figure 18.1 Gram stain of a cecal smear of a rabbit with *Clostridium spiroforme* infection, showing the typical spiral chains of cells.

part the active toxin. Clostridial binary toxins are responsible for enteric disease, inducing actin cytoskeleton disorganization through mono-ADP-ribosylation of globular actin, which induces cytoskeletal disarray.

CST is mouse lethal, dermonecrotic in guinea pigs, and neutralized by *C. perfringens* type E iota toxin antibodies. The *cst* genes have been cloned, allowing recombinant production of the enzyme (CSTa) and of the binding (CSTb) components of CST. CST has been shown to enter target cells via the lipolysis-stimulated lipoprotein receptor (LSR), which has also been recently identified as the host cell receptor of the binary toxins *C. difficile* transferase and *C. perfringens* iota toxin. CST, although not the related *Clostridium botulinum* C2 toxin, co-localizes with LSR during toxin uptake and trafficking to the endosomal compartments. The cell-binding (B) component of this AB toxin enters the cell via receptor-mediated endocytosis and once trafficked into the cytosol, the A component inhibits normal cell functions by mono-ADP-ribosylation of globular actin, which induces cytoskeletal disarray and death.

Pathogenesis

C. spiroforme is acquired by the fecal–oral route and colonizes the terminal small intestine and cecum, where it produces CST, which is considered to be the main virulence factor of this microorganism. The actin cytoskeleton is the target of several clostridial ADP-ribosyltransferases, including CST. ADP-ribosylation inactivates regulatory Rho proteins and damages the organization of the actin cytoskeleton. As noted, CST ADP-ribosylates actin monomers, inhibiting actin polymerization. Much less is known about B component binding to cell-surface receptors, and little is known about the details of toxin biochemistry, cellular uptake machinery, and host-cell responses following toxin-mediated disruption of the cytoskeleton.

Considerable further work is required to understand the detailed pathogenesis of infection, since this has not been investigated in any detail. No full-genome sequence of this organism has been completed to date, but it would no doubt be of immense value in providing the basis upon which to begin investigating the pathogenesis of infection by this neglected pathogenic *Clostridium*. The basis of the apparent restriction of this infection to lagomorphs (hares, rabbits) is one of many intriguing questions about this interesting and poorly investigated pathogen.

In the case series of rabbit enteritis, two or more potentially pathogenic organisms have frequently been identified, emphasizing that several different organisms may be acting in concert to produce clinical disease.

The similarity between *C. spiroforme* and anthrax toxins is of interest. Western blotting and ELISA show that the binding component of anthrax toxin shares epitopes with that of *C. spiroforme* toxin, which is closely related immunologically, but no functional complementation has been observed between iota toxin and anthrax toxin components. The binding components can form toxins active on macrophages only in combination with their respective enzymatic components. Agents which prevent acidification of endosomes do not have the same effects on anthrax toxin activity as they do on iota and *C. spiroforme* toxins. Therefore, the mechanisms of entry into the cells are presumably different. Since the binding components of anthrax toxins and iota toxin share a conserved putative translocation domain, these binding components could have a common mode of insertion into the cell membranes.

Epidemiology

C. spiroforme is not found in the intestine of normal rabbits, but is thought to be acquired from the environment. Considerable further work is, however, required to understand the detailed epidemiology of infection, including the main source(s) of infection for rabbits and the major risk factors for infection. In many cases, poor hygiene, antibiotic treatment, and carbohydrate overload have been apparently prominent influences on the development of disease. It has been postulated, although not definitely proved, that the normal gut flora acts as a microbial barrier, and disruption of this barrier by antibiotics, weaning, or other factors, is an important predisposing factor for *C. spiroforme* infection, as it is for *C. difficile* infection (CDI); this disease can also occur simultaneously in rabbits treated with broad-spectrum antibiotics.

Clinical signs

C. spiroforme infection may be acute, sub-acute, or chronic. All forms are characterized clinically by watery diarrhea, depression, and hypothermia, of variable duration. Dehydration and loss of condition are seen in chronic cases. Occasionally, terminal convulsions can be seen.

Gross changes

In acute cases, the carcasses are usually in good nutritional condition and soiling of the perineal region with feces is a common finding. Sub-acute and chronic cases are characterized by emaciated and dehydrated carcasses. The most significant gross lesions in all forms of the disease are in the gastrointestinal tract and consist of petechiae and ecchymoses on the cecal serosa, which may extend to the ileum and colon. The cecum is immensely dilated and has watery and sometimes hemorrhagic contents. The mucosa may be edematous, hemorrhagic, and occasionally covered by a fibrinous pseudomembrane (Figures 18.2 and 18.3).

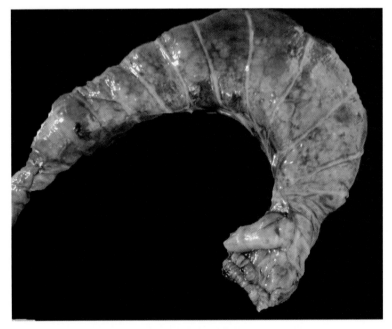

Figure 18.2 Cecum of a rabbit with presumptive *Clostridium spiroforme* infection showing severe serosal edema, congestion, and hemorrhage. Courtesy of the Pathology Group, Universidad CEU Cardenal Herrera, Spain.

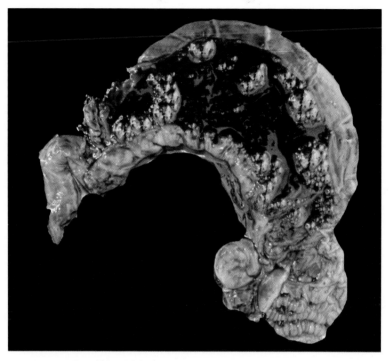

Figure 18.3 Cecum of a rabbit with presumptive *Clostridium spiroforme* infection showing hemorrhagic content. Courtesy of the Pathology Group, Universidad CEU Cardenal Herrera, Spain.

Microscopic changes

Microscopic examination of acute cases reveals necrosis of the superficial epithelium, with leucocytic and fibrinous exudation; the crypts and lamina propria tend to be spared. A large number of Gram-positive bacilli may be present on the surface of the necrotic epithelium and in the lumen. Congestion and hemorrhage of the submucosa are common. Attempts at regeneration via epithelial hyperplasia may be seen in sub-acute and chronic cases.

Diagnosis

A presumptive diagnosis may be achieved by noting appropriate clinical, gross, and microscopic changes, as described above. Typical, coiled, Gram-positive bacilli present on Gram-stained smears of intestinal mucosa (Figure 18.1) are strongly suggestive of *C. spiroforme* infection.

Isolation of *C. spiroforme* from intestinal contents of rabbits is diagnostic. This can be achieved by sampling the supernatant-pellet interphase of centrifuged specimens processed for routine toxin analysis. High-speed centrifugation at 20,000 x g for 15 minutes provides a rapid and effective means of separating this anaerobic pathogen from the majority of both indigenous and non-indigenous intestinal microbial flora. The unusual helically coiled, semicircular shape of the microorganism is considered, at least in part, responsible for this phenomenon. When cultivated on blood agar, *C. spiroforme* has a loosely coiled, spiral morphology, consisting of a uniform, end-to-end aggregation of semicircular cells. The identity of isolated cells can be tentatively confirmed by microscopic examination of Gram-stained smears (Figure 18.1). It is also possible to confirm the organism's identity by use of a PCR assay, with primers designed for the toxin gene. Detection of CST in cecal contents is also diagnostic, but no commercial ELISA or other immunological tests for the toxin are currently available for this purpose. Development of a multiplex quantitative PCR assay for use on feces or colonic contents of diarrheic rabbits to distinguish the various enteric pathogens of this species would be a considerable advance in this neglected field.

Treatment and prophylaxis

Probiotics are frequently used in the treatment of gastrointestinal diseases of rabbits based largely on anecdotal evidence of a beneficial effect rather than on scientific study. In one study to determine if probiotics could positively affect the fecal levels of *C. spiroforme*, oral administration of probiotic *Enterococcus faecium* was associated with a significant increase in fecal levels of *E. faecium*, but did not affect fecal levels of *C. spiroforme*. Antibiotic treatment should include narrow-spectrum orally administered antibiotics with activity against Gram-positive antibiotics; examples include penicillin and ampicillin, although macrolide and lincosamide activity is poor. Care should be taken not to administer drugs such as macrolides or lincosamides or extended spectrum cephalosporins that might interfere with the protective effect of the normal cecal and colonic microflora. Metronidazole is also effective *in vitro*.

Little work has been performed to understand the basis of immunity of rabbits to *C. spiroforme* infection and to develop effective immunization strategies. Investigations were conducted into an enterotoxemia caused by *C. spiroforme* responsible for significant losses in commercial rabbit farms in Western Australia. Two trials using laboratory- and farm-bred rabbits were performed to evaluate the protective value of a toxoid prepared from the supernatant of *C. spiroforme* cultures against intraperitoneal challenge with the trypsin-activated toxin of *C. spiroforme*. The trials showed clearly that a single vaccination at weaning (4 weeks) was protective against toxin but more complete and lasting protection was conferred following a second vaccination administered 14 days after the first. Adults showed similar levels of protective antibodies but did not appear to pass on this protection to their kits, although ELISA results indicated levels of antibody in kits from unvaccinated mothers to be lower than progeny from vaccinated mothers. However, antibody levels in kits from vaccinated mothers were low and did not protect against challenge with toxin. Further work is required on the development of effective immunization against *C. spiroforme* in rabbits.

Bibliography

Agnoletti, F., *et al.* (2009) A survey of *Clostridium spiroforme* antimicrobial susceptibility in rabbit breeding. *Vet. Microbiol.*, **136**: 188–191.

Aktories, K., *et al.* (1992) Mechanisms of the cytopathic action of actin-ADP-ribosylating toxins. *Mol. Microbiol.*, **6**: 2905–2908.

Barth, H., *et al.* (2004) Binary bacterial toxins: Biochemistry, biology, and applications of common *Clostridium* and *Bacillus* proteins. *Microbiol. Mol. Biol. Rev.*, **68**: 373–402.

Barth, H., *et al.* (2008) Binary actin-ADP-ribosylating toxins and their use as molecular Trojan horses for drug delivery into eukaryotic cells. *Curr. Med. Chem.*, **15**: 459–469.

Billington, S.J., *et al.* (1998) *Clostridium perfringens* type E animal enteritis isolates with highly conserved, silent enterotoxin gene sequences. *Infect. Immun.*, **66**: 4531–4536.

Borriello, S.P. and Carman, R.J. (1983) Association of iota-like toxin and *Clostridium spiroforme* with both spontaneous and antibiotic-associated diarrhea and colitis in rabbits. *J. Clin. Microbiol.*, **17**: 414–418.

Butt, M.T., *et al.* (1994) A cytotoxicity assay for *Clostridium spiroforme* enterotoxin in cecal fluid of rabbits. *Lab. Anim. Sci.*, **44**: 52–54.

Carman, R.J., *et al.* (1984) Experimental and spontaneous clostridial enteropathies of laboratory and free living lagomorphs. *Lab. Anim. Sci.*, **34**: 443–452.

Chowdhury, H.H., *et al.* (1999) Actin cytoskeleton depolymerization with *Clostridium spiroforme* toxin enhances the secretory activity of rat melanotrophs. *J. Physiol.*, **521** (Pt 2): 389–395.

Drigo, I., *et al.* (2008) Development of PCR protocols for specific identification of *Clostridium spiroforme* and detection of *sas* and *sbs* genes. *Vet. Microbiol.*, **131**: 414–418.

Ellis, T.M., *et al.* (1991) Evaluation of a toxoid for protection of rabbits against enterotoxaemia experimentally induced by trypsin-activated supernatant of *Clostridium spiroforme*. *Vet. Microbiol.*, **28**: 93–102.

Holmes, H.T., *et al.* (1988) Isolation of *Clostridium spiroforme* from rabbits. *Lab. Anim. Sci.*, **38**: 167–168.

Papatheodorou, P., *et al.* (2012) Identification of the cellular receptor of *Clostridium spiroforme* toxin. *Infect. Immun.*, **80**: 1418–1423.

Percy, D.H., *et al.* (eds) (2007) Pathology of Rabbits and Rodents, pp. 268–271. Blackwell Publishing, Ames, Iowa.

Perelle, S., *et al.* (1997) Immunological and functional comparison between *Clostridium perfringens* iota toxin, *C. spiroforme* toxin, and anthrax toxins. *FEMS Microbiol. Lett.*, **146**: 117–121.

Popoff, M.R., *et al.* (1988) *Clostridium spiroforme* toxin is a binary toxin which ADP-ribosylates cellular actin. *Biochem. Biophys. Res. Commun.*, **152**: 1361–1368.

Stiles, B.G., *et al.* (2011) Clostridial binary toxins: Iota and C2 family portraits. *Front Cell. Infect. Microbiol.*, **1**: 1–14.

Wigelsworth, D.J., *et al.* (2012) CD44 promotes intoxication by the clostridial iota-family toxins. *PLoS One*, **7**: e51356.

Yonushonis, W.P., *et al.* (1987) Diagnosis of spontaneous *Clostridium spiroforme* iota enterotoxemia in a barrier rabbit breeding colony. *Lab. Anim. Sci.*, **37**: 69–71.

Clostridial Histotoxic Infections

Blackleg

19

Camila C. Abreu and Francisco A. Uzal

Introduction

Blackleg (blackquarter, clostridial myositis) is an infectious disease of cattle and rarely of other ruminants, caused by *Clostridium chauvoei* and characterized mainly by necrotizing myositis. The disease has been reported in most parts of the world where livestock is raised, and although it can be prevented by vaccination, sporadic cases and occasional outbreaks still occur. Infection by *C. chauvoei* has also been reported in several other animal species although the pathogenesis in these species has not been fully elucidated.

Etiology

C. chauvoei is an anaerobic, Gram-positive, spore-forming rod, which has been known since 1887; the organism was named after J. B. A. Chauveau, a French scientist. *C. chauvoei* is usually found as single cells, sometimes in pairs and rarely in short chains. The Gram-positivity may be variable, particularly in old cultures, which may show many Gram-negative rods. *C. chauvoei* is peritrichously flagellated and almost all strains are motile. The spores are ovoid and may be central, subterminal, or, occasionally, terminal. Sporulation in *C. chauvoei* occurs readily. Oxidizing disinfectants, including iodine and chlorine, are fairly effective in destroying vegetative and sporulated forms of *C. chauvoei*. However, the spores are resistant to boiling and to the action of phenolic and quaternary ammonium disinfectants. Because of this, instruments used in post-mortem examinations of animals with blackleg should not be sterilized by this method.

Colonies of *C. chauvoei* on blood agar are usually 2 to 4 mm in diameter, slightly raised, whitish-gray, and with a glossy surface; they are usually semitransparent

Clostridial Diseases of Animals, First Edition. Francisco A. Uzal, J. Glenn Songer,
John F. Prescott and Michel R. Popoff.
© 2016 John Wiley & Sons, Inc. Published 2016 by John Wiley & Sons, Inc.

if examined within a day of incubation. As spores are formed, however, the colonies become opaque. The colonies are usually separated from each other and merge infrequently. Most colonies are circular and they may be surrounded by a narrow zone of hemolysis; this characteristic is dependent upon the strain and the source of the red blood cells in the media. Red blood cells of cattle, sheep, pigs, rabbits, and dogs are hemolysed by *C. chauvoei*, but erythrocytes of humans, horses, guinea pigs, and chickens are more resistant to hemolysis.

Most strains of *C. chauvoei* ferment several carbohydrates, but this microorganism can also grow on media without fermentable carbohydrates; in this case, energy is obtained from amino acid fermentation.

C. chauvoei and *Clostridium septicum* are difficult to distinguish from each other on the basis of their phenotypic characteristics. The most significant distinguishing characteristics include:

1 *C. chauvoei* ferments sucrose whereas *C. septicum*, with rare exceptions, does not;
2 *C. septicum* ferments salicin whereas *C. chauvoei* does not;
3 *C. septicum* may grow at 44 °C whereas *C. chauvoei* does not grow above 41 °C.

Both organisms can also be differentiated by PCR and sequencing of the 16S RNA gene and by MALDI TOF.

Several toxins and flagella are responsible for the virulence of *C. chauvoei*. A detailed description of the main virulence factors of *C. chauvoei* is presented in Chapter 4. Briefly, the following virulence factors have been identified so far: i) *C. chauvoei* toxin A (CctA), which is part of the *Staphylococcus aureus* α-hemolysin family; this toxin is thought to be essential for the hemolytic and cytotoxic activity of *C. chauvoei*; ii) cholesterol-dependent cytolysins, which can be involved in pathogenesis of gangrene lesions; iii) two different hyaluronidases; iv) a DNAse; and v) a neuraminidase. In addition, flagella are thought to contribute to the infectious process by providing *C. chauvoei* mobility, which allows the organism to spread. In fact, the flagella are considered to be so important for virulence that flagellar antigens have been considered good candidates for blackleg vaccines.

Epidemiology

Blackleg mainly affects cattle between 6 months and 2 years of age that are in good nutritional condition. Occasionally, cases in animals outside this age range may occur. Although little information is available in this regard, it is thought that the spores of *C. chauvoei* can survive for many years in the soil. Similarly, it is assumed that both spores and vegetative forms of this microorganism can be found in the feces of healthy or sick animals, although, again, little information is available in the scientific literature to support this claim. Blackleg is most commonly observed in pastured animals, although cases may also occur in housed animals fed silage, hay, or other feed. The great majority of blackleg cases occur in the wet season and there is a positive correlation between annual rainfall and incidence of blackleg. Although the reason for this correlation is not fully understood, it has been postulated that the rain may assist in the dissemination of spores and that water saturation favors anaerobiosis of the soil, which is required for germination and multiplication of *C. chauvoei* spores. Cases of blackleg have frequently been reported in non-vaccinated cattle, approximately a week after they were moved to a fresh, lush pasture, suggesting the acquisition of infection from the environment.

Occasionally, cases of blackleg have been described in sheep, although, in many of those cases, the port of entry of the infection was reported to be a skin or mucosal wound. Because of that, those cases should be considered *C. chauvoei*-associated gas gangrene (Chapter 20) rather than true blackleg cases (see pathogenesis below). Infections by *C. chauvoei* have also been reported in humans, deer, goats, pigs, mink, horses, freshwater fish, whales, frogs, hens, and in an oryx, although the pathogenesis in these species has not been determined.

Pathogenesis

The pathogenesis of blackleg has not been fully elucidated. The classical model states that the pathogenesis of this disease starts with ingestion of spores of *C. chauvoei*, which sometimes may undergo one or more replication cycles in the intestine before being absorbed into the bloodstream. Once absorbed, the spores are distributed via blood circulation to multiple tissues, including skeletal and cardiac muscle. When they reach the muscle, the spores of *C. chauvoei* are phagocytized by local macrophages, in the cytoplasm of which they may remain latent for long periods of time without harmful effects to the host. When, and if, the redox potential decreases in areas of muscle where spores are present, the spores germinate and proliferate, producing the virulence factors that are responsible for the clinical signs and lesions of blackleg. Although blunt trauma has been traditionally blamed for reduction of the redox potential in muscle, this has never been proved, and the cause of this redox potential reduction remains undetermined. It has been suggested that, in addition to blunt trauma, hypoxia associated with excessive exercise or other factors may also predispose spore germination. One suggestion is that the peak of blackleg with lush summer conditions is also associated with "gadding" or running of cattle to try to escape biting flies. This sudden exertion by unfit fattening cattle may result in local ischemic muscle damage through lactic acidosis. The latter explanation of ischemia or hypoxia would help explain the few cases in which lesions have apparently been seen in the heart but not in skeletal muscles. Because of this pathogenesis, blackleg is regarded as an "endogenous" infection, as opposed to the "exogenous" mechanism of malignant edema (Chapter 20) in which the spores or vegetative forms of the clostridial species involved gain access to the tissues via skin or mucosal wounds.

This long-believed model of pathogenesis does not explain, however, outbreaks of disease that seem to happen year after year in some areas, or those cases that have occurred soon after animals have been moved to new pastures believed to be contaminated with *C. chauvoei* spores or fed feedstuff that is heavily contaminated with this microorganism. Although these cases do not necessarily rule out the classical model of blackleg pathogenesis (in which the spores remain latent in muscle until the ideal conditions for germination are met), they suggest that other pathogenic mechanisms may also exist. It is possible, for instance, that when animals are exposed to large loads of *C. chauvoei*, bacteremia or sporemia ensues directly from the intestine. Why there is an apparent preference for muscle for this microorganism to colonize and grow remains to be determined.

The pathogenesis of heart lesions in cases of blackleg is not completely understood either. In an outbreak of blackleg in sheep in which cardiac, but not skeletal, muscle lesions were seen, it was hypothesized that one or more of the following predisposing factors might have been involved: stress-induced increased cortisol and catecholamine levels, toxicants such as ionophores and gossypol, and selenium and vitamin E deficiency. In cases in which heart and musculoskeletal lesions occur together, it is possible that the latter develops first and the toxemia-associated hypoxia acts as predisposing factor for the cardiac lesions. The pericarditis observed usually associated with heart lesions is likely secondary to local extension of myocardial injury, although it might also be a consequence of septicemia.

It has been suggested that blackleg can also be caused by germination of spores from other clostridia endogenously present in muscle, for example *Clostridium novyi*, *Clostridium septicum*, and *Clostridium sordellii*, and this disease is often called "pseudoblackleg", reserving the term blackleg for *C. chauvoei* infection.

Clinical signs

Most cases of blackleg are acute or sub-acute, although chronic cases may occasionally occur. In most acute cases, animals are found dead without clinical signs having been observed. In some of the acute and sub-acute cases in which clinical signs are evident, they include depression, lethargy, anorexia, and reluctance to move, which is followed by circulatory collapse and death. Swelling and crepitation of the affected area is evident when superficial muscles are affected, usually associated with lameness, most commonly in the rear legs. Lesions in deep muscles such as the diaphragm, sub-lumbar area, or the heart are usually not detected clinically. In the rare cases in which the tongue is affected, the local swelling may cause protrusion of this organ outside the mouth. In cases in which the heart is affected, signs of congestive heart failure such as jugular vein distension and brisket edema may be seen. Other clinical signs associated with heart lesions of blackleg include increased diffuse lung sounds, abnormal breathing patterns, and pericardial friction rub. An excess of pericardial fluid may be observed ultrasonographically.

The clinical signs in sheep are similar to those in cattle. Sudden death was observed in lambs with *C. chauvoei* myocarditis.

Gross changes

Carcasses of animals dying of blackleg are usually in very good nutritional condition. In most cases, the large muscles of the rear quarters are affected, with the muscles of the front quarters and other skeletal muscles being less frequently involved. Although lesions in the heart were traditionally considered unusual, a recent study from California suggests that they are rather common, with the great majority of cases having lesions in both skeletal muscles and the heart. In the study referred to, only 3% of cases had lesions in the heart but not in the skeletal musculature. It was speculated that in that retrospective study, all cases might have had skeletal muscle lesions but that these were missed in some animals.

When superficial skeletal muscles are affected, swelling can often be seen externally, with the overlying skin being stretched and usually dark. Crepitation can be felt by palpation in the subcutaneous tissue of affected areas. The subcutaneous tissues and fasciae in affected areas are usually expanded by serosanguineous fluid in which many gas bubbles are present. Cut sections of affected muscles show discoloration ranging from dark red to black, and edema in the periphery of the lesions. The center of the lesions is dry, friable, dark red to black, and presents many small cavities associated with the presence of gas bubbles (Figure 19.1). Usually, a sweet odor, typically reminiscent of rancid butter, emanates from the affected tissues.

The gross lesions in the myocardium are similar to those in the skeletal muscle, and they can affect the walls of any of the chambers of the organ (Figure 19.2). They may be focal or multifocal. Pericarditis is frequently present; in these cases, the pericardium is diffusely congested and hemorrhagic and may be covered by a thin layer of fibrin (Figure 19.3); the two layers of the pericardial sac may be adhered to each other by fibrin. The presence of an excess of sero-sanguineous fluid in the pericardial sac is common. Fibrinous endocarditis is occasionally observed in areas associated with myocardial lesions. Fibrinous pleuritis affecting

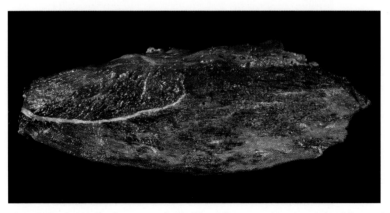

Figure 19.1 Skeletal muscle of a steer with blackleg. The tissue shows multifocal hemorrhage, necrosis, and many small cavities due to the presence of gas bubbles. Courtesy of S.S. Diab.

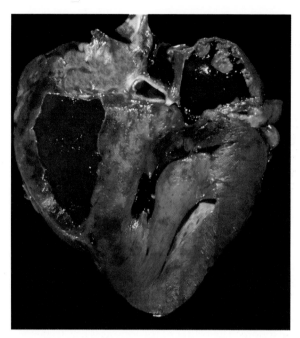

Figure 19.2 Heart of a steer with blackleg. The myocardium shows several dark areas of hemorrhage and necrosis.

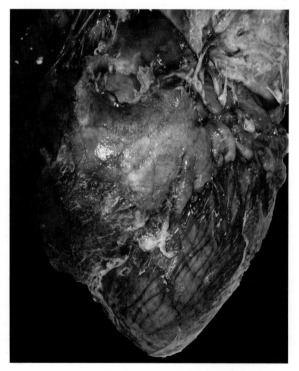

Figure 19.3 Heart of a steer with blackleg showing fibrinous pericarditis. The pericardial sac has been opened and the epicardium is visible. Courtesy of S.S. Diab.

the pleura adjacent to the heart can occasionally be seen. The lungs are almost always congested and edematous, and may show multifocal hemorrhage.

The gross lesions in sheep resemble those described in cattle.

Microscopic changes

The microscopic lesions of blackleg are, with only a few exceptions, very similar in both cardiac and skeletal muscle. The affected muscular fibers of both skeletal and cardiac muscle are swollen, hypereosinophilic, vacuolated, and fragmented; they show loss of cross striations, and hypercontraction bands are frequently seen (Figure 19.4). Some of the fragmented myofibers may be infiltrated by neutrophils, which, as the lesions progress, are progressively being replaced by macrophages, plasma cells, and lymphocytes. The interstitium is usually expanded by hemorrhage and proteinaceous edema. Leucocyte infiltration composed mostly of neutrophils, but also a few lymphocytes and plasma cells, is not a prominent feature of blackleg, although it tends to be more marked in later stages of the disease. Interstitial vessels may contain fibrin thrombi (Figure 19.5) and arteries and arterioles may show fibrinoid necrosis, with intramural infiltration of neutrophils. Large numbers of Gram-positive rods, single or in clusters, many of which contain a central, subterminal or, rarely, terminal spore, can be seen free in the interstitium (Figure 19.6), frequently surrounding affected

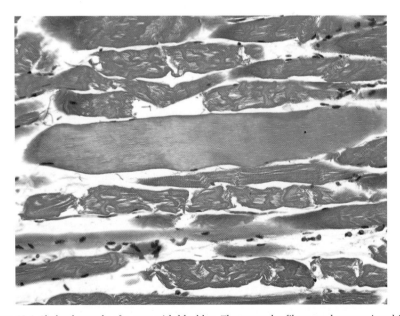

Figure 19.4 Skeletal muscle of a cow with blackleg. The muscular fibers are hypereosinophilic and show loss of cross striations; hypercontraction bands, vacuolation, and fragmentation are also seen. HE, 250x.

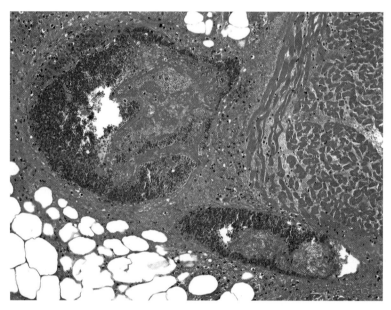

Figure 19.5 Skeletal muscle of a cow with blackleg showing thrombosis. The interstitium surrounding affected blood vessels shows neutrophilic infiltration and edema. HE, 250x.

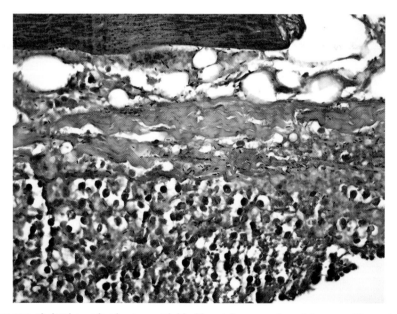

Figure 19.6 Skeletal muscle of a steer with blackleg. A large number of Gram-positive rods are present in the interstitium. Gram, 600x.

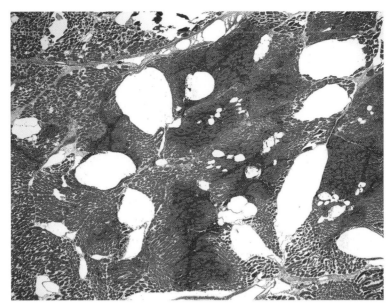

Figure 19.7 Skeletal muscle of a steer with blackleg showing diffuse hemorrhage and multifocal vacuoles caused by accumulation of gas in the tissues. HE, 40x.

vessels. Although the vascular changes can be observed in both skeletal and cardiac muscles, they are more prevalent in the latter. Large, empty vacuoles, representing spaces created by gas bubbles, are usually present in the interstitium (Figure 19.7). Microscopic lesions in the pericardial sac or pleura are characterized by fibrinosuppurative inflammation with hemorrhages and occasional vascular changes similar to those described in muscle.

The microscopic lesions of clostridial myocarditis in sheep are very similar to those in cattle.

Diagnosis

A presumptive diagnosis of blackleg can be made based on clinical history, clinical signs, and gross and microscopic changes. However, a final diagnosis should be based on identification of *C. chauvoei* in affected tissues. Detection of *C. chauvoei* can be achieved by anaerobic culture, fluorescent antibody test (FAT), PCR, or immunohistochemistry (IHC). Samples for culture should be collected as soon as possible after death, as invasion of other anaerobes from the gut occurs soon after death, which confuses cultural procedures. Differentiation between *C. chauvoei* and *C. septicum* is difficult due to morphological and biochemical similarities between these organisms. Identification of isolated strains is usually performed by conventional biochemical procedures, PCR or MALDI TOF. FAT is usually performed on tissue smears, although a few reports on the successful use

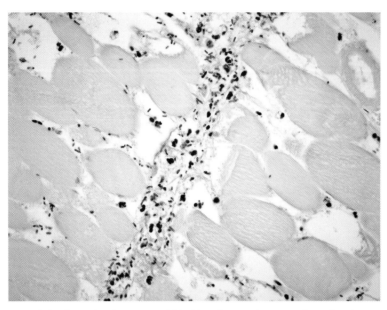

Figure 19.8 Skeletal muscle of a steer with blackleg showing large numbers of rods positively stained for *Clostridium chauvoei*. Streptavidine peroxidase, 600x.

of FAT on tissues that had been fixed for short periods of time in formalin have been published. IHC is performed on formalin-fixed tissues, which has the advantage of allowing the association of the microorganism with tissue morphology and lesions (Figure 19.8). Identification of *C. chauvoei* in animals with no lesions compatible with blackleg should not be considered diagnostically significant, as the spores of this microorganism can be present in the muscles of healthy cattle. A sandwich ELISA for detection of the flagellin of *C. chauvoei* has been used for detection of this microorganism, although this test is not currently commercially available.

"Pseudoblackleg", presumably caused by endogenous activation of spores of other histotoxic clostridia, can be differentiated by the means described above. *C. septicum* is a notorious post-mortem invader, so care must be taken to recognize where this may complicate the microbiologic diagnosis.

Prevention and treatment

Vaccination is the most important method currently available to prevent blackleg and pseudoblackleg, and this procedure forms part of the management of many cattle-producing operations worldwide. Most blackleg vaccines are bacterins produced from formalin-inactivated cultures of virulent strains of *C. chauvoei*, including bacterial cells and culture supernatant. These vaccines are generally available in polyvalent formulation, together with *C. novyi, C. septicum,* and *C. sordellii*, the agents of gas gangrene and pseudoblackleg. However, although there is abundant literature on the evaluation of *C. chauvoei* vaccines *in vivo* in cattle and other animal species, describing measurement of antibody titers and other features such as local reactions, there are very few articles describing clinical trials evaluating vaccine efficacy to prevent disease in cattle. Nevertheless, the limited studies published on this topic show that vaccination with *C. chauvoei* vaccines is close to 100% effective in preventing blackleg after natural exposure, and between 50% and 100% effective in protecting cattle from experimental challenge.

Initial vaccination against blackleg is recommended at 2 months of age, followed by a booster four to six weeks later. Boosters annually or every six months, depending on the severity of the problem in the area or ranch, are advisable until 2 years of age, after which vaccination is usually no longer necessary.

Although most current blackleg vaccines consist of whole cultures of *C. chauvoei*, the specific antigens critically responsible for inducing protective immunity are unknown. Guinea pigs vaccinated with recombinant CctA were highly protected against challenge with a virulent strain of *C. chauvoei*, suggesting that this toxin is a promising candidate to develop novel vaccines against blackleg.

Bibliography

Assis, R.A., *et al.* (2005) Immunohistochemical detection of Clostridia species in paraffin-embedded tissues of experimentally inoculated guinea pigs. *Pesq. Vet. Bras.*, **25**: 4–8.

Assis, R.A., *et al.* (2007) Detection of several clostridia by a direct fluorescent antibody test in formalin-fixed, paraffin-embedded tissues. *Arq. Bras. Med. Vet. Zootec.*, **59**: 1319–1322.

Bagge, E., *et al.* (2009) Detection and identification by PCR of *Clostridium chauvoei* in clinical isolates, bovine faeces and substrates from biogas plant. *Acta Vet. Scand.*, **51**: 8.

Falquet, L., *et al.* (2013) Draft Genome Sequence of the Virulent *Clostridium chauvoei* Reference Strain JF4335. *Genome Announc.*, **1**: e00593–13.

Frey, J., *et al.* (2012) Cytotoxin CctA, a major virulence factor of *Clostridium chauvoei* conferring protective immunity against myonecrosis. *Vaccine*, **30**: 5500–5505.

Frey, J., *et al.* (2015) Patho-genetics of *Clostridium chauvoei*. *Res. Microbiol.*, **166**: 384–392.

Glastonbury, J.R., *et al.* (1988) Clostridial myocarditis in lambs. *Aust. Vet. J.*, **65**: 208–209.

Groseth, P.K., *et al.* (2011) Large outbreak of blackleg in housed cattle. *Vet. Rec.*, **169**: 339.

Hogg, R., *et al.* (2009) Clostridial myocarditis in a scimitar-horned oryx. *Vet. Rec.*, **165**: 356.

Kojima, A., *et al.* (2000) Cloning and expression of a gene encoding the flagellin of *Clostridium chauvoei*. *Vet. Microbiol.*, **76**: 359–372.

Kojima, A., *et al.* (2001) Rapid detection and identification of *Clostridium chauvoei* by PCR based on flagellin gene sequence. *Vet. Microbiol.*, **78**: 363–371.

Langford, E.V. (1970) Feed-borne *Clostridium chauvoei* infection in mink. *Can. Vet. J.*, **11**: 170–172.

Mudenda Hang'ombe, B., *et al.* (2006) Purification and sensitivity of *Clostridium chauvoei* hemolysin to various erythrocytes. *Comp. Immunol. Microbiol. Infect. Dis.*, **29**: 263–268.

Nagano, N., *et al.* (2008) Human fulminant gas gangrene caused by *Clostridium chauvoei*. *J. Clin. Microbiol.*, **46**: 1545.

Popoff, M.R. (2014) Clostridial pore-forming toxins: Powerful virulence factors. *Anaerobe*, **30**: 220–238.

Prukner-Radovcic, E., *et al.* (1995) *Clostridium chauvoei* in hens. *Avian Pathol.*, **24**: 201–206.

Sasaki, Y., *et al.* (2002) Phylogenetic analysis and PCR detection of *Clostridium chauvoei*, *Clostridium haemolyticum*, *Clostridium novyi* types A and B, and *Clostridium septicum* based on the flagellin gene. *Vet. Microbiol.*, **86**: 257–267.

Sathish, S., *et al.* (2008) Molecular characterization of the diversity of *Clostridium chauvoei* isolates collected from two bovine slaughterhouses: Analysis of cross-contamination. *Anaerobe*, **14**: 190–199.

Smith, L.D.S., *et al.* (1984) *Clostridium chauvoei*. In: Smith, L.D.S. and Williams, B.L. (eds) *The Pathogenic Anaerobic Bacteria*, 3rd edition, pp. 164–175. Charles C. Thomas, Springfield, IL.

Snider, T.A., *et al.* (2011) Pathology in practice. Myocarditis and epicarditis. *J. Am. Vet. Med. Assoc.*, **238**: 1119–1121.

Sojka, J.E., *et al.* (1992) *Clostridium chauvoei* myositis infection in a neonatal calf. *J. Vet. Diagn. Invest.*, **4**: 201–203.

Useh, N.M., *et al.* (2003) Pathogenesis and pathology of blackleg in ruminants: The role of toxins and neuraminidase. A short review. *Vet. Q.*, **25**: 155–159.

Useh, N.M., *et al.* (2006) Relationship between outbreaks of blackleg in cattle and annual rainfall in Zaria, *Nigeria. Vet. Rec.*, **158**: 100–101.

Usharani, J., *et al.* (2015) Development of a recombinant flagellin based ELISA for the detection of *Clostridium chauvoei*. *Anaerobe*, **33**: 48–54.

Uzal, F.A. (2012) Evidence-based medicine concerning efficacy of vaccination against *Clostridium chauvoei* infection in cattle. *Vet. Clin. North Am. Food Anim. Pract.*, **28**: 71–77.

Uzal, F.A., *et al.* (2003) PCR detection of *Clostridium chauvoei* in pure cultures and in formalin-fixed, paraffin-embedded tissues. *Vet. Microbiol.*, **91**: 239–248.

Uzal, F.A., *et al.* (2003) Outbreak of clostridial myocarditis in calves. *Vet. Rec.*, **152**: 134–136.

Van Vleet, J.F., *et al.* (2007) Muscle and tendon. In: Maxie, M.G. (ed.) *Jubb, Kennedy, and Palmer's Pathology of Domestic Animals*, 5th edition, Vol. **1**, pp. 185–280. Saunders, Philadelphia.

Vilei, E.M., *et al.* (2011) Genetic and functional characterization of the NanA sialidase from *Clostridium chauvoei*. *Vet. Res.*, **42**: 2.

Weatherhead, J.E., *et al.* (2012) Lethal human neutropenic enterocolitis caused by *Clostridium chauvoei* in the United States: Tip of the iceberg? *J. Infect.*, **64**: 225–227.

20 Gas Gangrene (Malignant Edema)

Rodrigo O. S. Silva, Francisco A. Uzal, Carlos A. Oliveira Jr, and Francisco C. F. Lobato

Introduction

Gas gangrene, also called malignant edema, is a necrotizing clostridial infection of soft tissue that affects ruminants, horses, pigs, and occasionally other mammalian and avian species worldwide. We prefer the name gas gangrene because this is the term used in human medicine and is a more modern and well-established descriptive term. The disease is caused by one or more of the following clostridia: *Clostridium septicum*, *Clostridium chauvoei*, *Clostridium novyi* type A, *Clostridium perfringens* type A, and *Clostridium sordellii*. These agents are ubiquitous, and can be found in the environment and in the intestine of healthy animals and humans.

Etiology

A thorough description of the agents of gas gangrene and their toxins is presented in Chapters 3 and 4, respectively. Briefly, alpha-toxin (ATX), a β-pore-forming member of the aerolysin family, is considered the main virulence factor of *C. septicum*. *C. perfringens* type A is associated with enteric and histotoxic diseases of humans and animals. As an etiological agent of gas gangrene, *C. perfringens* type A is more prevalent in humans than in animals. Reversed genetics have demonstrated that alpha toxin (CPA) is the major virulence factor for *C. perfringens* type A gas gangrene. *C. chauvoei* is best known as the etiological agent of blackleg in ruminants (Chapter 19), but it may also be involved in cases of gas gangrene. Toxin A (CctA), an α-hemolysin, is considered to be the main virulence factor of *C. chauvoei*. *C. sordellii*'s lethal and hemorrhagic toxins (TcsL and TcsH, respectively) are the main virulence factors responsible for gas gangrene associated with this

Clostridial Diseases of Animals, First Edition. Francisco A. Uzal, J. Glenn Songer, John F. Prescott and Michel R. Popoff.
© 2016 John Wiley & Sons, Inc. Published 2016 by John Wiley & Sons, Inc.

microorganism. The alpha-toxin (TcnA) is considered the main virulence factor for type A *C. novyi*-associated gas gangrene. These five histotoxic clostridia produce spores that are variably resistant to heat, alcohol and acid pH, but then germinate returning to the vegetative form when exposed to an appropriately anoxic environment with the necessary nutrients and temperature. The spores are essential for the survival and maintenance of these agents and are directly linked to the epidemiology of gas gangrene.

Epidemiology

The incidence of gas gangrene seems to be higher in ruminants and horses than in other animal species. This, however, may be due to the environment in which these animals live and the way they are managed, rather than differences in species susceptibility. Cases of gas gangrene may occur in individuals of any age, including neonates; no breed or gender predisposition has been reported.

The clostridial agents of gas gangrene, including their spores, are ubiquitous, most of them being commonly isolated from the intestinal content of animals and the environment, mostly from soils rich in organic matter and high humidity. Soils that become flooded seasonally are more commonly contaminated by these microorganisms than are dry soils. The presence of wild or domestic animal feces and/or animal carcasses in the pastures can increase the level of soil contamination.

In several parts of the world, *C. septicum* is considered the most prevalent cause of gas gangrene. However, this microorganism is also a frequent post-mortem invader, and its presence should be cautiously interpreted in animals that have been dead for a while, since invasion of tissues by *C. septicum* present in the intestine may start very soon after death or even during the agonal period. Association between two or more of the histotoxic clostridia is not unusual as the cause of gas gangrene, and may further be complicated by the presence of aerobic bacteria such as *E. coli*.

Gas gangrene occurs sporadically, but outbreaks may also occur, mostly associated with injection of contaminated products or lack of hygiene during medical or surgical procedures. The disease is highly lethal.

Pathogenesis

Based on the limited current knowledge about gas gangrene of animals, it is thought that the pathogenesis of the disease is similar in all animal species. The disease starts with contamination of wounds with spores or vegetative forms of one or more of the clostridial species responsible for the disease, which are usually in the environment. Aerobic bacterial contamination can sometimes help render the local environment more anoxic and encourage the germination of spores. As is the case for tetanus, deep wounds or traumatic injuries help establish the anoxic environment required for the growth of clostridia.

The most frequent means of entry of these agents in animals include vaccination, parturition, shearing, branding, neutering, docking, and blood extraction. Gas gangrene can also occur in foals and sporadically in ruminants as a result of umbilical infections, while in rams, gas gangrene caused by *C. novyi* type A is commonly associated with fights (head butting), a condition sometimes known as "big head". Cases of gangrenous mastitis have been described in cattle and sheep. In sheep, some of these cases were associated with excessive vacuum from the milking machine. The reduced redox potential caused by anoxia associated with traumatic or deep wounds, or by local irritants in the case of some injection wounds, and the presence of metabolites from decomposing protein commonly found in these initial tissue lesions contribute to germination of spores and proliferation of vegetative clostridia.

In addition to the main virulence factors mentioned earlier in this chapter for the agents of gas gangrene, most strains of the histotoxic clostridia produce numerous tissue-degrading enzymes such as collagenases, DNAses, hyaluronidases, and neuraminidases, and pore-forming toxins, which also contribute to tissue damage, nutrient acquisition, and evasion of host defenses, thus allowing the spread of infection. Most of the toxins produced by the histotoxic clostridia act first locally, producing tissue necrosis which, in turn, provides an ideal environment for further multiplication of these microorganisms and further production of toxins, which eventually gain access to the systemic circulation, producing toxemia, shock, and death. Bacteremia may also occur, and the agents of gas gangrene can be found in several distant organs. In some cases, intravascular hemolysis can also occur as a consequence of toxemia, mainly when *C. perfringens* type A is involved.

Although contaminated wounds are the most common port of entry for the agents of malignant edema in animals, some cases of gas gangrene in which no previous trauma has been identified have been described in humans and a non-human primate. The pathogenesis of this infection is not fully understood and it is believed that the agent, commonly *C. perfringens*, gains access to the bloodstream via a damaged mucosal barrier, thus reaching muscles and other organs. The pathogenesis of these infections may also be similar to that of blackleg, and involve germination of endogenous spores present in these tissues or previously healthy animals.

Clinical signs

Clinical signs are similar in most animal species. The disease is almost always acute, although occasionally sub-acute and chronic cases can occur. A few hours post infection, the area surrounding the port of entry shows swelling and erythema; this lesion is usually painful and hot. As time passes, and progress is usually rapid, there is increasing swelling associated with subcutaneous edema and emphysema; the latter becomes evident as crepitation on palpation. The skin is taut and diffusely red or black with bruises and suffusions. Depression, tachycardia, muscle tremors, and hyperthermia are almost always present. When a limb is affected, the animal shows reluctance to move and lameness, followed by recumbency. In later stages of the disease, the affected area becomes cold, the pain disappears due to the necrosis of local nerve endings, and sub-normal body temperatures are common. In most cases, death occurs by toxemia and systemic shock between a few hours to 2–4 days after the onset of clinical signs. Occasionally, animals are found dead without clinical signs having been observed. Rare cases of chronic disease with death occurring up to 30 days post infection have been reported. In these cases, treatment with penicillin G may have delayed the usual rapid progression of disease and localized the infection to necrotic tissue; the outcome is inevitably usually fatal, either because of the progression of disease or through euthanasia.

Despite the similarity of clinical signs in all species, a few specific forms of the disease have been described. In rams, fighting injuries can lead to a clinical condition called "big head", a specific form of gas gangrene characterized by a non-gaseous, non-hemorrhagic, edematous swelling of the head, face, and neck of young individuals. This form is typically associated with *C. novyi* type A, but *C. sordellii* or *C chauvoei* can also be involved. Post-parturient gas gangrene of cattle, a form of necrotizing vulvo-vaginitis and metritis usually described in first-calf-heifers, is characterized by vulvar swelling that starts 1 to 3 days after calving, accompanied by hyperthermia and depression, and culminates in recumbency and death. In avian gas gangrene, affected animals present depression, anorexia, and ataxia due to toxemia. This form of the disease is typically produced by *C. septicum*.

Gross changes

Gross changes related to gas gangrene in most animal species are similar and, regardless of the clostridial species involved, include mainly diffuse hemorrhagic and gelatinous subcutaneous edema and emphysema (Figure 20.1). The underlying muscles are not always affected, but when they are, they show multifocal to diffuse areas of dark red, gray, or blue discoloration (Figures 20.2 and 20.3). Serosal and sub-endocardial hemorrhages, congested and edematous spleen, lungs, and liver are frequently observed as a consequence of the severe toxemia that characterizes this disease.

Cases of gas gangrene in which *C. septicum* or *C. perfringens* are involved are usually characterized by severe systemic changes and rapid dissemination of these organisms from the port of entry. Marked gas production is also commonly reported when *C. perfringens* is the etiological agent. Cases associated with *C. chauvoei*, *C. sordellii*, or *C. novyi* type A tend to be more focal.

In post-parturient gas gangrene of cattle, diffuse perineal and perivaginal gelatinous and hemorrhagic edema is common, which sometimes extends to adjacent musculature. Petechiation of serous membranes is a common finding, while multifocal areas of necrosis and ulceration are observed in vulvar, vaginal, and uterine mucosae, which might be covered by a fibrinous pseudomembrane.

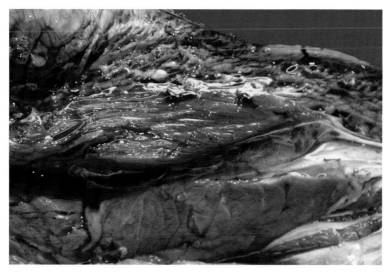

Figure 20.1 Gas gangrene produced by *Clostridium novyi* in a 2-month-old calf following castration. Note the severe subcutaneous edema, emphysema, and hemorrhage.

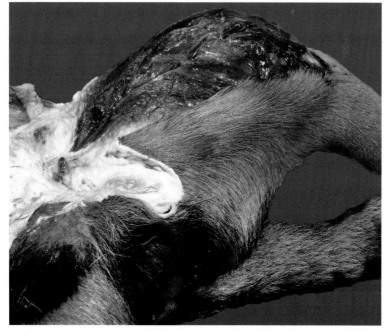

Figure 20.2 Gas gangrene caused by *Clostridium septicum* in a 10-month-old male Rottweiler dog. Note edema, hemorrhage, and dark red discoloration of affected muscle.

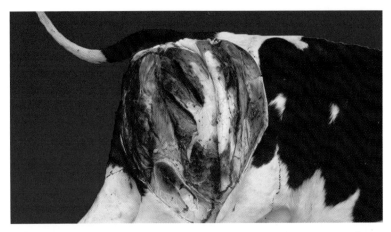

Figure 20.3 Gas gangrene caused by *Clostridium septicum* in a steer after intramuscular injection with a contaminated needle. Note the dark red discoloration of affected muscles indicating hemorrhage and necrosis.

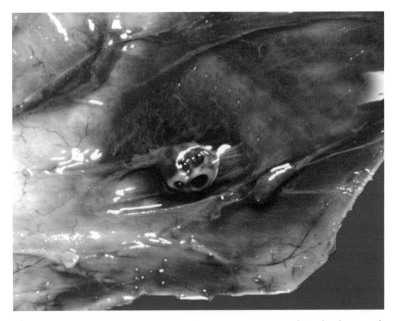

Figure 20.4 Omphalophlebitis caused by *Clostridium septicum* in a newborn lamb. Note the internal umbilical remnant showing edema, swelling, and hemorrhage.

Cases of omphalophlebitis caused by *C. septicum*, *C. sordellii*, or *C. perfringens* have been described in foals and lambs. The internal umbilical remnant commonly shows swelling, lack of elasticity, and hemorrhage (Figure 20.4). Edema in abdominal muscles and subcutaneous tissue around the navel is common, and hemorrhage can be seen in parietal peritoneum and serosal surfaces of the abdominal organs. The peritoneal fluid is commonly reddish and foul smelling. Concomitant cases of uroperitoneum are common. Gangrenous mastitis in sheep and cattle is characterized by a clear line of demarcation between affected and unaffected tissue that can be seen externally (Figure 20.5) and severe edema and hemorrhage of the subcutaneous tissue and mammary gland (Figure 20.6). The rare chronic cases of gas gangrene described are characterized by extensive loss of tissue, usually with unsuccessful regeneration attempts (Figure 20.7).

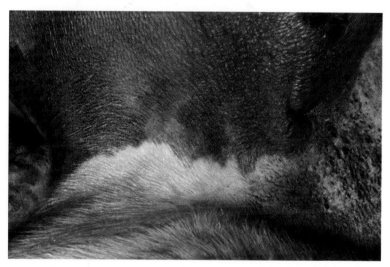

Figure 20.5 Gangrenous mastitis in a ewe due to *Clostridium novyi*. Note the clear line of demarcation between the skin overlying the gangrenous mammary gland and the surrounding normal-looking skin. *Staphylococcus aureus* was also isolated from the mammary gland in this case.

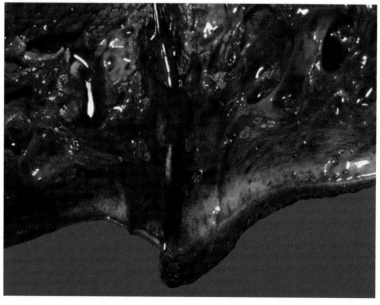

Figure 20.6 Gangrenous mastitis in a ewe due to *Clostridium novyi* (same animal as in Figure 20.5). Note severe subcutaneous edema, which is also affecting the adjacent mammary gland.

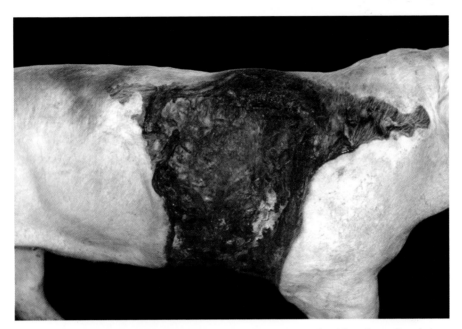

Figure 20.7 Chronic gas gangrene caused by *Clostridium septicum, Clostridium chauvoei*, and *Clostridium sordellii* in a pig. The port of entry in this case was not determined. Courtesy of J.M. Benoit.

Microscopic changes

As is the case for gross changes, the microscopic changes in gas gangrene are very similar among animal species, regardless of the clostridial species involved. These changes are characterized by edema, hemorrhage, vasculitis, and thrombosis in subcutaneous tissue, which may extend to the fasciae and muscular tissue (Figure 20.8). The infiltration of inflammatory exudate, mostly composed of neutrophils, in subcutaneous tissue and musculature may vary from minimal to very marked. Typically, little or no inflammatory infiltrate is present in lesions produced by *C. perfringens* type A, a phenomenon which is a consequence of the leukostatic action of CPA. Abundant Gram-positive bacilli with central, subterminal, or occasionally terminal spores, single or in clusters, are usually seen within areas of edema or hemorrhage. Filamentous bacilli may be seen when *C. septicum* is involved. Necrosis of adjacent skeletal muscle similar to that seen in cases of blackleg (Chapter 19) may be observed.

In post-parturient gas gangrene of cattle, ulcers and necrosis could be seen in the vagina, vulva, and uterus. The ulcer beds are commonly infiltrated by large numbers of inflammatory cells, cell debris, and fibrin. In clostridial omphalophlebitis of horses and other species, severe inflammation is observed in umbilical vessels, urachus, and other tissues of the umbilical cord. Diffuse edema and congestion are common findings in all tissues around the navel.

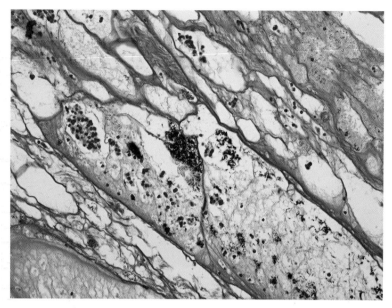

Figure 20.8 Subcutaneous tissue of a cow with malignant edema by *Clostridium septicum*. There is severe edema distending the connective tissue, and large clusters of intralesional bacilli.

Diagnosis

A presumptive diagnosis of gas gangrene may be established based on clinical signs and gross and microscopic changes. Gas gangrene must be differentiated from other acute diseases of ruminants, such as anthrax, bacillary hemoglobinuria, snake bites, and intoxication by several plants or drugs. Post-mortem examination and collection of samples for diagnostic work-up must be performed as soon as possible after death to avoid false positive results due to invasion of muscle and other tissues by clostridial species originating in the intestine. Examination of smears from affected subcutaneous tissue and/or muscle stained with Gram, in which large Gram-positive rods are observed, provides strong supportive evidence for a presumptive diagnosis of malignant edema.

Confirmation of the diagnosis should rely on identification of the clostridia involved by anaerobic culture, fluorescent antibody test (FAT) (Figures 20.9 and 20.10), PCR, and/or immunohistochemistry (Figure 20.11) in tissues with lesions compatible with gas gangrene. Isolated organisms can be identified by conventional biochemical techniques, PCR, or by MALDI TOF. Cultural procedures may be complicated by the invasive potential of *C. septicum*, which grows very rapidly and, during transportation or culture, often overgrows other clostridia present in the specimens. Examination of smears from fresh tissues by FAT helps avoid this issue by providing an assessment of the clostridial species present at the time of sample collection. For this reason, it is important to prepare the smears at the time of necropsy and/or sample collection rather than

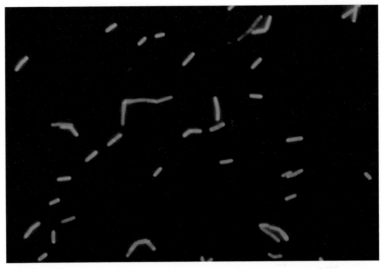

Figure 20.9 Direct fluorescent antibody test for *Clostridium septicum* on a smear of muscle from a calf with malignant edema. 400x.

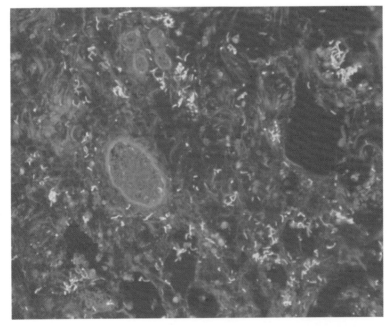

Figure 20.10 Direct fluorescent antibody test for *Clostridium septicum* on formalin-fixed, paraffin-embedded, subcutaneous tissue of a cow with malignant edema. 200x.

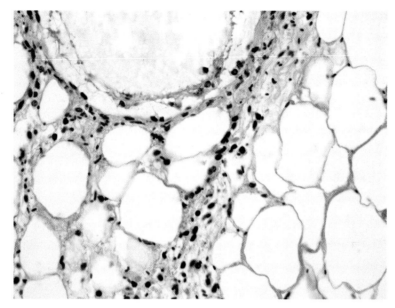

Figure 20.11 Immunohistochemistry (streptavidin-biotin peroxidase) for *Clostridium septicum* in the fascia of a sheep with malignant edema. 400x.

once the samples arrive at the laboratory. Immunohistochemistry has been used successfully to detect all the clostridial species involved in malignant edema on formalin-fixed tissues (Figure 20.11). Demonstration of these organisms in tissues from animals with no compatible lesions is not diagnostic, as some of these clostridia can invade tissues very soon after death.

Treatment, control, and prophylaxis

Because most cases of gas gangrene in ruminants are acute with a short clinical course, there is frequently no time to start treatment. When possible, affected animals should receive procaine penicillin G, an antibiotic with outstanding activity against the etiological agents of gas gangrene. In valuable animals, in addition to the antibiotic treatment recommended for ruminants, anti-inflammatory drugs, fluid therapy, and incisions of the skin over the affected muscles to drain exudates and gas, and washing these wounds with hydrogen peroxide and iodine solution are often recommended. However, even when treated early, studies report survival rates lower than 80% for horses and lower than 50% for ruminants.

Considering that the spores of all the clostridial species responsible for gas gangrene are extremely resistant to environmental conditions and several disinfectants, and that those species are frequently found in soil and as part of the microbiota of animals, the eradication of any of the etiological agents of gas gangrene is not possible. Prevention and control should, therefore, be based on immunization of the animals, on strict hygienic measures including surgical hygiene, on navel treatment with antiseptics, and avoidance of soil or fecal contamination of wounds. Proper carcass disposal helps reduce soil contamination with clostridia, but preventing predisposition is the key to controlling infection. Systematic vaccination of ruminants with a combination of bacterins and toxoids against the five *Clostridium* species involved in gas gangrene results in a marked reduction of the incidence of this disease. Animals aged between 4 and 6 months, or younger in areas where gas gangrene is endemic, should receive two doses of the vaccine against gas gangrene, with an interval of four weeks between the immunizations. An annual booster is recommended.

Bibliography

Aronoff, D.M. (2013) *Clostridium novyi, C. sordellii,* and *C. tetani*: Mechanisms of disease. *Anaerobe*, **24**: 98–101.

Awad, M.M., *et al.* (1995) Virulence studies on chromosomal alpha-toxin and theta-toxin mutants constructed by allelic exchange provide genetic evidence for the essential role of alpha-toxin in *Clostridium perfringens*-mediated gas gangrene. *Mol. Microbiol.*, **15**: 191–202.

Awad, M.M., *et al.* (2001) Synergistic effects of alpha-toxin and perfringolysin O in *Clostridium perfringens*-mediated gas gangrene. *Infect. Immun.*, **69**: 7904–7910.

Carter, G.P., *et al.* (2014) Regulation of toxin production in the pathogenic clostridia. *Mol. Microbiol.*, **91**: 221–231.

Farias Lobato, D.F., *et al.* (2014) Acute myonecrosis in horse caused by *Clostridium novyi* type A. *Braz. J. Microbiol.*, **45**: 221–224.

Kennedy, C.L., *et al.* (2005) The α-toxin of *Clostridium septicum* is essential for virulence. *Mol. Microbiol.*, **57**: 1357–1366.

Odani, J.S., *et al.* (2009) Malignant edema in postpartum dairy cattle. *J. Vet. Diagn. Invest.*, **21**: 920–924.

Ortega, J., *et al.* (2007) Infection of Internal Umbilical Remnant in Foals by *Clostridium sordellii*. *Vet. Pathol.*, **44**: 269–275.

Peek, S.F., *et al.* (2003) Clostridial myonecrosis in horses (37 cases 1985–2000). *Equine Vet. J.*, **35**: 86–92.

Ribeiro, M.G., *et al.* (2012) Myonecrosis by *Clostridium septicum* in a dog, diagnosed by a new multiplex-PCR. *Anaerobe*, **18**: 504–507.

Sasaki, Y., *et al.* (2001) Tetracycline-resistance genes of *Clostridium perfringens, Clostridium septicum* and *Clostridium sordellii* isolated from cattle affected with malignant edema. *Vet. Microbiol.*, **83**: 61–69.

Stevens, D.L., *et al.* (2012) Life-threatening clostridial infections. *Anaerobe*, **18**: 254–259.

Uzal, F.A., *et al.* (2014) Towards an understanding of the role of *Clostridium perfringens* toxins in human and animal disease. *Future Microbiol.*, **9**: 361–377.

Uzal, F.A., *et al.* (2015) Animal models to study the pathogenesis of human and animal *Clostridium perfringens* infections. *Vet. Microbiol.*, **179**: 23–33.

Verherstraeten, S., *et al.* (2015) Perfringolysin O: The Underrated *Clostridium perfringens* toxin? *Toxins*, **7**: 1702–1721.

Willoughby, D.H., *et al.* (1996) Periodic recurrence of gangrenous dermatitis associated with *Clostridium septicum* in a broiler chicken operation. *J. Vet. Diagn. Invest.*, **8**: 259–261.

Yasuda, M., *et al.* (2015) A case of nontraumatic gas gangrene in a common marmoset (*Callithrix jacchus*). *J. Vet. Med. Sci.*, Epub ahead of print.

21 Gangrenous Dermatitis in Poultry

H. L. Shivaprasad

Introduction

Gangrenous dermatitis (GD) is a common disease of broiler chickens and turkeys caused by various species of anaerobic and aerobic bacteria, including several clostridial species. The disease is characterized by a sudden increase in mortality and lesions in the skin, subcutaneous tissue, and the underlying muscles, usually over the keel, abdomen, thigh, and wings. GD is a disease of considerable economic significance in poultry and occurs throughout the world.

GD has also been called cellulitis and clostridial dermatitis, especially in turkeys, as well as gangrenous dermatomyositis, blue wing disease, and avian malignant edema, amongst others, in broiler chickens. The disease is most common in commercial broiler chickens and turkeys raised on re-used deep-litter production systems. GD can result in increased condemnation rates and downgrading of the carcasses at processing plants. GD should be distinguished from cellulitis in broiler chickens caused by *Escherichia coli*, which is characterized by fibrinonecrotic inflammation of the subcutaneous tissue.

Etiology

Various anaerobic and aerobic bacteria have been associated with GD. These include mainly *Clostridium septicum* and *Clostridium perfringens* type A, and, occasionally *Clostridium sordellii*, *Staphylococcus aureus*, *E. coli*, *Pseudomonas aeruginosa*, and others. However, most of the outbreaks of GD have been associated with *C. septicum* and *C. perfringens*, either alone or in combination with some of the aerobic bacteria mentioned above acting as secondary contaminants. There is

Clostridial Diseases of Animals, First Edition. Francisco A. Uzal, J. Glenn Songer, John F. Prescott and Michel R. Popoff.

experimental evidence that *C. septicum* is more significant than *C. perfringens* in causing GD based on subcutaneous inoculation in turkeys.

C. septicum and *C. perfringens* are found in the environment, especially in the soil and litter. *C. perfringens* is part of the normal flora of the intestines of many animals, including chickens and turkeys. *C. septicum* has also been isolated from the intestine of normal animals including chickens. *C. septicum* produces at least four major toxins, namely alpha, beta, delta, and gamma (Chapter 4). Alpha toxin, a cytolysin, is a lethal toxin which is considered the critical virulence factor for GD.

Multilocus sequence typing (MLST) analysis of numerous isolates of *C. septicum* from poultry has revealed a highly conserved core genome. All strains of *C. perfringens* produce alpha toxin (CPA), while some of them may also produce other toxins, including NetB (Chapter 5). The role of the individual toxins of *C. perfringens* type A in the pathogenesis of GD is not known although it is thought that, as is the case for all the diseases produced by this microorganism, GD is mediated by one or more of the toxins produced by *C. perfringens*, with CPA likely playing the most critical role.

Epidemiology

GD occurs most commonly in market-age broiler chickens (> 35 days) and turkeys (> 13–16 weeks). GD has been known to occur in the same farms in successive flocks. The mode of transmission is not well understood but it is thought that the bacteria are transmitted through a break in the skin or ingestion of contaminated feed and/or water. Breaks in the skin of chickens and turkeys are common due to scratching by toe nails and biting by pen mates, and may be exacerbated by aggression between the birds. Factors such as overcrowding, poor and wet litter conditions, increased humidity, reduced resting of buildings between broods of birds, poor hygienic conditions, contaminated equipment, use of contaminated animal byproducts in the feed, multi-age birds on the ranch/farm, failure to remove dead birds in a timely manner, and contaminated feed and water can all predispose GD, likely because of the build-up of clostridial pathogens in the environment. Administration of dexamethasone, an immunosuppressive drug, has been shown to promote high incidence of GD in turkeys, and supports the notion that "stress" may be a further predisposing factor. GD has also been known to occur more often in males than in females, perhaps because they are larger or more aggressive, and to be more prevalent in certain strains or breeds; the disease is seen more often in spring.

GD can also occur secondarily to various immunosuppressive diseases such as infectious bursal disease caused by Birnavirus and chicken infectious anemia caused by Circovirus, both in chickens, and hemorrhagic enteritis caused by group II Adenovirus in turkeys.

Feeds containing growth-promoting antibiotics have also been known to be associated with outbreaks of GD. There is also anecdotal evidence that the use of ionophores to control coccidia can predispose the birds to GD. It is speculated that ionophores disturb the normal intestinal flora, resulting in overgrowth of *C. septicum* and *C. perfringens*, which are then absorbed into the bloodstream and reach the skin, where they cause GD.

Pathogenesis

The pathogenesis of GD is poorly understood. The so-called "outside-in" theory suggests that a break in the skin of birds provides an optimal environment for colonization from the contaminated environment of *C. septicum* and/or *C. perfringens* of the skin, with subsequent invasion of the subcutis and underlying muscles, causing the typical lesions of the disease. It is assumed that the disease is mediated by one or more toxins produced by these bacteria which, as noted, may act synergistically. Another theory, called "inside-out", suggests that pathogenic bacteria and/or their toxins enter the circulation though a damaged intestinal wall and localize in the skin, resulting in the lesions of GD, but this theory seems far less likely.

It has been demonstrated that chickens with GD have lower T-cell and B-cell mitogen-stimulated lymphoproliferation, higher levels of nitric oxide and α-1-acid glycoprotein, a greater number of MHC class II intradermal and intraepithelial lymphocytes, and increased levels of mRNAs encoding pro-inflammatory cytokines and chemokines in skin compared to GD-free chickens.

Clinical signs

Because of the acute onset of the disease there may be no clinical signs observed in the affected birds. When observed, clinical signs consist of depression, lack of coordination, lateral recumbency, inappetence, leg weakness, ataxia, and high fever. Fluid accumulation or edema can be observed in the lower abdomen and inner thighs. Mortality in a flock is usually low, although it can be variable, ranging from a few dead birds per day to 3% per day. However, morbidity and mortality as high as 60% have been reported in some flocks.

Gross changes

Gross lesions generally involve the breast, lower abdomen, inner thighs, and occasionally the neck, head, and tail. The typical lesion is characterized by large areas of moist skin which can be featherless and dark to reddish-purple, or green (Figure 21.1), with multifocal ulcerations. Subcutaneous accumulation of serosanguinous fluid with or without emphysema can also be observed (Figure 21.2). Underlying muscles are discolored and their appearance can range from pale to dark red or black (Figure 21.3) with occasional white streaks. The

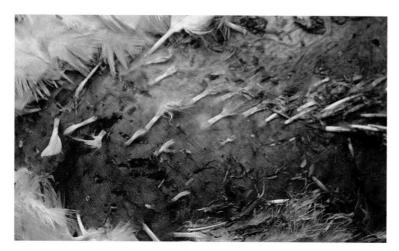

Figure 21.1 Gangrenous dermatitis in a 14-day-old turkey showing wet and dark skin.

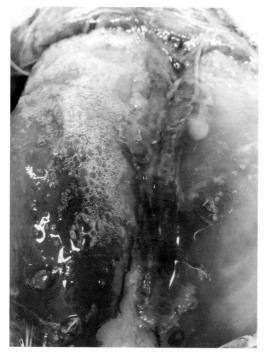

Figure 21.2 Gangrenous dermatitis in a 38-day-old broiler chicken showing subcutaneous accumulation of serosanguinous fluid with gas bubbles (emphysema).

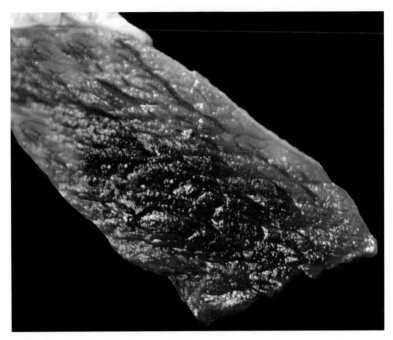

Figure 21.3 Dark discoloration due to hemorrhage in the muscle of a turkey with gangrenous dermatitis.

muscles can be crepitant due to the presence of gas in the interstitium. In one experiment, 11 of 14 turkey poults inoculated subcutaneously with *C. septicum* died within 12 hours of inoculation and were found to have developed fibrinous pericarditis, pleuritis, and peritonitis, and generalized vascular congestion, but no cellulitis. In another experiment, 10-week-old turkeys given an isolate of *C. septicum* intravenously developed cellulitis followed by death within 36 hours.

Microscopic changes

In uncomplicated cases of gangrenous dermatitis caused by *C. septicum* or *C. perfringens*, the most consistent lesion is proteinaceous, acidophilic subcutaneous edema (Figure 21.4), in which numerous large, Gram-positive rods are seen (Figure 21.5). The underlying skeletal muscles show various degrees of degeneration and necrosis, with large numbers of Gram-positive bacilli, but usually without a significant inflammatory infiltrate (Figure 21.6).

In cases complicated with *S. aureus*, fibrinous exudate mixed with heterophils and numerous Gram-positive cocci are present in the dermis. There is often necrosis of the epidermis, with frequent ulceration and inflammation in the dermis and subcutis (Figure 21.7).

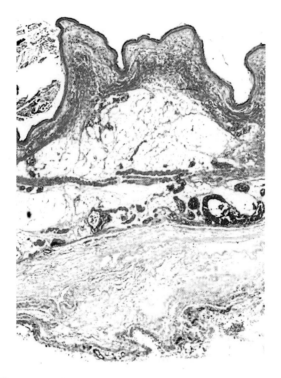

Figure 21.4 Serofibrinous exudate and emphysema in the subcutis of a broiler chicken with gangrenous dermatitis. HE, 40x.

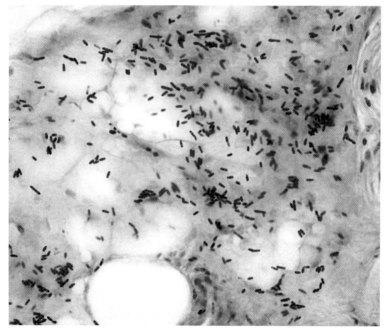

Figure 21.5 Large numbers of Gram-positive rods in the subcutaneous serofibrinous exudate of a broiler chicken with gangrenous dermatitis. HE, 400x.

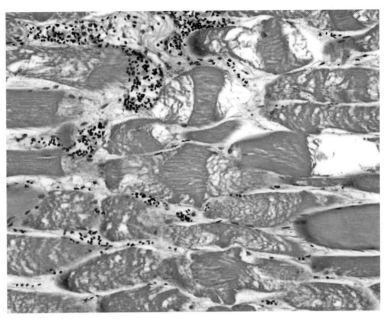

Figure 21.6 Skeletal muscle of a chicken with gangrenous dermatitis, showing degeneration, necrosis, and mild inflammatory infiltrate. HE, 200x.

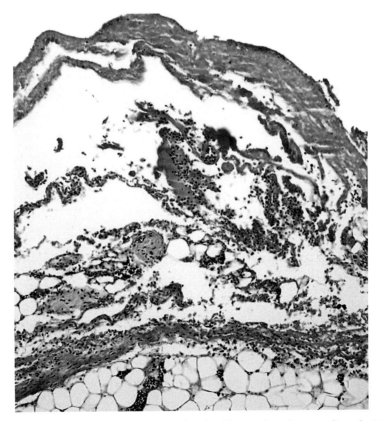

Figure 21.7 Gangrenous dermatitis produced by *Clostridium septicum*, but complicated with *Staphylococcus aureus* infection in a chicken. There is necrosis of the epidermis with ulceration, and inflammatory infiltrate in the dermis and subcutis. HE, 100x.

Diagnosis

A presumptive diagnosis of GD in a flock can be made based on a history of sudden increase in mortality, coupled with clinical signs and the characteristic skin lesions. The presence of Gram-positive bacilli on impression smears of the serosanguineous exudate adds support to the presumptive diagnosis. Confirmation of GD should be based on detection of the involved microorganisms in the subcutis and/or underlying muscle by culture, fluorescent antibody test, and/or immunohistochemistry (Figure 21.8). Concomitant immunosuppressive diseases such as infectious bursal disease and chicken infectious anemia in chickens, and hemorrhagic enteritis in turkeys, can predispose the birds to GD and should therefore also be investigated.

Control, treatment, and prophylaxis

Currently there are no vaccines commercially available to prevent GD. Experimentally, bacterins or toxoids of *C. septicum* given subcutaneously to turkeys at 1 day or 6 weeks of age have been shown to reduce losses due to GD. Similarly, a mixed clostridial bacterin containing *C. chauvoei* and *C. septicum* given subcutaneously to 1-day-old broiler chicks also reduced losses due to GD.

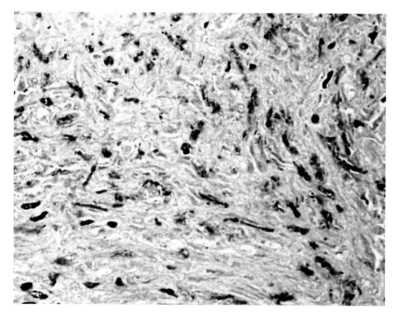

Figure 21.8 Immunohistochemistry (streptavidin-biotin peroxidase) for *Clostridium septicum* in the subcutaneous tissue of a broiler chicken with gangrenous dermatitis.

A non-cytolytic alpha-toxin recombinant protein of *C. septicum* given to 3-day-old turkey poults followed by another vaccination after five weeks, provided 78% to 95% protection after subcutaneous challenge with *C. septicum* 81 days later.

GD can be treated effectively with many antibiotics including chlortetracycline, oxytetracycline, erythromycin, and penicillin in the water, or with chlortetracycline in the feed. However, in outbreaks predisposed by immunosuppressive viral diseases and other factors, antibiotic treatments are ineffective. This is why prevention of immunosuppressive diseases and other predisposing factors is critical to avoid outbreaks of GD.

In antibiotic-free flocks, water treatment with copper sulfate or drinking water acidification with citric or propionic acid have been used to reduce, but not eliminate, GD. There is considerable scope to reduce the well-established environmental predisposing factors described earlier.

Bibliography

Carr, D., *et al.* (1996) Excessive mortality in market-age turkeys associated with cellulitis. *Avian Dis.,* **40**: 736–741.

Cervantes, H.M., *et al.* (1988) Staphylococcus-induced gangrenous dermatitis in broilers. *Avian Dis.,* **32**: 140–142.

Clark, S., *et al.* (2010) Clostridial dermatitis and cellulitis: An emerging disease of turkeys. A Review. *Avian Dis.,* **54**: 788–794.

Hofacre, C.L., *et al.* (1988) Subcutaneous clostridial infection in broilers. *Avian Dis.,* **30**: 620–622.

Huff, G.R., *et al.* (2013) Dexamethasone immunosuppression resulting in turkey clostridial dermatitis: A retrospective analysis of seven studies, 1998–2009. *Avian Dis.,* **57**: 730–736.

Kim, D.K., *et al.* (2012) Genome-wide differential gene expression profiles in broiler chickens with gangrenous dermatitis. *Avian Dis.,* **56**: 670–679.

Lancto, C.A., *et al.* (2014) A noncytolytic α toxin recombinant protein protects turkeys against *Clostridium septicum* challenge. *Avian Dis.,* **58**: 566–571.

Lee, K.W., *et al.* (2012) *Clostridium perfringens* alpha-toxin and NetB toxin antibodies and their possible role in protection against necrotic enteritis and gangrenous dermatitis in broiler chickens. *Avian Dis.,* **56**: 230–233.

Li, G., *et al.* (2010a) An outbreak of gangrenous dermatitis in commercial broiler chickens. *Avian Pathol.,* **39**: 247–253.

Li, G., *et al.* (2010b) Immunopathology and cytokine responses in commercial broiler chickens with gangrenous dermatitis. *Avian Pathol.,* **39**: 255–264.

Neumann, A.P., *et al.* (2009) MLST analysis reveals a highly conserved core genome among poultry isolates of *Clostridium septicum*. *Anaerobe,* **15**: 99–106.

Neumann, A.P., *et al.* (2010) Quantitative real-time PCR assay for *Clostridium septicum* in poultry gangrenous dermatitis associated samples. *Mol. Cell Probes,* **24**: 211–218.

Opengart, K. (2013) Gangrenous Dermatitis. In: Swayne, D.E. (ed.) *Diseases of Poultry,* 13th edition, pp. 957–960. Wiley-Blackwell, Ames, Iowa.

Rosenberger, J.K., *et al.* (1975) The roles of the infectious bursal agent and several avian adenoviruses in the hemorrhagic-aplastic-anemia syndrome and gangrenous dermatitis. *Avian Dis.,* **19**: 17–29.

Tellez, G. *et al.* (2009) Evidence for *Clostridium septicum* as a primary cause of cellulitis in commercial turkeys. *J. Vet. Diagn. Invest.,* **21**: 374–377.

Thachil, A.J., *et al.* (2010) Role of *Clostridium perfringens* and *Clostridium septicum* in causing turkey cellulitis. *Avian Dis.*, **54**: 795–801.

Thachil, A.J., *et al.* (2013) Vaccination of turkeys with *Clostridium septicum* bacterin-toxoid: Evaluation of protection against clostridial dermatitis. *Avian Dis.*, **57**: 214–219.

Thachil, A.J., *et al.* (2014) Effects of dexamethasone immunosuppression on turkey clostridial dermatitis. *Avian Dis.*, **58**: 433–436.

Wilder, T.D., *et al.* (2001) Differences in the pathogenicity of various bacterial isolates used in an induction model for gangrenous dermatitis in broiler chickens. *Avian Dis.*, **45**: 659–662.

Willoughby, D.H., *et al.* (1996) Periodic recurrence of gangrenous dermatitis associated with *Clostridium septicum* in a broiler chicken operation. *J. Vet. Diagn. Invest.*, **8**: 259–261.

22 Bacillary Hemoglobinuria

Mauricio Navarro, Fernando Dutra Quintela, and Francisco A. Uzal

Introduction

Bacillary hemoglobinuria (BH), also known as red water disease, is a highly acute and usually fatal disease that occurs mostly in cattle. The disease is less frequently seen in sheep, and has rarely been reported in horses, pigs, and elk. It has been described in several countries of North and South America, Europe, and Oceania, where it can be sporadic or endemic.

Etiology

BH is caused by *Clostridium haemolyticum* (also sometimes referred to as *Clostridium novyi* type D), a Gram-positive, motile, and sporulated rod, which is considered one of the most strict anaerobic pathogenic clostridia. *C. haemolyticum* produces several toxins, of which beta toxin, a phospholipase C, is the main virulence factor. A description of the toxins produced by *C. haemolyticum* is presented in Chapter 4. Briefly, beta toxin is highly hemolytic and induces disruption of capillary endothelium and necrosis of hepatocytes. This toxin is antigenically closely related to the beta toxin of *Clostridium novyi* type B. Other toxins of *C. haemolyticum* are a tropomyosinase and a lipase, known as eta and theta toxins, respectively; the role of these two toxins in the virulence of the microorganism is probably minor, although little information is available in this regard.

Epidemiology

The morbidity of BH varies between 0.25% and 12%, but the lethality can reach 80% to 100%. The geographic distribution of the disease is dependent both on the soil characteristics and on the presence of liver flukes.

Clostridial Diseases of Animals, First Edition. Francisco A. Uzal, J. Glenn Songer,
John F. Prescott and Michel R. Popoff.

In most cases, BH occurs sporadically, but it may be endemic in areas where fascioliasis abounds. Therefore, the main determining factor for the incidence of the disease is the number of liver fluke metacercariae present on pastures where animals graze.

BH may occur at any time during the year, but most cases occur in summer and early fall. Dry weather conditions may induce animals to concentrate on portions of the pastures infested with liver flukes, including areas surrounding small ponds, drains, dams, swamps, and other bodies of water, thus being exposed to an increased intake of metacercariae. For these reasons, the disease is far more frequently seen on pasture-grazing cattle rather than in intensively reared animals. BH occurs mostly in animals older than 1 year, although cases can occasionally be seen in younger animals. Affected animals are usually in good nutritional condition and BH is most frequently seen in animals recently introduced to an infected area. No apparent sex or breed predisposition has been determined. Clinically healthy animals may eliminate spores through feces and urine, thus contaminating pastures. The movement of flood or drainage water may also spread the microorganism, and decomposing carcasses of dead animals due to BH represent a potential additional source of infection.

Pathogenesis

The spores of *C. haemolyticum* are found in soil, where they are very resistant to environmental conditions and can survive for several years, especially in poorly drained pastures with alkaline water pH, usually 8.0 or higher. Spores are ingested by animals and absorbed from the intestine into the bloodstream, reaching the liver via portal circulation. It is thought that in the liver, the spores are phagocytized by Kupffer cells, in the cytoplasm of which they can survive for long periods of time. Spores of *C. haemolyticum* have also been found in the intestine, kidney, and bone marrow of healthy cattle.

In the great majority of cases, BH occurs after initiating hepatic damage largely attributable to liver flukes, mainly *Fasciola hepatica*, although other trematodes including *Fascioloides magna* and *Dicrocoelium dendriticum* may also be involved. When immature forms of liver flukes penetrate into the liver, the necrosis and hemorrhage associated with migration create the anaerobic conditions allowing for spore germination and bacterial multiplication, with consequent production of toxins. Large quantities of beta toxin result in hemolysis. In addition, activation of the arachidonic acid cascade, production of thromboxane and leukotrienes, platelet aggregation, and increase in capillary permeability are thought to be consequences of the action of beta toxin. Both hepatocyte necrosis and thrombus formation due to endothelial disruption contribute to the development of a large focus of coagulative necrosis. This focus is probably a consequence of both ischemia related to thrombosis and of the direct action of beta toxin on the hepatocytes. Hemolysis results in hemoglobinuria and jaundice, two of the main clinical features of the disease, and in severe hypoxia that leads to hemoglobinuric nephrosis.

Sporadically, BH occurs in animals free from liver flukes. In those cases, the initial germination of the spores of *C. haemolyticum* has been suggested to be associated with a variety of insults, including *Fusobacterium necrophorum* and *Cysticercus tenuicollis* infection, liver biopsies, telangiectasia, metabolic disturbances, and reduced hepatic blood circulation associated with pressure of the pregnant uterus against the liver. However, the role of these predisposing factors in the development of BH has not been definitively determined.

Clinical signs

Most clinical signs of BH in cattle are a consequence of the severe hemolytic anemia characteristic of this condition, which may be acute or sub-acute. In range farming conditions, animals may be found dead without clinical signs having been observed. The clinical course in the acute form of the disease lasts between 10 and 12 hours, whereas the clinical course in sub-acute cases may last 3 to 4 days. The latter is less common. Both forms of BH are clinically characterized by hemoglobinuria, jaundice, and high initial fever (40–41 °C) which drops rapidly just before death. Animals become lethargic and there is an abrupt decrease in rumination, milk production, and defecation, increased heart rate, severe dyspnea, and blood in the feces. Hematological changes are characterized by a marked reduction in hematocrit, red blood cell count, and hemoglobin concentration, accompanied by initial leukocytosis. The latter reverts quickly into leukopenia as a consequence of the severe toxemia. Death results from severe hemolysis-associated anoxia and toxemia.

Clinical signs in other species are essentially similar to those seen in cattle.

Gross changes

Carcasses of animals dying of BH present with dehydration, varying degrees of jaundice, and the perineal region and tail soiled with dark, liquid feces. The subcutaneous tissue is diffusely edematous and presents widespread multifocal petechiae and ecchymoses, which also extend to the fascia and muscles. In the great majority of cases of BH, a large and usually single area of necrosis delimited by a hyperemic rim, frequently visible on the diaphragmatic surface of the liver (Figure 22.1), is considered a pathognomonic finding. Less frequently, additional smaller foci of necrosis may also be present around the main lesion or widespread in the liver parenchyma. The foci of necrosis are usually pale and roughly conical with their base on the surface of the liver (Figure 22.2), and of variable consistency, with some of them being very friable. They can vary in size, reaching up to 30-cm diameter, and they are sometimes covered with fibrin (Figure 22.1). The rest of the liver is usually slightly friable, orange-tan, congested, and may show a diffuse acinar pattern. Bile ducts may be thickened, suggesting previous infestation by liver flukes; however, lesions attributable to these parasites may

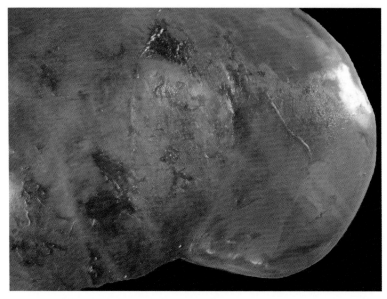

Figure 22.1 External surface of the liver of a cow with bacillary hemoglobinuria. A large, single focus of necrosis surrounded by a hyperemic rim is affecting the liver. A layer of fibrin is present over the area of necrosis. Courtesy of E. Paredes.

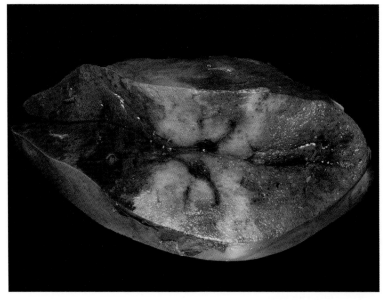

Figure 22.2 Section of the liver of a cow with bacillary hemoglobinuria. A well-delimited, roughly conical, and pale focus of necrosis is observed. Courtesy of E. Paredes.

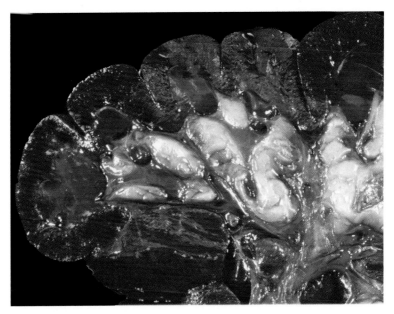

Figure 22.3 Kidney of a cow with bacillary hemoglobinuria. The renal cortex and medulla are diffusely dark, suggesting hemoglobinuric nephrosis. Jaundice in adipose tissue is also evident. Courtesy of E. Waters.

sometimes not be present. Severe petechiation and ecchymoses are usually seen on most serosas and on the endocardium. An excess of hemoglobin-stained fluid is frequently found in the pericardial sac, and in the thoracic and abdominal cavities. Large quantities of bright red blood clots can be found in the lumen of the small and large intestines. The lungs are edematous and the spleen is usually enlarged and pulpy. The urinary bladder is filled with dark red urine and the kidneys are usually dark to frankly black (Figure 22.3) and friable, and they may show numerous petechiae under the capsule.

Gross changes in other species are poorly documented, but are thought to be very similar to those seen in cattle.

Microscopic changes

The most typical and almost pathognomonic microscopic change is found in the liver and consists of focally extensive coagulative necrosis. A rim of inflammatory cells, mainly composed of viable and degenerated neutrophils, and fewer lymphocytes and plasma cells surrounds the necrotic tissue (Figure 22.4). Large numbers of Gram-positive rods, singly or in clusters, many with subterminal spores, are visible in sinusoids of necrotic areas, mostly along the inner margin of the leukocytic rim (Figure 22.5). In the area of necrosis, the hepatocytes are usually dissociated and present acidophilic cytoplasm, with pyknotic nuclei.

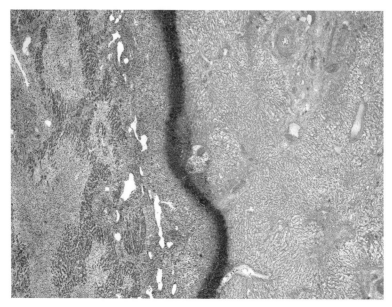

Figure 22.4 Liver of a cow with bacillary hemoglobinuria. An area of coagulative necrosis (right) is delimited by a narrow band of dense, leukocytic infiltrate, mainly composed of degenerated neutrophils. A more normal-looking area of liver parenchyma is observed on the left. HE, 40x.

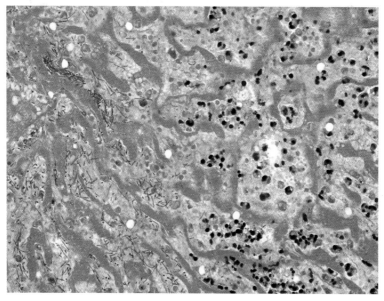

Figure 22.5 Liver of a cow with bacillary hemoglobinuria. Large numbers of rods are observed in the sinusoids between necrotic hepatocytes, at the periphery of the area of necrosis, and close to the band of leukocytic infiltrate. HE, 400x.

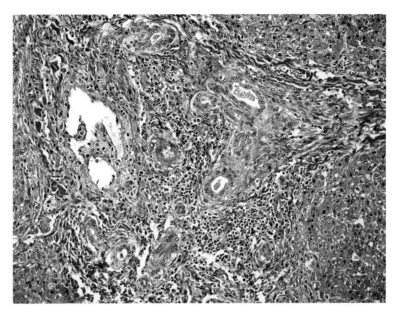

Figure 22.6 Liver of a cow with bacillary hemoglobinuria. Portal area showing bile duct hyperplasia, fibrosis, and mixed inflammatory infiltrate consistent with *Fasciola hepatica* infestation. HE, 200x.

Many outlines of erythrocytes and debris are observed in sinusoids. The walls of blood vessels across the main lesion are necrotic and many are partially to totally obstructed by fibrin thrombi. In the liver outside the necrotic foci, mild to moderate bile duct hyperplasia, periportal lymphoplasmacytic inflammation, and fibrosis may be observed (Figure 22.6); these changes are thought to be associated with previous liver fluke migration. Most of the liver shows variable degrees of centrilobular degeneration and necrosis, likely a consequence of the hypoxic state associated with the severe anemia characteristic of this disease. Vascular alterations including intimal necrosis, congestion, and hemorrhages are frequently seen in the liver and occasionally in other tissues. The spleen is severely congested, and macrophages are distended with intracytoplasmic hemosiderin; multifocal areas of necrosis containing neutrophils are usually observed in red and white pulp.

The intestinal mucosa is usually diffusely congested, and multifocal or diffuse hemorrhages involving one or several layers of the intestine may be seen. The kidneys show marked distention of the glomerular spaces and tubular lumen by a homogeneous or globular acidophilic substance consistent with hemoglobin. The renal tubules show epithelial degeneration and necrosis with variable amounts of intracytoplasmic, eosinophilic granules and protein casts formed mostly by hemoglobin inside the lumen (hemoglobinuric nephrosis) (Figure 22.7).

As with gross changes, descriptions of microscopic lesions in species other than cattle are scant and are usually assumed to be the same as in cattle.

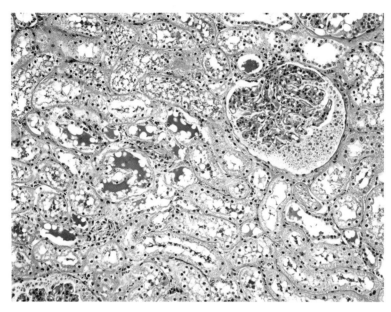

Figure 22.7 Kidney of a cow with bacillary hemoglobinuria. The glomerular space and tubular lumen are distended by an eosinophilic substance consistent with hemoglobin. Small globules of the same substance are also present in the lumen of the tubular epithelium, which shows evidence of degeneration and occasionally necrosis. HE, 200x.

Diagnosis

A presumptive clinical diagnosis of BH can be made based on the history and clinical signs, including the sudden onset of disease in animals usually grazing in liver-fluke-infested areas, and the production of red urine, anemia, and high body temperature that rapidly drops. Hemolytic anemia, hemoglobinuria, and variations on leukocytic response can be determined by clinical pathology, and this supports the clinical diagnosis. At necropsy, a still presumptive, but highly suggestive diagnosis of BH may be established based on the presence of the characteristic focus of necrosis in the liver, coupled with the consequences of hemolysis, including jaundice, dark kidneys, hemoglobinuria, and hemorrhages throughout the body. Microscopic examination of the liver adds certainty to the gross presumptive diagnosis, as does recognition of large numbers of bacteria with clostridial morphology on a Gram stain. Confirmation is achieved by demonstration of *C. haemolyticum* in the liver by culture, PCR, FAT, or immunohistochemistry in animals with clinical, gross, and microscopic changes suggestive of BH. Because of the fastidious nature of *C. haemolyticum*, isolation is not easy, and failure to isolate this organism does not preclude a diagnosis of BH. Once isolated, identification of *C. haemolyticum* can be achieved by conventional biochemical techniques and also by PCR, using specific primers targeting the 16S rDNA sequence or the beta toxin gene. MALDI-TOF mass spectrometry has been recently incorporated into the list of tests available to identify this microorganism.

Because *C. haemolyticum* may be found in the liver of a small number of clinically healthy animals, demonstration of this microorganism in animals without typical hepatic lesions should not be considered diagnostic for BH.

Treatment and control

BH is usually acute, with most animals dying within a few hours of disease onset. Because of this, there is usually not enough time to initiate treatment and even in those cases in which this is attempted, the success rate is low. Procaine penicillin G is the antibiotic treatment of choice but is unlikely to be effective in affected animals because of the acuteness of the disease process. It may be of more value in preventing disease in animals at risk during an outbreak, before they are vaccinated.

Vaccination is an effective method of protecting cattle against BH. Bacterin/toxoids against *C. haemolyticum* are commercially available in mono- and polyvalent preparations. Two initial doses four to six weeks prior to the expected peak of occurrence of the disease are recommended. This should be followed by an annual booster for the rest of the life of the animals. In areas with a high incidence of BH, a booster every six months is suggested. Because the disease is rarely observed in animals younger than 1 year old, vaccination before this age is not frequently applied.

Where the disease is associated with liver flukes, reducing parasitic burden or preventing fluke infestation is also considered very effective in reducing the incidence of BH. This is achieved by treating the animals with fasciolicides and reducing the access of animals to swampy or poorly drained pastures. Although controlling the intermediate host of liver flukes has been suggested as a way to help prevent BH, there are currently no effective methods to achieve this under extensive conditions. When possible, carcasses of animals that have died from BH should be removed from pastures to prevent contamination with spores.

Bibliography

Ahourai, P., *et al.* (1990) Bovine bacillary hemoglobinuria (*Clostridium haemolyticum*) in Iran. *J. Vet. Diagn. Invest.*, **2**: 143–144.

Bender, L.C., *et al.* (1999) Bacillary hemoglobinuria in a free-ranging elk calf. *J. Zoo. Wildl. Med.*, **30**: 293–296.

Hauer, P.J., *et al.* (2004) Cloning and molecular characterization of the beta toxin (phospholipase C) gene of *Clostridium haemolyticum*. *Anaerobe*, **10**: 243–254.

Hauer, P.J., *et al.* (2006) Evidence of the protective immunogenicity of native and recombinant *Clostridium haemolyticum* phospholipase C (beta toxin) in guinea pigs. *Vaccine*, **24**: 124–132.

Janzen, E.D., *et al.* (1981) Bacillary hemoglobinuria associated with hepatic necrobacillosis in a yearling feedlot heifer. *Can. Vet. J.*, **22**: 393–394.

Oaks, J.L., *et al.* (1997) Apparent *Clostridium haemolyticum/Clostridium novyi* infection and exotoxemia in two horses. *J. Vet. Diagn. Invest.*, **9**: 324–325.

Olander, H.J., *et al.* (1966) Bacillary hemoglobinuria: Induction by liver biopsy in naturally and experimentally infected animals. *Path. Vet.*, **3**: 421–450.

Pearson, E.G. (2009) Diseases of the hepatobiliary system. In: Smith, B.P. (ed.) *Large Animal Internal Medicine*, 4th edition, pp. 893–924. Mosby Elsevier, St. Louis, MO.

Randhawa, S.S., *et al.* (1995) An outbreak of bacillary haemoglobinuria in sheep in India. *Trop. Anim. Hlth Prod.*, **27**: 31–36.

Sasaki, Y., *et al.* (2001) Phylogenetic positions of *Clostridium novyi* and *Clostridium haemolyticum* based on 16S rDNA sequences. *Int. J. Syst. Evol. Microbiol.*, **51**: 901–904.

Shinozuka, Y., *et al.* (2011) Bacillary hemoglobinuria in Japanese black cattle in Hiroshima, Japan: A case study. *J. Vet. Med. Sci.*, **73**: 255–258.

Stalker, M.J., *et al.* (2007) Liver and biliary system. In: Maxie, M.G. (ed.) *Jubb, Kennedy and Palmer's Pathology of Domestic Animals*, 5th edition, Vol. **2**, pp. 297–388. Elsevier, Philadelphia.

Stogdale, L., *et al.* (1984) Bacillary hemoglobinuria in cattle. *Comp. Cont. Edu. Practic. Vet.*, **6**: 284–290.

Takagi, M., *et al.* (2009) Successful treatment of bacillary hemoglobinuria in Japanese Black Cows. *J. Vet. Med. Sci.*, **71**: 1105–1108.

Uzal, F.A., *et al.* (1992) Bacillary haemoglobinuria diagnosis by the peroxidase-antiperoxidase (PAP) technique. *J. Vet. Med.*, **39**: 595–598.

Van Kampen, K.R., *et al.* (1969) Experimental bacillary hemoglobinuria II. Pathogenesis of the hepatic lesion in the rabbit. *Path. Vet.*, **6**: 59–75.

Vine, N., *et al.* (2006) Bacillary hemoglobinuria in dairy cows. *Vet. Rec.*, **159**: 160.

Infectious Necrotic Hepatitis

Mauricio Navarro and Francisco A. Uzal

Introduction

Infectious necrotic hepatitis (INH), also known as black disease, is an acute and highly lethal disease of sheep caused by *Clostridium novyi* type B. It may also affect cattle, and rarely horses and dogs. The disease is clinically and pathologically similar to bacillary hemoglobinuria (BH) and therefore only those aspects that are specific to INH will be emphasized here. Readers should refer to Chapter 22 for common features of these two diseases.

Etiology

C. novyi is an anaerobic, Gram-positive, spore-forming rod, which is classified into four types (A, B, C, and D) based on the production of toxins, which are fully described in Chapter 4. Briefly, *C. novyi* type A produces alpha toxin (TcnA), which is thought to be the main virulence factor of this microorganism, and gamma toxin, a non-lethal phospholipase. *C. novyi* type A is responsible for gas gangrene of man and animals, acting alone or in combination with other clostridia. *C. novyi* type B produces mainly TcnA and beta toxin, which are thought to be the main virulence factors of the microorganism. However, the molecular Koch postulates have not been fulfilled and the definitive role of these toxins in the virulence of *C. novyi* type B remains, therefore, unconfirmed. The beta toxin of *C. novyi* type B is serologically indistinguishable from the beta toxin produced by *C. haemolyticum* (also known as *C. novyi* type D). TcnA is edema-inducing and lethal, while beta toxin is necrotizing and hemolytic, but is not usually produced in lethal amounts. The spores of *C. novyi* type B are very resistant to environmental factors and, as with *C. haemolyticum*, they can presumably remain latent in

Clostridial Diseases of Animals, First Edition. Francisco A. Uzal, J. Glenn Songer,
John F. Prescott and Michel R. Popoff.
© 2016 John Wiley & Sons, Inc. Published 2016 by John Wiley & Sons, Inc.

phagocytic cells of ruminants and possibly other species, mainly in the liver, but also in the spleen and bone marrow; the microorganism can also be found in soil and as part of the intestinal microbiota. Finally, *C. novyi* type C is nontoxigenic and nonpathogenic.

Pathogenesis

The pathogenesis of INH is similar to that of BH (Chapter 22). Both diseases are associated with initiating hepatic damage, usually induced by the migration of the immature forms of *Fasciola hepatica* and other liver flukes such as *Dicrocoelium dendriticum* and *Fascioloides magna*, which creates the anaerobic conditions for the germination of the spores and the proliferation of *C. novyi* type B, with the consequent production of toxins. In INH, the released TcnA acts on the actin cytoskeleton and the vimentin and tubulin systems of cells, inducing irreversible changes in cell morphology; additionally, the glycosyltransferase activity of TcnA has a role in modifying several small GTP-binding proteins (Chapter 4). Capillary endothelium is particularly affected by these mechanisms, which result in cell instability followed by an extensive infiltration of fluid into the connective tissue. Although the high resemblance between beta toxin in *C. novyi* type B and *C. haemolyticum* suggests a similar mechanism of virulence for these two microorganisms, the beta toxin gene is far less expressed in *C. novyi* type B than in *C. haemolyticum*.

Epidemiology

INH has been reported in many countries and it occurs mostly in regions where liver fluke, the main predisposing factor, is endemic. However, as in the case of BH, INH has been described occasionally in animals without the presence of these parasites. In those cases, other causes of liver damage have been suggested, although their role in predisposing INH has not been demonstrated conclusively. Suggested predisposing factors include *Cysticercus tenuicollis*, *Thysanosoma actinioides*, telangiectasia, liver abscesses, fatty changes, and plant toxins. INH affects mainly adult animals, usually in good nutritional condition, with no apparent breed or sex predisposition. INH rarely occurs in young individuals. The risk for developing the disease is always present, especially in regions with liver fluke, given the distribution of *C. novyi* type B in the microbiota of soil and digestive tract of animals.

Clinical signs

In sheep, INH is a highly acute disease and because of that, affected animals die within a few hours of disease onset and frequently without clinical signs being observed. When clinical signs are seen, they are non-specific and include weakness, reluctance to move, drowsiness, anorexia, hyperthermia, tachypnea, tachycardia, and recumbency. As with several other infectious diseases of sheep, affected animals tend to get separated from the flock. Unlike BH, sheep suffering from INH do not manifest significant jaundice or hemoglobinuria, and this difference seems to be related to the small amount of beta toxin produced by *C. novyi* type B. Clinico-pathological changes are characterized by signs of toxemia and include neutrophilia with a left shift, metabolic acidosis, azotemia, and an increase in liver and muscle enzymes.

In cattle, signs of INH are mostly similar to those seen in sheep, although constipation and blood in feces may also be present.

Descriptions of INH in horses are limited. The few cases described in this species were characterized by variable degrees of jaundice, tachypnea, hematuria, and, rarely, neurological signs, including ataxia and head tilt. It is not clear why jaundice is observed in horses and not in ruminants but this phenomenon may be related to the higher susceptibility of horses to the action of *C. novyi* beta toxin.

Gross changes

In general, gross changes in sheep and cattle that die of INH are essentially similar to those described for BH, with a few exceptions. The lesions associated with hemolytic anemia, which are characteristic of BH, are usually not seen in cases of ruminants with INH. The most characteristic gross change is observed in the liver and is very similar to the hepatic changes in BH, with the difference that in INH the foci of necrosis tend to be smaller and multiple (Figure 23.1). Carcasses of sheep dying of INH decompose very quickly. In most cases of INH, striking

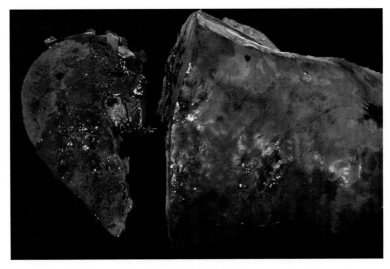

Figure 23.1 Liver of a sheep with infectious necrotic hepatitis. Multiple well-delimited and pale foci of necrosis are evident. Courtesy of G. Riffkin.

hemorrhagic subcutaneous edema and congestion are present in ventral areas. The latter give the carcass a dark appearance, from which the name "black disease" originated. Horses with black disease present single or multifocal foci of hepatic necrosis, accompanied by toxemic changes and varying degrees of jaundice.

Microscopic changes

In sheep, cattle, and horses with INH, microscopic lesions in the liver and most other organs are indistinguishable from those seen in BH, although kidney lesions are not usually observed in cases of INH, either in sheep or cattle; these lesions have only been described in horses.

Diagnosis

The tests and diagnostic criteria for INH are those described for BH (Chapter 22). As in BH, a diagnosis of INH cannot be established based solely on detection of *C. novyi* type B alone in the liver, since the microorganism can be present in this organ in small numbers of healthy animals.

Treatment and control

Ante-mortem diagnosis of INH in sheep is unusual, but in the rare cases in which this occurs, or when a post-mortem diagnosis has been established in other animals of the flock, treatment of sick animals with high doses of procaine penicillin in addition to supportive care may be attempted. Nevertheless, antibiotics may be ineffective due to well-advanced toxin production.

As in the case of BH, vaccination against *C. novyi* type B and control of liver fluke infestation is effective as a means of preventing or reducing the incidence of INH.

Bibliography

Bagadi, H.O., *et al.* (1973) An epidemiological survey of infectious necrotic hepatitis (black disease) of sheep in southern Scotland. *Res. Vet. Sci.,* **15**: 49–53.

Bagadi, H.O., *et al.* (1973) Experimental studies on infectious necrotic hepatitis (black disease) of sheep. *Res. Vet. Sci.,* **15**: 53–61.

Bagadi, H.O. (1974) Infectious necrotic hepatitis (black disease) of sheep. *Vet. Bull.,* **44**: 385–388.

Belyi, Y., *et al.* (2010) Bacterial toxin and effector glycosyltransferases. *Biochim. Biophys. Acta,* **1800**: 134–143.

Borrmann, E., *et al.* (1999) Detection of *Clostridium novyi* Type B alpha toxin by cell culture systems. *FEMS Immunol. Med. Mic.,* **24**: 275–280.

Pearson, E.G. (2009) Diseases of the hepatobiliary system. In: Smith, B.P. (ed.) *Large Animal Internal Medicine*, 4th edition, pp. 893–924. Mosby Elsevier, St. Louis, MO.

Robles, C.A., *et al.* (2000) Black disease in merino sheep infected with *Thysanosoma actinioides* in the Patagonia region, Argentina. *Arch. Med. Vet.*, **32**: 93–99.

Stalker, M.J., *et al.* (2007) Liver and biliary system. In: Maxie, M.G. (ed.) *Jubb, Kennedy and Palmer's Pathology of Domestic Animals*, 5th edition, Vol. **2**, pp. 297–388. Elsevier, Philadelphia.

Sweeney, H.J., *et al.* (1986) Infectious necrotic hepatitis in a horse. *Equine Vet. J.*, **18**: 150–151.

Uzal, F.A., *et al.* (1996) Un caso de hepatitis infecciosa necrosante en oveja sin *Fasciola hepatica*. *Rev. Med. Vet.*, **77**: 377–379.

Whitfield, L.K., *et al.* (2015) Necrotic hepatitis associated with *Clostridium novyi* infection (black disease) in a horse in New Zealand. *New Zeal. Vet. J.*, **63**: 177–179.

24 Tyzzer's Disease

Karina C. Fresneda and Francisco R. Carvallo Chaigneau

Introduction

Tyzzer's disease is an infectious disease caused by *Clostridium piliforme*. The disease is named after Ernest Tyzzer, who, in 1917, initially described this condition as a fatal epizootic diarrheal disease of Japanese waltzing mice. It affects a wide variety of domestic and non-domestic animal species, including humans. The most susceptible species are horses, rabbits, and laboratory animals. There is neither an effective treatment nor commercial vaccines available to prevent this disease.

Etiology

Clostridium piliforme is a Gram-negative, spore-forming, obligate intracellular, filamentous, pleomorphic, and motile bacterium. Vegetative organisms are 0.3 to 0.5 μm in diameter and 8 to 10 μm in length, with very thin (10–15 nm diameter) peritrichous flagella. The spores measure 0.5 to 1.0 μm in diameter, and they have thick coats (80–200 nm). This microorganism may develop subterminal spores, which are not, however, easily seen in tissue sections. The rods appear in bundles within the cytoplasm of hepatocytes and enterocytes. *C. piliforme* has never been cultured on artificial media and it grows only in tissue culture or in fertile eggs. It stains positively with silver, methylene blue, and thionine stains and it is PAS positive.

Although formerly known as *Bacillus piliformis*, 16S rRNA gene sequencing led to assignment of this microorganism to the genus Clostridium and the designation of *Clostridium piliforme*. The phylogenetic tree suggests that the closest

Clostridial Diseases of Animals, First Edition. Francisco A. Uzal, J. Glenn Songer, John F. Prescott and Michel R. Popoff.
© 2016 John Wiley & Sons, Inc. Published 2016 by John Wiley & Sons, Inc.

relatives of this organism are *Clostridium coccoides*, *Clostridium oroticum*, *Clostridium clostridiformis*, *Clostridium symbiosum*, and *Clostridium aminovalericum*.

C. *piliforme* is relatively labile in the vegetative phase, but its spores may survive for long periods in the environment, including contaminated bedding, where it can remain infectious for at least one year, although some reports indicate that spores can remain viable in the environment for up to five years. The spores of C. *piliforme* are resistant to heating up to 60 °C for 30 min, 80 °C for 15 min, and to exposure to 70% ethanol, 3% cresol, 4% chlorhexidine, 0.037% formaldehyde, 0.4% peracetic acid, 0.015% sodium hypochlorite, 1% iodophol, or 5% phenol.

Epidemiology

Neonates and juvenile individuals are usually more susceptible to Tyzzer's disease than adults. Predisposing factors such as stress, overcrowding, dietary imbalances, coprophagia, poor sanitary management, parasitism, sulfonamide and corticosteroid administration may lead to the clinical presentation of the disease.

Foals, lagomorphs, and laboratory animals appear to be the most susceptible species, presenting low morbidity and high mortality. In addition, this disease has also been reported, among others, in red pandas, white-tailed deer, cattle, dogs, cats, cotton-top tamarins, coyotes, snow leopards, gray foxes, servals, and in several avian species like weaver birds. A human case was described in an immunosuppressed patient infected with Human Immunodeficiency Virus.

The disease in horses, which is considered one of the most susceptible species, has been reported in North America, Australia, Europe, and Africa. The ingestion of spores from the environment is the most likely route of infection, although this has not been confirmed. Fecal shedding of C. *piliforme* in adult horses has been demonstrated, and this led to the belief that coprophagia may play an important role in the infection of foals. Vertical transmission does not occur under natural conditions, although intrauterine transmission has been demonstrated in mice and in rats treated with prednisolone during the last week of pregnancy. Colostral transfer of antibodies to C. *piliforme* has been demonstrated in horses.

Pathogenesis

Very little is known about the pathogenesis of C. *piliforme* infection. The proposed theory of mode of transmission is fecal–oral, by ingestion of spores from an environment contaminated by feces. Following oral exposure, most immunocompetent animals clear the infection within a few weeks. However, in permissive individuals, C. *piliforme* proliferates in the intestinal mucosa, specifically in the ileum, colon, and cecum, producing necrosis and sloughing of enterocytes. Entry to the portal circulation results in subsequent dissemination to the liver and other organs, predominantly the myocardium. The organism is shed in feces.

The incubation period of the disease may be as long as seven days. Experimentally, in hamsters inoculated with infected liver homogenates, organisms and lesions are detectable in the mucosa of the small and large intestine by three days post inoculation, and multiple lesions and bacilli may be present in the liver by day 6 to 8 post exposure. Depletion of neutrophils or natural killer cells in experimentally infected mice increases the severity of disease, but macrophage depletion does not appear to influence the susceptibility to, or the course of, the disease.

Clinical signs

The young of many animal species can contract Tyzzer's disease, and show similar clinical signs, with only a few differences that are discussed later in this chapter. Most animal species have icterus and dehydration; fecal staining of the perineum may also be observed, although this is not a consistent finding.

In foals, Tyzzer's disease is a fatal infection, occurring mainly between 1 and 4 weeks of age, with either no clinical signs or acute signs of enterohepatic disease. In adults, the mortality is lower. When observed, clinical signs are of short duration and include lethargy, weakness, anorexia, fever, hypothermia, varying degrees of watery diarrhea, abdominal pain, dehydration, tachycardia, vomiting, jaundice, seizures, and coma.

Sudden death or outbreaks of profuse watery diarrhea are the main clinical signs in rabbits and mice.

Gerbils and rats are very susceptible to the disease, and in addition to the clinical signs mentioned above for all species, they may show ruffled hair coat and hunched posture.

Clinical signs reported in kittens are diarrhea of approximately five days' duration, head tilt, and vacant staring, which rapidly progress to depression and collapse.

The disease in a weaver bird consisted of incapacity to fly or perch, and neurological signs including head tilt, torticollis, and rolling onto its back.

Clinico-pathologic findings

Biochemical findings are similar in all species and include hypoglycemia, hypoalbuminemia, hypoproteinemia, hyperbilirubinemia, and elevated hepatic enzymes, such as aspartate aminotransferase (AST), alanine aminotransferase (SGPT), alkaline phosphatase, and lactate dehydrogenase (LDH). Foals may also present elevated serum fibrinogen. Non-regenerative anemia, leukocytosis, or leukopenia can be present.

Gross changes

Although a triad of lesion locations (intestine, liver, and heart) is frequently mentioned in the literature, the changes and distribution of lesions are variable among species. With a few differences, similar gross lesions are observed in all the affected animal species. In foals, the most significant finding is hepatomegaly with numerous 1- to 5-mm-diameter pale foci, dispersed throughout the parenchyma (Figures 24.1 and 24.2). Hepatic and mesenteric lymph nodes can be markedly enlarged and edematous. Intestinal lesions are characterized by congestion of the ileum, cecum, and colon. In the heart, one or many pale, round to linear foci can be identified, although lesions in this organ are usually only visible microscopically. In addition, splenomegaly and icterus (Figure 24.3) may be evident, and multifocal hemorrhages can be identified in the lung, diaphragm, and small and large intestines.

In rats, a pronounced dilation (three to four times its normal diameter) of the ileum (megaloileitis), together with transmural inflammation is described.

In cats, gross lesions can be absent or restricted to the colon, with the presence of gray, pasty feces and occasional blood.

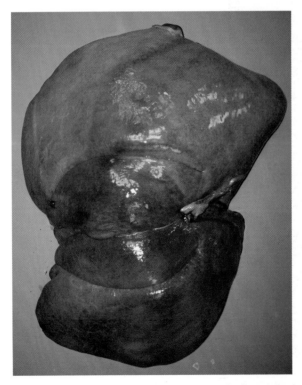

Figure 24.1 Liver of a foal with Tyzzer's disease. The liver is markedly enlarged, with multifocal to coalescing white foci. Courtesy of F.A. Uzal.

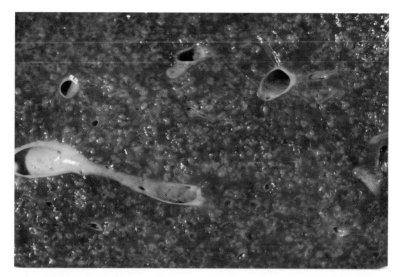

Figure 24.2 Cross-section of the liver of a foal with Tyzzer's disease. Multiple pale foci of necrosis are dispersed throughout the parenchyma. Courtesy of F.A. Uzal.

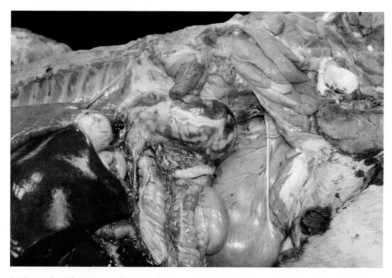

Figure 24.3 Foal with Tyzzer's disease showing diffuse icterus. Courtesy of F.A. Uzal.

Microscopic changes

As with the clinical signs and gross lesions, microscopic changes are similar in all the species. Hepatic lesions consist of random, multifocal coagulation or caseous necrosis; these foci are frequently infiltrated by large numbers of neutrophils (Figures 24.4 and 24.5). In chronic cases, these lesions may

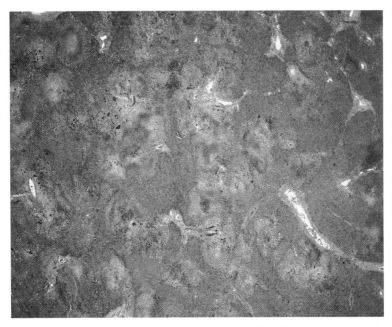

Figure 24.4 Liver of a foal with Tyzzer's disease. Multiple random foci of necrosis are observed. HE, 40x. Courtesy of F.A. Uzal.

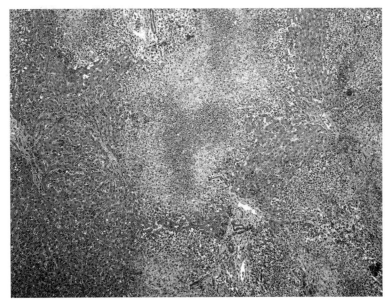

Figure 24.5 Higher magnification of Figure 24.4. A focus of coagulative necrosis with a large number of viable and degenerated neutrophils admixed with eosinophilic cell debris is observed. HE, 100x. Courtesy of F.A. Uzal.

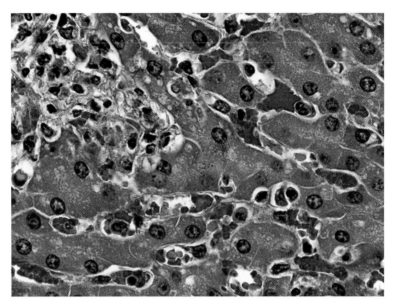

Figure 24.6 Liver of a foal with Tyzzer's disease. Multiple filamentous bacteria are seen in the cytoplasm of a hepatocyte. HE, 400x. Courtesy of F.A. Uzal.

progress to granulomas, with occasional fibrosis and mineralization. Filamentous bacteria are identified at the margins of the necrotic area, in the cytoplasm of viable hepatocytes (Figure 24.6). These microorganisms may be faintly seen on HE-stained sections but are very evident on Giemsa- or Steiner-stained sections (Figure 24.7). Although colitis and myocarditis have been described in most of the species, in horses they are rarely seen. When present, in horses or other species, multiple foci of degeneration, necrosis, inflammation, and edema are evident in the mucosa and muscularis mucosa of the intestine (Figure 24.8). Lymphatics can be dilated with cellular debris. Bacteria can be identified most frequently in enterocytes (Figures 24.9 and 24.10), and occasionally in smooth muscle cells and neurons of the Auerbach plexus. In the heart, multifocal myocyte degeneration and necrosis, and acute inflammation, with intrasarcoplasmic bacteria, are characteristic. Occasionally, the lesions progress to granulomatous myocarditis.

Megaloileitis in the rat is characterized by segmental transmural necrosis and predominantly mononuclear inflammation. In gerbils, intestinal necrosis and inflammation of smooth muscle and Peyer's patches have been described. Bacteria can also invade other organs and evoke an inflammatory response, such as suppurative encephalitis.

Tyzzer's disease has been described in a lorikeet and a cockatiel, both < 2 weeks of age. In both cases, there was necrotizing hepatitis and myocarditis, and numerous bacteria were identified in the muscular layers of the gizzard and occasionally in the intestinal mucosa and muscular layers.

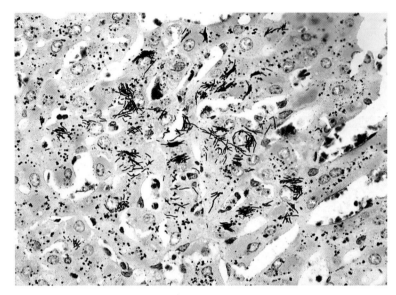

Figure 24.7 Liver of a rabbit with multiple intracytoplasmic filamentous bacteria. Steiner stain, 400x. Courtesy of F.A. Uzal.

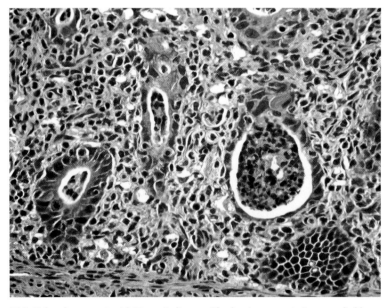

Figure 24.8 Colon from a cat with Tyzzer's disease. The lamina propria is expanded by numerous mononuclear cells, and the crypts are dilated with necrotic debris. HE, 600x.

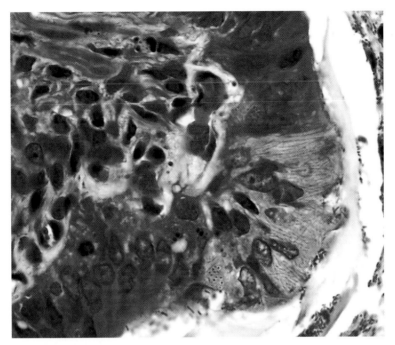

Figure 24.9 Small intestine of a rabbit with Tyzzer's disease. Numerous filamentous bacilli are seen in the cytoplasm of enterocytes. Cross-sections of those bacilli are also seen. HE, 100x. Courtesy of S.S. Diab.

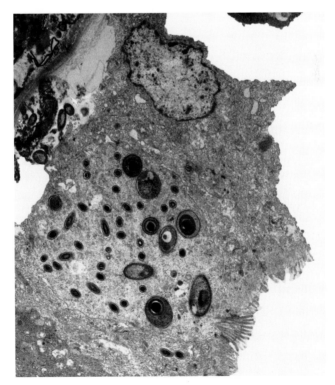

Figure 24.10 Transmission electron micrograph of the colon of a cat with Tyzzer's disease. A crypt enterocyte contains numerous transverse, longitudinal, and oblique sections of both vegetative cells and spores. Uranyl acetate and lead citrate stain, 6000x.

In a weaver bird with Tyzzer's disease, extensive areas of hypercellularity and rarefaction, and multiple microabscesses were observed in the brain.

Diagnosis

A presumptive diagnosis of Tyzzer's disease can be reached based on gross observations. A definitive diagnosis, however, should be based upon the histologic demonstration of hepatic, intestinal, and/or myocardial lesions and the presence of bacteria in the cytoplasm of affected cells. Using appropriate special stains, such as Giemsa, Periodic acid Schiff, and silver-based stains (such as Steiner's and Warthin Starry), it is possible to identify long, intracytoplasmic filamentous bacteria, either singly or in clusters, which are characteristic of the disease. This provides sufficient evidence on which to base a diagnosis of Tyzzer's disease.

Detection of the organism by PCR, immunohistochemistry, or, less frequently, by culture in embryonated eggs, is also diagnostic. The most commonly used PCR amplifies a 196 bp DNA fragment of the *C. piliforme* 16S rRNA. Another useful tool for visualization of *C. piliforme* is transmission electron microscopy, in which vegetative cells and spores can be recognized in the cytoplasm of affected cells.

Treatment

Because of the peracute or acute nature of the disease, the intracellular parasitism and the development of spores, treatment for Tyzzer's disease is rarely effective. In foals, dextrose and broad spectrum antibiotics given intravenously were successful if applied soon after the onset of the disease. Additional supportive therapy, which has some value, includes intravenous dimethyl sulfoxide, anti-ulcer prophylaxis, and parenteral nutrition. However, in the majority of cases, foals respond temporarily to this treatment and then rapidly deteriorate and succumb to the disease. Due to the impossibility of cultivating this bacterium *in vitro* using conventional cultural methods, antimicrobial susceptibility patterns were determined in embryonated eggs. Penicillin, tetracycline, erythromycin, and streptomycin were effective against this microorganism.

Prevention and control

No commercial vaccine is available for Tyzzer's disease. Because *C. piliforme* is a spore-forming organism, control requires that special care be taken with the environment. Good hygiene may be beneficial for decreasing the likelihood that disease will occur. It is also recommended that all foals receive adequate passive transfer of immune globulins soon after birth. In lab animals, it is especially recommended to keep them free of spores and to control opportunities for cage-to-cage spread.

Bibliography

Brooks, J.W. *et al.* (2006) *Clostridium piliforme* infection in two farm-raised white-tailed deer fawns (*Odocoileus virginianus*) and association with copper toxicosis. *Vet. Pathol.*, **43**: 765–768.

Dürre, P. (2009) The Genus Clostridium. In: Goldman, E. and Green, L.H. (eds) *Practical Handbook of Microbiology*, 2nd edition, pp. 339–353. CRC Press, Boca Raton, FL.

Feldman, S., *et al.* (2006) Ribosomal RNA sequences of *Clostridium piliforme* isolated from rodent and rabbit: Re-examining the phylogeny of the Tyzzer's disease agent and development of a diagnostic polymerase chain reaction assay. *J. Am. Assoc. Lab. Anim. Sci.*, **45**: 65–73.

Ganaway, J.R., *et al.* (1971) Tyzzer's disease of rabbits: Isolation and propagation of *Bacillus piliformis* (Tyzzer) in embryonated eggs. *Infect. Immun.*, **3**: 429–437.

Ganaway, J.R., *et al.* (1971) Tyzzer's disease. *Am. J. Pathol.*, **64**: 717–730.

Headley, S.A., *et al.* (2009) Diagnostic exercise: Tyzzer's disease, distemper, and coccidiosis in a pup. *Vet. Pathol.*, **46**: 151–154.

Ikegami, T., *et al.* (1999) Naturally occurring Tyzzer's disease in a calf. *Vet. Pathol.*, **36**: 253–255.

Ikegami, T., *et al.* (1999) Enterocolitis associated with dual infection by *Clostridium piliforme* and feline panleukopenia virus in three kittens. *Vet. Pathol.*, **36**: 613–615.

Langan, J., *et al.* (2000) Tyzzer's disease in red panda. *J. Zoo. Wildl. Med.*, **31**: 558–562.

Maczulak, A.E., *et al.* (2011) Clostridium. In: Maczulak, A.E. and Ruskin, R.H. (eds) *Encyclopedia of Microbiology*, pp. 168–173. Facts on File Publisher, New York.

Mete, A., *et al.* (2011) *Clostridium piliforme* encephalitis in a weaver bird (*Ploceus castaneiceps*). *J. Vet. Diagn. Invest.*, **23**: 1240–1242.

Niepceron, A., *et al.* (2010) Development of a high-sensitivity nested PCR assay for the detection of *Clostridium piliforme* in clinical samples. *Vet. J.*, **185**: 222–224.

Nimmo-Wilkie, J.S., *et al.* (1985) Colitis due to *Bacillus piliformis* in two kittens. *Vet. Pathol.*, **22**: 649–652.

Percy, D.H., *et al.* (2007) Mouse. In: Percy, D.H. and Barthold, S.W. (eds) *Pathology of Laboratory Rodents and Rabbits*, 3rd edition, pp. 3–124. Blackwell Publishing, Ames, IA.

Poonacha, K.B. (1997) Naturally-occurring Tyzzer's disease in a serval (*Felis capensis*). *J. Vet. Diagn. Invest.*, **9**: 82–84.

Quinn, P.J., *et al.* (2011) Clostridium species. In: Quinn, P.J. *et al.* (eds) *Veterinary Microbiology and Microbial Disease*, 2nd edition, pp. 233–249. Wiley-Blackwell Publishing Ltd, Ames, IA.

Raymond, J.T., *et al.* (2001) Tyzzer's disease in a neonatal rainbow lorikeet. *Vet. Pathol.*, **38**: 326–327.

Sassevielle, V., *et al.* (2007) Naturally-occurring Tyzzer's disease in cotton-top tamarins (*Saguinus oedipus*). *J. Am. Assoc. Lab. Anim. Sci.*, **57**: 125–127.

Sellon, D.C. (2007) Systemic clostridial infections, Tyzzer's Disease. In: Sellon, D.C. and Long, R.W. (eds) *Equine Infectious Diseases*, pp. 367–372. Saunders Elsevier, St Louis, MI.

Songer, J.G., *et al.* (2005) Anaerobic gram positive rods and cocci. In: Songer, J.G. and Post, K.W. (eds) *Veterinary Microbiology: Bacterial and fungal agents of animal diseases*, pp. 261–286. Saunders Elsevier, St. Louis, MI.

Swerczek, T. (2013) Tyzzer's disease in foals: Retrospective studies from 1969 to 2010. *Can. Vet. J.*, **54**: 876–880.

Timoney, J.F., *et al.* (1988) *Hagan and Bruner's Microbiology and Infectious Diseases of Domestic Animals*, 8th edition, pp. 206–213. Comstock Publishing Associates, a division of Cornell University Press, Ithaca, NY and London.

Wobeser, G., *et al.* (2009) Tularemia, plague, yersiniosis, and Tyzzer's disease in wild rodents and lagomorphs in Canada: A review. *Can. Vet. J.*, **50**: 1251–1256.

Zachary, J.F. (2005) Mechanisms of microbial infections. In: Zachary, J.F. and McGavin, M.D. (eds) *Pathologic Basis of Veterinary Disease*, 5th edition, pp. 147–241. Elsevier Mosby, St. Louis, MI.

Clostridial Neurotoxic Infections

25 Tetanus

Michel R. Popoff

Introduction

Tetanus is a neurologic disease characterized by spastic paralysis. It is caused by a toxin, tetanus toxin (TeNT), which is produced by an environmental and sporulating anaerobic bacterium, *Clostridium tetani*. See Chapters 2, 3, and 7 for a description of the agent and the toxin.

Epidemiology

Tetanus is the result of wound contamination with *C. tetani* spores acquired from the environment. Deep wounds with a little exposure to air and the presence of necrotic tissue, both ensuring anaerobic conditions, favor spore germination. *C. tetani* spores germinate at low oxidation–reduction potential (Eh 10 mV or less) at neutral pH. In traumatized tissues with acidic pH due to local ischemia and anoxia, germination and *C. tetani* growth can occur at higher oxidation–reduction potential (until Eh 85 mV at pH 6.5). *C. tetani* is not an invasive pathogen but rather the presence of necrotic cells provides nutrients for the growth of *C. tetani*. Experimentally, *C. tetani* infection has been reproduced by intramuscular injection of spores with a necrotizing reagent such as calcium chloride.

In *in vitro* cultures, *C. tetani* spores can germinate in a wide range of Eh from −100 mV to +580 mV, but subsequent vegetative growth cannot be obtained with Eh above +300 mV.

Details of local colonization by *C. tetani* are not yet fully characterized. In addition to TeNT, *C. tetani* produces tetanolysin, a hemolysin from the cholesterol-dependent cytolysin family, the prototype of which is the perfringolysin of *C. perfringens*. Tetanolysin may facilitate local tissue colonization and resistance

Clostridial Diseases of Animals, First Edition. Francisco A. Uzal, J. Glenn Songer, John F. Prescott and Michel R. Popoff.
© 2016 John Wiley & Sons, Inc. Published 2016 by John Wiley & Sons, Inc.

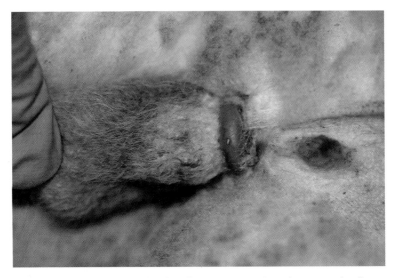

Figure 25.1 Scrotum of a lamb that developed tetanus approximately two weeks after castration with a rubber ring. Courtesy of F.A. Uzal.

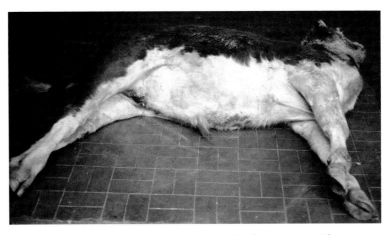

Figure 25.2 Tetanus in a steer that developed a few weeks after castration. Observe generalized rigidity of the body. Courtesy of F.A. Uzal.

to macrophages of *C. tetani* during the early steps of wound tetanus, since tetanolysin is able to form pores and to induce membrane damage in macrophages.

Tetanus occurs after contamination of a wound, and this can sometimes be small and difficult to find. Tetanus may even develop after healing of the wound. Wounds in parts of the body in contact with the soil are most at risk of producing tetanus. Examples include accidental wounds or punctures with prickly plants of the end of the limbs, the lower side of the trunk, and the abdomen.

The umbilicus is a common source of tetanus in newborns, notably in lambs and foals. Surgical and other wounds can be contaminated with *C. tetani* spores: these include castration (Figures 25.1 and 25.2), tail docking, ear surgery, injections such as vaccinations, or wounds incurred during shearing. Puerperal tetanus occurs after contamination of the vaginal mucosa and uterus during difficult delivery.

Clinical signs

Although all animal species are susceptible to tetanus, there is considerable variability in susceptibility among species. The most susceptible species are horses, guinea pigs, monkeys, sheep, mice, goats, and humans, whereas carnivores such as cats and dogs are less vulnerable, and birds are resistant (Table 25.1). Unlike other ruminants, cattle are quite resistant. Interestingly, poikilothermic animals such as frogs are resistant to tetanus intoxication when maintained at low temperature (below 18 °C) despite large amounts of TeNT in the circulating body fluids, but are susceptible when exposed to higher temperatures (27 °C and above). The protective effects of cooling have been attributed to a retardation of binding rate of TeNT on target neurons and the inhibition of its action.

Tetanus is characterized by hyperactivity of voluntary muscles, leading to rigidity and tetanic spasms (see Figures 25.2 and 25.4). Rigidity consists of tonic, involuntary, and prolonged muscle contractions, whereas spasms are shorter-lasting muscle contractions, usually triggered by sensory stimulations (reflex spasms) such as touch, light, or noise.

Table 25.1 Sensitivity of animal species to tetanus toxin. Relative minimum lethal doses compared to guinea pig lethal dose for various animal species

Species	Minimum lethal dose
Guinea pig	1
Horse	0.5
Monkey	2–4
Sheep	2
Mouse	2–6
Goat	12
Rabbit	4–900
Dog	300–480
Cat	960–1200
Goose	6000
Pigeon	6000–24,000
Hen	180,000
Human	10

Two forms of tetanus can be distinguished: generalized ("systemic") and local tetanus. In the generalized form, an increasing spasticity of the muscles of mastication occurs initially, and is followed by a progressive spastic paralysis of the muscles of the trunk, upper and lower limbs. Rigidity of the masseter and temporal muscles (trismus) leads to an inability to open the mouth. Later, generalized tetanic spasms develop. Spastic paralysis of the extensors of the neck and back is accompanied by opisthotonus. Neonatal tetanus is a generalized form in newborns less than 1 month old.In local tetanus, the muscles of the infected region become painful and then spastic. Local tetanus is more likely to be observed in those animal species, such as dogs, that are relatively resistant to the toxin.

The autonomic nervous system is also affected with episodes of tachycardia, hypertension, and sweating alternating with bradycardia and hypotension. Death occurs because of respiratory failure due to the spastic paralysis of the diaphragm, laryngeal, and other respiratory muscles. Disease may last for weeks.

Horses
Tetanus is common in non-immunized horses. Different forms of tetanus can be observed in horses. In the acute form, the symptoms of spastic paralysis rapidly spread from the head (muscles of mastication, ears, third eyelid) to the respiratory muscles and then to the limbs. Generalized convulsions are accompanied by crisis of sudation. Death can occur in one to two days because of respiratory failure. In the sub-acute forms, the symptoms develop in one to three weeks, and some animals may recover. Hyperesthesia and prolapse of the third eyelid are common early signs. Eating and swallowing are difficult because of paralysis of the mastication muscles. The nostrils are flared and the ears are held stiffly in a vertical position. The muscles of the neck, back, and tail will be very tense, so that the tail is often raised vertically. The limbs become stiff and the head is in an opisthotonus position. The body is in extension, with a global feature comparable to that of a wooden horse. The look of the horse is anxious and expresses pain. The face is tense due to trismus. The respiration is fast and the respiratory movements painful. The pulse is normal, although, during the crisis of tetanic spasm, the pulse and respiration are faster.

In localized tetanus, the muscle contractions are less intense and localized to a group of muscles such as those of a limb. This form can last for several weeks and the animals can recover.

Cattle
The symptoms are comparable to those observed in horses, but the reflex hyperexcitability is less pronounced. The first sign is of global stiffness (Figure 25.2), with a deviation of the tail to one side. Later, the head and neck go into extension. The ears are stiff and point backwards; prolapse of the third eyelid can also be observed (Figure 25.3). Bloat is common. Trismus is pronounced. In severe disease, the thoracic and abdominal muscles are spastic, and respiration is painful and loud. Severely affected animals die of respiratory failure in five to nine days.

Sheep

The predominant symptom is a stiffness of the limbs with a rigid gait. Feeding is difficult or impossible due to the contraction of the masticatory muscles. The ears are stiff, in a horizontal position, and the third eyelid is prolapsed. Then, animals go into in lateral recumbency (Figure 25.4). The tail is also stiff. Several newborn lambs within a flock can be affected by tetanus following umbilical contamination.

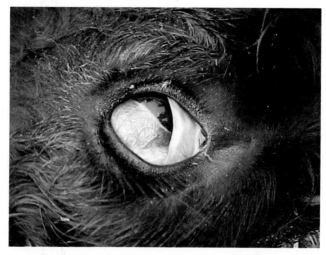

Figure 25.3 Third eyelid prolapse in a steer with tetanus. Courtesy of F.C. Faria Lobato.

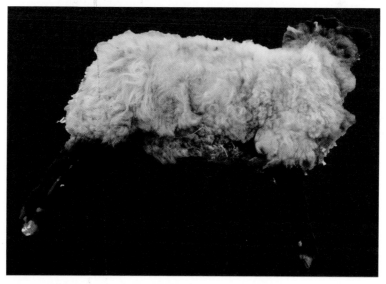

Figure 25.4 Lamb with tetanus. The animal is in lateral recumbency and shows stiffness of the limbs. Courtesy of F.A. Uzal.

Swine

Tetanus in pigs is most often generalized and fatal, and observed mainly in piglets. Affected animals have difficulty in walking, and do so with a stiff gait. Disease usually develops rapidly, with tetanic spasms of skeletal muscles. Feeding is difficult or impossible because of trismus. The ears stand stiffly on the head. Respiration is fast and shallow.

Dogs and cats

Tetanus in these species is rare and the disease is usually mild. The incubation period is five to ten days in dogs. The localized form is more common in cats than in dogs, since cats are more resistant to TeNT. Spastic paralysis is observed in certain groups of muscles, particularly trismus, stiff limbs, and body stretching of the body because of the large spinal extensor muscle spasm. Muscle spasms are relatively mild. The ears are commonly upwardly erect and close together, and the skin of the forehead is often wrinkled because of muscle tension.

Gross and microscopic changes

No gross or microscopic changes, except those related to the entry wound, when found, are seen in the carcasses of animals dying of tetanus.

Diagnosis

The diagnosis of tetanus is essentially based on the clinical observation of the characteristics of spastic paralysis. No circulating TeNT can usually be found in the blood of animals with tetanus.

The biological confirmation of tetanus can be obtained by evidence of *C. tetani* in the wound responsible for the entry of the pathogen. However, the wound is, in many cases, no longer obvious in the clinical phase of the disease. *C. tetani* can be detected by a Gram stain of infected wound material, in which case the presence of Gram-positive (and sometimes Gram-negative) rods with terminal spores is characteristic of the organism (Figure 25.5). In addition, PCR can be done on wound material or after enrichment culture of wound debris in complex liquid medium for anaerobic bacteria. *C. tetani* can also be isolated on blood agar plates. Since *C. tetani* is a highly motile bacterium, plate-containing dense agar (20 to 30 g per L) is recommended in order to obtain isolated colonies.

Prophylaxis, treatment, and control

Medical prevention consists of immunization with formaldehyde-inactivated TeNT. Two injections at 3–4 weeks' interval are required to induce effective immunity. In humans, this is usually repeated every ten years. However, the

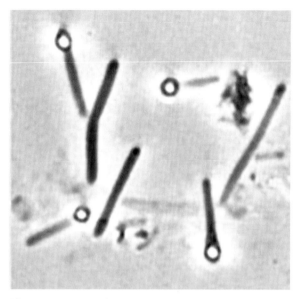

Figure 25.5 *Clostridium tetani*. Terminal spores are observed in several rods, giving the typical drumstick appearance to the organism. Unstained phase contrast microscopy, 600x.

recommendation for animals at risk, such as horses, is usually for more frequent immunization.

No specific treatment is available for tetanus. TeNT antibodies prevent free TeNT from entering neurons via the serum, but toxin which has been taken up into neuronal cells cannot be accessed by anti-toxin antibodies.

Wound debridement and cleaning, antibiotic use, and injection of TeNT immunoglobulin are recommended when a risk of tetanus is suspected. Penicillin G and metronidazole are the antibiotics of choice to treat infection, but will not affect existing disease. Non-specific treatment includes sedation and muscle relaxation, and nursing care (feeding, maintaining hydration, preventing soiling).

Interestingly, botulinum toxin has been successfully used to counterbalance the muscle rigidity of tetanus.

Measures of good hygiene, notably disinfection of wounds such as the umbilicus wound, are important in the prevention of tetanus. Surgical interventions must, of course, be performed with sterilized materials and in appropriate conditions of hygiene.

Bibliography

Acke, E., *et al.* (2004) Tetanus in the dog: Review and a case report of concurrent tetanus with hiatal hernia. *Irish Vet. J.*, **57**: 593–597.

Green, S.L., *et al.* (1994) Tetanus in the horse: A review of 20 cases (1970 to 1990). *J. Vet. Intern. Med.*, **8**: 128–132.

Hachisuka, Y., *et al.* (1982) The effect of oxidation–reduction potential on spore germination, outgrowth, and vegetative growth of *Clostridium tetani, Clostridium butyricum,* and *Bacillus subtilis. Microbiol. Immunol.,* **26**: 803–811.

Hassel, B. (2013) Tetanus: Pathophysiology, treatment, and the possibility of using botulinum toxin against tetanus-induced rigidity and spasms. *Toxins,* **5**: 73–83.

Keyel, P.A., *et al.* (2011) Macrophage responses to bacterial toxins: A balance between activation and suppression. *Immunol. Res.,* **50**: 118–123.

Popoff, M.R. and Bouvet, P. (2009) Clostridial toxins. *Future Microbiol.,* **4**: 1021–1064.

Rethy, L., *et al.* (1997) Human lethal dose of tetanus toxin. *Lancet,* **350**: 1518.

Wright, G.P. (1955) The neurotoxins of *Clostridium botulinum* and *Clostridium tetani. Pharmacol. Rev.,* **7**: 413–465.

Botulism

Caroline Le Maréchal, Cédric Woudstra,
and Patrick Fach

Introduction

Botulism is a severe, flaccid neuroparalytic disease of humans and animals. Animal botulism was first described at the beginning of the 20th century, although it is thought to have occurred long before that. It affects most mammals, birds, and fish. Animal botulism is a major environmental and economic concern, mainly because of the high mortality rate during outbreaks. It is considered to be a zoonosis, as it may be a source of food-borne botulism for humans. It is also considered a potential bioterrorism threat.

Etiology

Botulism can be caused by one of seven different neuroparalytic toxin subtypes (A to G). These botulinum neurotoxins (BoNTs) are produced by anaerobic, Gram-positive clostridia, mainly *Clostridium botulinum*. All BoNT subtypes act at the neuromuscular junction, blocking the release of acetylcholine and leading to flaccid paralysis. BoNT types A, B, E, and, more rarely, type F, are mainly responsible for human botulism, whereas toxin types C and D and their mosaic variants are mostly involved in animal botulism worldwide. Cases of animal botulism caused by BoNT types A, B, and E have also been reported.

BoNTs are proteins of approximately 150 kDa, composed of two subunits linked by a disulfide bond: a light chain (50 kDa) and a heavy chain (100 kDa). The light chain is a zinc protease that cleaves the SNARE protein, interfering with the exocytotic cell mechanism and preventing release of acetylcholine in the synaptic cleft. The heavy chain is involved in binding to the receptor on the neuronal membrane and the translocation of the light chain into nerve cells.

Clostridial Diseases of Animals, First Edition. Francisco A. Uzal, J. Glenn Songer,
John F. Prescott and Michel R. Popoff.
© 2016 John Wiley & Sons, Inc. Published 2016 by John Wiley & Sons, Inc.

BoNTs are absorbed from the intestine by binding to receptors on the apical surface of gut epithelial cells. Absorption may also occur in the stomach. Then, BoNTs reach the nerve endings via the bloodstream. Binding of type C BoNT to the receptor is ganglioside-dependent, but binding of type D toxin is not.

C. botulinum strains can be divided into four groups based on their genotypic and phenotypic characteristics. Group I and II strains are mainly involved in human disease, while group III strains are associated with animal disease. Sequences of several *C. botulinum* group III strains have been published recently and revealed that *C. botulinum* group III strains, *C. novyi*, and *C. haemolyticum* are closely related. Given these genetic results, it has been suggested that a new genotypic name be created, *C. novyi sensu lato* for *C. botulinum* group III, *C. novyi*, and *C. haemolyticum*. Group IV strains produce the type G toxin and have been reclassified as the new species *Clostridium argentinense*.

Group III strains produce type C, D, and mosaic toxin types C/D and D/C. These toxins are encoded by genes carried by bacteriophages in plasmids. These pseudolysogen circular plasmid prophages do not integrate into the genome. Mosaic toxins were first described in 1996. The mosaic-type gene comprises two-thirds of one gene and one-third of the other gene. Type C/D BoNTs are composed of the light chain of type C toxin and the heavy chain of the type D toxin; type D/C toxin consists of the light chain of type D toxin and the heavy chain of the type C toxin.

BoNTs are produced during vegetative growth. Suitable growth conditions include anaerobiosis, the presence of a protein source, sufficient temperature (25–42 °C), and moisture. *C. botulinum* is not able to synthesize some essential amino acids, so high protein substrates are essential. Decaying matter, such as decomposing cadavers or other rotting organic matter, offers ideal conditions for growth of *C. botulinum*. This microorganism can survive extreme environmental conditions; spores remain viable for years.

Pathogenesis

Two main routes of exposure to BoNTs have been identified:
1 Ingestion of preformed toxins in food, water, or carrion.
2 *In vivo* production of BoNTs – so-called toxico-infection.
Ingestion of preformed toxins has been considered the main exposure route in cases of animal botulism. However, it seems that *in vivo* production of BoNTs has also to be considered as a route of exposure. Cattle, horses, and poultry are more likely to be affected by this form of botulism. In Japan, it has recently been suggested that bovine botulism results from ingestion of spores that germinate, multiply, and produce BoNT in the bovine gastrointestinal tract. It has been suggested that avian botulism (especially in broiler chickens) is mainly due to BoNT production in the cecum, as a high level of type C toxin is necessary to induce botulism (106.3 mouse lethal doses [MLD/kg] for 8-week-old broilers) and such levels of toxins are not found in the environment, supporting the theory of *in vivo* toxin production.

Occurrence and prevalence of animal botulism

Animal botulism is not a notifiable disease in most countries. Lack of accurate knowledge of outbreaks likely results in underestimation of the incidence of animal botulism. In addition, difficulties in evaluating cases of the disease include limited knowledge of the disease by some veterinary practitioners and lack of laboratories performing diagnostic analyses. Botulism is classified as an emerging disease in Europe at present, and sporadic, sometimes massive outbreaks have been reported around the world in recent years. This increase in the number of cases in the last decade may be linked to the decrease in antibiotic use in animal feed.

Mosaic forms are the most common BoNTs causing animal botulism in Europe and in Japan. It is not known whether mosaic types are emerging or if their recent identification is due to the availability of more specific detection methods. Table 26.1 presents the occurrence of BoNT types involved in affected species during botulism outbreaks.

Birds

BoNT C/D seems to be the prevalent type involved in avian botulism in Europe and the Americas at the moment. It has also been reported in Japan. Tools allowing the identification of mosaic BoNTs have been developed recently. Mosaic BoNTs may be involved in avian botulism in other parts of the world, but this has not been confirmed. Birds are considered to be fairly resistant to type D BoNT (approximately 320,000 MLD/kg are required to produce disease in poultry), but some D or D/C outbreaks have been reported in poultry. Type E avian botulism outbreaks are also reported, mainly around the North American Great Lakes, where it causes large-scale mortality among birds and fish. Some type E

Table 26.1 Occurrence of BoNT types in animal botulism

Animal species	BoNT type	Occurence
Fur animals (mink, fox)	C, C/D	++++
	A, E	+
Cattle	D, D/C	++++
	C/D, C	++
	A, B	+
Birds	C, C/D	++++
	E, D	++
	A	+
Equine	C, D	+++
	B	+
	A	+
Fish	E	?

botulism outbreaks were also described in broiler flocks in France in the 1990s, but no type E outbreak in poultry flocks has been reported in the literature since then.

Gallinaceous birds are more susceptible to type C/D BoNT than to type C. The LD_{50} for type C BoNT in chickens via intravenous inoculation is 16,000 MLD/kg, in peafowl 2700 MLD/kg, in turkeys 320 MLD/kg, and in pheasants 60 MLD/kg.

Type C botulism has been diagnosed in water birds in at least 28 countries around the world, although it is rare in the tropics. Botulism has already been reported in 264 bird species representing 39 families. It often affects waterfowl but sometimes also fish-eating birds, and it is the most significant disease of migratory birds, notably waterfowl and shorebirds. Millions of birds have been killed by botulism type C during outbreaks in Canada or the USA, and outbreaks with losses exceeding 50,000 birds have been commonly reported. The effect of botulism on local populations can be significant and may cause important declines in some endangered species, impeding conservation efforts. For example, nearly 15% of the western population of American white pelicans died during a botulism outbreak in 1996.

Botulism outbreaks are also reported in poultry production units. An increase in the number of outbreaks in poultry farms, notably in broilers, was reported in Sweden, Denmark, Norway, and France in 2007 and 2008. For example, according to the French epidemiological surveillance network for poultry, 121 botulism outbreaks were reported in 2007 in France, whereas only 28 cases were reported in 2006. In broilers and turkeys, 87 cases were reported between 2000 and 2006, while 393 cases were reported between 2007 and 2011. Production types mostly affected by botulism are broiler chickens and turkeys, but outbreaks in pheasants, layer hens, ducks, geese, and guinea fowl have also been reported. Not all avian species are susceptible to BoNTs; many of the carrion-eating species are resistant.

Cattle

Botulism in cattle was first described in South Africa in 1920. Bovine botulism outbreaks have been reported throughout the world (Europe, North and South America, Africa, Oceania, and Asia). Types D and D/C are the most common BoNT types involved in bovine botulism. Mosaic type D/C exhibits higher toxicity for cattle than BoNTs C or D. Botulism outbreaks due to type B have also been reported in the Netherlands and the USA, but they are less frequent. BoNT types C and D are often related to contamination of feed by carcasses of poultry, wild birds, or other animals, whereas type B is more associated with improperly stored silage previously contaminated by soils containing *C. botulinum* type B spores.

Oral administration of 22.5 MLD/kg of type D BoNT can induce the disease in cattle. This species is 12.88 times more sensitive to BoNT type C toxin than mice, on a per kilogram basis. An estimated 1 g of BoNT can potentially kill

400,000 adult cows. The cattle intravenous median lethal dose is 0.388 ng per kg. Large numbers of mortalities occur during outbreaks, with rates varying from 8% to 80%. The highest mortalities are seen during the first week of the outbreaks but losses can continue for more than three weeks thereafter.

Twelve outbreaks of botulism were reported in dairy and beef cattle between 2008 and 2012 in Italy. In the Netherlands, botulism is estimated to affect about 20 dairy herds each year. Clinical botulism outbreaks were confirmed in 1108 German cattle herds between 1995 and 2010. In the United Kingdom, between 20 and 30 cases per year are reported in cattle. In Sweden, seven cases were diagnosed during the last ten years. At least eight outbreaks were reported between 2004 and 2007 in Japan.

Visceral or chronic botulism has been reported in Germany and Denmark. It is allegedly associated with toxico-infection, in which BoNT are produced *in situ* within the gastrointestinal tract. The existence of this specific clinical form of botulism is controversial.

Horses

Botulism in horses is mainly attributed to *C. botulinum* toxin types A, B, and C. In the USA, *C. botulinum* type B toxin causes more than 85% of equine botulism cases. Type B is endemic in the mid-Atlantic region and Kentucky, whereas type A is endemic in states west of the Mississippi River. *C. botulinum* type C is uncommon in horses in the USA. On the contrary, types C and D are most common in Europe, except in the Netherlands where type B is encountered more frequently than either type C or type D. Type D is more common in South America and South Africa. The most common form of equine botulism is forage poisoning, an emerging problem in Europe, which is linked to the use of grass silage as feed. Horses are highly sensitive to BoNTs; often, horses are susceptible to less than a single mouse MLD. This leads to a very low rate of laboratory confirmation of diagnosis with the mouse bioassay.

Equine grass sickness has been suggested as being associated with *C. botulinum* type C intoxication, but this association has not been confirmed and the etiology of this disease remains unclear.

Fur animals

Fur animal botulism outbreaks are mainly caused by type C toxins, but rare outbreaks caused by types A and E have also been reported. Botulism is considered a major hazard in fur animal production. Mink, foxes, and ferrets are most often affected, and large outbreaks have been reported. For example, in 2002, 52,000 foxes from 83 breeding farms in Finland were affected.

Fish

Fish are susceptible to *C. botulinum* type E toxin. The lethal dose for coho salmon is 90 MLD and mortality is observed at 50 MLD for round goby. BoNT E is responsible for visceral toxicosis of catfish (VTC). VTC causes large losses to the catfish industry, up to 37.8% of total loss in some years. Few data are available about the impact of botulism on fish populations or the prevalence of this disease on fish farms. However, type E spores are routinely ingested by healthy fish without any germination.

Other animal species

Few reports exist on botulism in dogs, although they are known to be sensitive to the disease. Cats are reported to seem resistant. Only one paper reports type C botulism in a group of cats after being fed pelican carrion. Botulism in pigs is rare and they are also relatively resistant.

Botulism has been reported in sheep and goats, with clinical signs similar to those in cattle, mostly in England, Wales, Australia, the USA, and South Africa. Such outbreaks are uncommon in the UK (14 were reported between 1999 and 2007).

Epidemiology

Source of contamination

The source for initial proliferation of group III *C. botulinum* is typically unknown. However, several routes of contamination have been suggested, including:

1 Contamination of feed or water by cadavers, where optimal conditions for *C. botulinum* growth and toxin production are present.
2 Cross-contamination among various forms of animal production (for example, poultry manure is considered a risk factor when used as bedding or feed for cattle, notably because of the risk of accidental inclusion of poultry cadavers that may constitute a source of BoNTs).
3 Environmental contamination, illustrated by recurrent botulism outbreaks in waterbirds in places where spores are present in the sediment found at the bottom of lakes and other inland bodies of water.
4 Unbalanced feed ration or bad quality feed (with presence of glyphosphate residues, for instance), inducing a change in intestinal microbiota and allowing the growth of *C. botulinum* in the gastrointestinal tract.

Healthy carriage

Many hypotheses about the origin of animal botulism outbreaks are based on the idea that *C. botulinum* is a normal inhabitant of the intestinal tract of healthy animals. Several studies have been conducted to determine the characteristics of such asymptomatic carriage by animals. *C. botulinum* has been detected in pig feces in 24% of the examined samples in a German study, 76% in a Japanese study, 62% in a Swedish study, and 3% in a Finnish study. In these studies, BoNT types B, E, and C were identified. Type C was found in the kidney and liver of healthy swine. *C. botulinum* has also been detected in porcine, equine, bovine, and caprine tonsils. Botulism is rare in pigs, but the data mentioned above indicate that pigs can be reservoirs. Particular attention should be paid to preventing cross-contamination between pigs and poultry and pigs and cattle.

Healthy carriage in cattle has also been reported. Prevalence varies substantially from one study to another, including 73% of type B and less than 5% of types E and F in bovine fecal samples in a Swedish study, 13% in cattle feces in a Dutch study, and 0–4% of fecal samples in two German studies, respectively. Most of these studies have focused on the presence of BoNT associated with human botulism outbreaks, and further investigations are needed to evaluate the healthy carriage of group III *C. botulinum*. The possibility of *C. botulinum* being part of the normal cattle microflora is a controversial topic in the veterinary literature. Some authors consider that *C. botulinum* is part of the enteric microflora, while others suggest that the presence of these bacteria in feces of healthy animals is rare.

C. botulinum is apparently not part of the normal gastrointestinal flora of the horse. Healthy carriage in birds is also a controversial topic. *C. botulinum* is reported to be a normal member of the avian gut flora but very few studies have clearly demonstrated its presence in the gastrointestinal tracts of birds. For example, *C. botulinum* spores have been detected in the gastrointestinal tracts of more than 50% of healthy mallards in a marsh with a history of botulism outbreaks. The organism has also been found in the proventriculus, gizzard, duodenum, and small intestine of unaffected birds during a botulism outbreak in a broiler chicken flock.

Two studies have recently been conducted to evaluate such carriage in broilers using real-time PCR. Both studies showed that none of the investigated flocks was positive for *C. botulinum* types C or C/D. The difficulty in detection of *C. botulinum* in the avian gut may be because of the low level of bacteria, at least under the detection limit of available methods.

In summary, it seems that birds can be healthy carriers of *C. botulinum* spores (notably after a botulism outbreak) but that normal carriage in broilers is nonexistent or extremely low, under the detection limit of available methods. It is likely that an outbreak is preceded by a recent introduction of spores to the flock. The spores may cause disease directly, or may multiply in birds that die of an unrelated cause.

Fish can also be healthy carriers of *C. botulinum* spores. Prevalence of *C. botulinum* in trout varies from 5–100% in winter and from 80–100% in summer. Tilapia have been implicated as the source of type C BoNT in pelican botulism outbreaks in California. These fish actually harbor *C. botulinum* capable of producing toxin in their gastrointestinal tracts without producing disease in the fish. They consume large amounts of sediment, which may explain the presence of toxin-producing *C. botulinum* in their intestines. Spores of *C. botulinum* type C are widely distributed in marsh sediments.

Data about asymptomatic carriage of group III *C. botulinum* are scarce, especially in cattle and poultry production. New information on this topic will be very helpful in understanding the epidemiology and pathogenesis of animal botulism.

Environmental conditions favorable for botulism outbreaks

Temperature

Whatever the animal species, botulism is often reported to be seasonal, with an increase in the number of outbreaks during summer and fall, when ambient conditions are near the optimal temperature for bacterial growth. For example, this is typically reported in wild bird outbreaks, for which warm temperatures are also often associated with initiation of botulism. Incidence of botulism outbreaks increases during very hot summers. Occasional winter and spring outbreaks have also been reported in some countries.

Water and feed pH

Water and feed pH are also reported as being risk factors for the germination of *C. botulinum* spores and BoNT production. Many of the large epizootics of wild bird botulism have occurred in areas of alkaline waters in western North America. The risk of botulism outbreaks has been reported to be increased when water pH is between 7.5 and 9.0, redox potential is negative, and water temperature is above 20 °C. In cattle, forage botulism occurs when pH (> 4.5), moisture, and anaerobic conditions within the forage allow the proliferation of *C. botulinum*. Animal feed without acidification is amenable to production of *C. botulinum* spores and toxin production. Silage with a pH above 4.5 is typically considered risky.

Risk factors associated with avian botulism

Risk factors in poultry production

In poultry, poor biosafety, no acidification or chlorination of water, and a lack of pest control have been reported as risk factors for botulism. The following conditions may also be considered risk factors:
- A high mortality rate in a flock with a prior history of botulism; *C. botulinum* spores can persist for several years in the environment;
- Poor hygiene conditions in the poultry house;
- High animal density, which contributes to a rapid propagation of an outbreak within the flock;
- Poor feed storage conditions;
- The presence of cadavers within or adjacent to the poultry house, and the corresponding spread of insects;
- Botulism in farm pets;
- High daily weight gain;
- Warm and stormy weather;
- The presence of wild waterfowl and water adjacent to the poultry house.

The increase in the number of botulism outbreaks in poultry in Europe in 2007 and 2008 was potentially linked to feed. The presence of *C. botulinum* spores was indeed demonstrated in feed samples collected from four outbreaks on Swedish farms. During a recent European workshop about animal botulism in Europe, feed, rice hulls used as litter, decomposing carcasses, rodents, soil, and hay packaged in plastic were mentioned as potential sources of *C. botulinum* spores.

Risk factors in wild birds

Foraging behavior seems to be one of the most important risk factors for development of wild bird botulism. Filter feeding and dabbling waterfowl, shorebirds that feed near the surface of wetland soils, and sediment- and fish-eating birds are at greater risk than other waterfowl.

Some outbreaks have been associated with landfills. The presence of ideal conditions in landfills for *C. botulinum* growth (notably rotting organic matter and a rise in temperature due to the composting effect) may then induce spore germination followed by BoNT production. It is also thought that *C. botulinum* spores are passively transferred from landfills contaminated by spores to other locations. Environmental factors that contribute to initiation of avian botulism outbreaks include low water levels, water-level fluctuations, water quality, and the presence of vertebrate and invertebrate carcasses and rotting vegetation in ponds and other water reservoirs. Type C is highly prevalent in some wetland sediments (60% of samples from a marsh with a prior history of botulism were culture positive, as compared to 6% in lakes with no history of the disease).

Role of invertebrates in avian botulism

Type C BoNT and group III *C. botulinum* strains may be found in invertebrate organisms. The carcass-and-maggot cycle is a well-known scenario through which botulism outbreaks occur in waterfowl when maggots and other invertebrates are consumed by wild aquatic birds. Maggots collected from carcasses of animals dead from botulism carried BoNTs. These highly toxic maggots perform cascades of intoxications when birds consuming maggots develop botulism and die. The carcasses attract flies for egg laying, resulting in an increase of toxic maggots that leads to further botulism outbreaks. Although it has been suggested that BoNT production may occur in dead invertebrate organisms, there is no direct evidence that this occurs. Invertebrates can also carry *C. botulinum* spores and transfer them from place to place. This has been shown experimentally for necrophagous flies that can transfer *C. botulinum* spores between two points and excrete them up to 24 hours after exposure, playing a role in botulism outbreaks. Slugs can also excrete spores in feces for up to four days, while the spores persist in slug carcasses for longer periods of time. Slugs may be involved in silage contamination by *C. botulinum* spores. Recently, chironomids (a type of midget) collected in the Great Lakes region of the US, where avian botulism occurs regularly, were found to be carrying type E strains of *C. botulinum*. Their contamination may be due to the presence of *C. botulinum* spores and vegetative cells in cladophora (a type of green alga), which is a food source for larvae of chironomids. Larvae of chironomids are important food sources for fish and for birds, which might be exposed to botulism by eating these larvae. After a botulism outbreak, darkling beetles collected in affected poultry houses were often culture positive for *C. botulinum*. This suggests that darkling beetles could be reservoirs and carriers of *C. botulinum*. These beetles feed on bird droppings, bird carcasses, and litter, which could explain why they harbor *C. botulinum*. Poultry eat darkling beetles and can thus become infected. In conclusion, insects can be carriers of *C. botulinum* spores and, therefore, insect control is crucial in the management of avian botulism.

Risk factors associated with fur botulism

Botulism outbreaks in fur-producing animals are typically associated with food poisoning. Fur animal feed is mainly composed of poultry, swine, and bovine slaughter by-products, fishery by-products, fur animal cadavers, animal fat, and cereals. The fur animal food chain is highly contaminated by *C. botulinum*, notably by type C toxin-producing strains, and these animals are widely exposed to these strains.

Risk factors associated with bovine botulism

In cattle, type B botulism is typically associated with grass-fed animals, while types C and D cases are more often related to carcass-contaminated feed. The latter are also grown on decomposing plant material.

Contamination of feed and water by rotting organic matter containing BoNTs or BoNT-producing clostridia is often incriminated in cattle botulism outbreaks. Type C is usually associated with decomposing carcasses, such as cats or waterfowl. Grain, hay, or silage can be contaminated by rooting organic matter during harvesting or storage. Silage that is not properly stored (allowed to rot, for example) provides ideal conditions for *C. botulinum* growth (moisture, high temperature, anaerobiosis). The pH of silage has to be less than 4.5 to avoid growth of *C. botulinum* spores. Use of mixing and distributing feeders increases the risk of dissemination of contaminated feed to all animals, even if only a small quantity of feed is contaminated. Types D and C bovine botulism have also often been associated with poultry litter used as feed or bedding. The practice is no longer allowed in the USA, but the recent emergence of bovine botulism in England, Wales, and Northern Ireland has been associated with broiler litter. In Northern Ireland, for instance, most cases have been linked to the spreading of broiler litter on pastures, and 85% of outbreaks have occurred when cattle were at pasture. Equipment such as trailers or tractor buckets used for removing litter from broiler houses could play a role in the transfer of spores from poultry production to cattle production. Botulism can also occur as a result of pica in cattle. This behavior originates when phosphorus and/or calcium-deficient cattle develop a depraved appetite, gnawing on bone to compensate for those deficiencies. This has been notably described in Australia, South Africa, Brazil, and Argentina.

Molecular epidemiology

Molecular epidemiological investigations of *C. botulinum* strains allow better characterization of the organism at the genetic level. There is little information in this regard about group III strains. This could be explained by the difficulty of isolating group III *C. botulinum* strains. There is actually no selective medium, and group III *C. botulinum* strains are known to grow poorly in mixed culture and on agar plates. The instability of the phage carrying the BoNT gene in laboratory conditions is also problematic, and this phage is easily lost during isolation procedures. One complete genome and twelve draft genomes from avian strains are available. Analysis of these genomes showed that the chromosome is highly conserved and that genetic diversity is observed in the plasmidosome of the isolates. This minor genetic diversity among the chromosomes has also been described by comparison of the group III isolates via classical molecular techniques. New typing methods should be designed to compare group III strains and perform epidemiological investigations when needed. A PCR-based method should be developed to compare strains while avoiding the need for isolation.

Pulsed-field gel electrophoresis (PFGE), randomly amplified polymorphic DNA (RAPD), and amplified fragment length polymorphism (AFLP) have been used to compare group III *C. botulinum* strains. Type D-C strains isolated from the bovine gastrointestinal tract in Japan were compared by PFGE after digestion with *Sac*II. This revealed that at least two strains of different origin were involved in bovine botulism outbreaks in Japan. On the other hand, studies revealed an apparently common pulsotype involved in avian botulism in Sweden and in Spain. RAPD analysis is a fast and simple PCR-based DNA fingerprinting method, but with the major drawback of poor reproducibility due to non-specific primer binding. This technique was used to compare avian isolates, and results match those obtained by PFGE analysis. AFLP is a useful technique in epidemiological investigations. This has been tested in a study comparing all *C. botulinum* groups and strains isolated from a type C bovine botulism outbreak. Using this method, *C. botulinum* strains clustered according to toxin type, source, and, for some profiles, to geographic location.

Molecular epidemiological studies regarding group III *C. botulinum* are, thus, scarce, and further investigations are needed to provide efficient tools that will allow a better understanding of animal botulism epidemiology.

Clinical signs

Clinical signs of animal botulism are often strongly indicative but not specific. Avian botulism has to be differentiated from lead, selenium, or ionophore intoxication and from other diseases with neurological symptoms such as Newcastle's disease, Marek's disease, and avian influenza. Differential diagnosis for ruminants includes calcium deficiency, tick paralysis, and intoxications such as those by magnesium and ionophores. Botulism in most mammalian species is characterized by progressive, symmetrical, and flaccid paralysis, which often starts in the hindquarters with weaknesses, muscle tremors, stumbling, and recumbency, and is usually fatal. Weakness progresses from the hindquarters to the forequarters, head, and neck. Disease ranges from peracute to chronic forms. Some cases may present as sudden death. Clinical signs appear from 18 hours to 17 days after exposure. This is faster for monogastrics than for ruminants, in which no signs may be observed for several days after exposure.

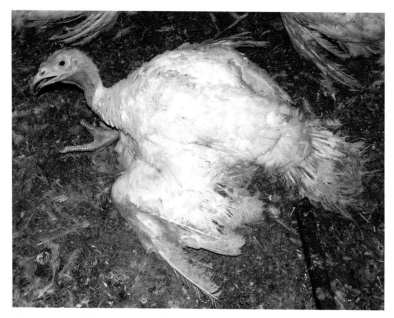

Figure 26.1 Turkey with typical signs of botulism: paralysis of legs, wings, and neck. Courtesy of R. Souillard.

Clinical signs in birds

Generalized flaccid paralysis is characteristic of avian botulism, with loss of motor control, flight, and ambulation. Wing muscles are usually affected first. Typically, the nictitating membrane is paralyzed. Then, birds are unable to lift their heads, a typical sign called "limber neck" (Figure 26.1). Death usually results from drowning (for water birds) or respiratory failure. Birds, especially gulls, may walk on their tarsometatarsi. Diarrhea may also be observed, notably in broilers. C2 toxin may cause necrotic changes in the intestinal mucosa, with fluid accumulation in the intestine.

Clinical signs in cattle

Reluctance to move, digestive disorders (constipation or signs of colic) (Figure 26.2), weakness in the hind limbs resulting in recumbency, often followed by dysphagia, are the initial signs of botulism in cattle. Dysphagia can be explained by a decrease in tone and strength of masseter, tongue (Figure 26.3), and pharyngeal muscles. The complete inability to eat or drink and tongue paralysis are the next signs of botulism. Some signs may differ between type C or D botulism and type B. The most distinct signs of type C or D intoxication are paralysis in the muscles of the tail and of the hind part of the body, which leads to recumbency. The disease caused by *C. botulinum* type B is characterized clinically by indigestion, diarrhea, hypersalivation, and dehydration.

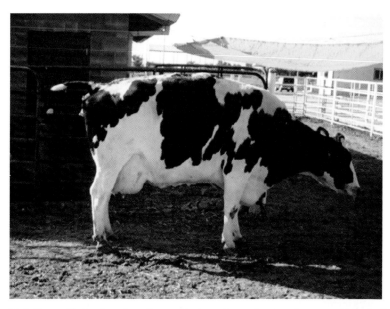

Figure 26.2 Cow suffering from botulism with signs of constipation. Courtesy of R. Moeller.

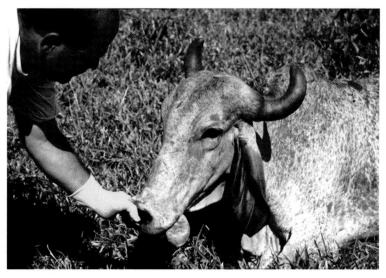

Figure 26.3 Tongue paralysis in a cow with botulism. Courtesy of I. Dutra.

Another clinical form of cattle botulism, called visceral botulism, has been described recently. It is linked to intestinal proliferation of *C. botulinum*. Visceral botulism symptoms are indigestion (constipation alternating with diarrhea), chronic laminitis, engorged veins, edema of ventral areas, retracted abdomen, emaciation, and apathy.

Clinical signs in horses

In adult horses, the first sign of botulism can be mild abdominal discomfort, generally followed by muscle weakness and dysphagia. Botulism in horses is also characterized by decreased tail, eyelid, and tongue tone. This can lead to recumbency and difficulty in rising, lifting the head, and breathing. Mydriasis is also common, notably in type C equine botulism. Horses with type A or B botulism may have more dysphagia than in type C. The shaker foal syndrome can be compared to infant botulism in humans. The initial signs are long periods of lying down and muscle tremors. Lethargy and weakness increase as the disease progresses and respiratory difficulties occur. Other signs are very similar to the ones observed in adults, but they develop more slowly.

Clinical signs in fur animals

Paralysis of the hind legs, followed by general paralysis and recumbency are typical signs of botulism in fur animals. The progression of the disease can be very rapid; it is common to find dead animals within two to three hours of the appearance of clinical signs.

Clinical signs in fish

An increase in mortality is the first sign of a botulism outbreak in fish. This is followed by agitation and paralysis of the fins, ending with paralysis of the tail. Loss of the ability to swim and a tendency to sink to the bottom of the pond or pool are also reported.

Clinical signs commonly observed in catfish with so-called visceral toxicosis include erratic swimming and progressive muscular weakness leading to death.

Gross and microscopic changes

Botulism is characterized by the absence of specific gross or microscopic lesions. This can be used as a presumptive diagnostic criterion. Occasionally, hemorrhagic lesions can be observed in the jejunum, especially in cattle. These lesions may be due to the action of C2 toxins by *C. botulinum*. Such lesions are not specific enough to be used for diagnostic confirmation. In catfish, internal lesions include chylous or clear fluid in the coelomic cavity, intussusception of the intestinal tract, reticular pattern in the liver, congested spleen, and eversion of the stomach into the oral cavity. Edema of the nuchal ligament has been described in horses with type A and C botulism; this is thought to be a consequence of the inability of horses to keep the head up due to weakness of the neck muscles.

Prophylaxis and control

Prevention of animal botulism can be achieved by:
• Providing safe and high quality feed and water;
• Properly storing animal feed;

- Preventing access to animal carcasses;
- Disinfestation and rodent control;
- Avoiding water contamination by dying or dead animals;
- Avoiding exposure of animals to poultry litter (as feed, bedding material, or on pastures);
- Vaccination;
- Supplementation of protein and phosphorus to cattle to prevent pica (bone gnawing) in areas of phosphorus deficiency.

Poultry litter is a major risk factor for cattle botulism because of the risk of carcasses present within the litter. Therefore, farmers are advised to pay particular attention when using such litter. It is, in particular, advised to prevent cattle from grazing on pasture treated with broiler litter in the same year. The increasing use of farm equipment, such as silage cutters or feeders to mix and distribute feeds, notably in cattle farms, may be a new risk factor for botulism, given that contamination can be disseminated during distribution. Feed ingredients should be properly stored, and silage used in ruminant rations should be of high quality.

The most efficient measure to prevent avian botulism outbreaks (in wildlife or on farms) is the daily removal of carcasses to prevent clostridial growth and BoNT accumulation. One of the main problems with botulism is the recurrence of the disease. Cleaning and disinfection are also key to preventing recurrence.

Vaccination is efficient in preventing animal botulism. It induces generation of neutralizing antibodies against BoNTs. Formalin-inactivated toxoids are commercially available for cattle, sheep, horses, goats, and mink. Vaccines developed for mink are also efficiently used for birds, notably for pheasants. To achieve immunization, toxoids should generally be injected twice or more to develop sufficient protection.

In Europe, only mink are routinely vaccinated; horses and cattle are vaccinated only during outbreak situations. In some countries where botulism is endemic, cattle are routinely vaccinated against type C and D toxins; Israel and Australia are examples of this. In France, vaccination is highly recommended at the beginning of an outbreak to limit the number of affected animals within a flock or herd.

Vaccination is not widely used to prevent avian botulism. A simpler method is required, as the number of animals to be vaccinated is high and available vaccines often require at least two injections. Induction of protection is influenced more by time and number of doses than by the amount of toxoid, adjuvants, and routes. Study of these factors will be key to the development of a single-dose vaccine that could be better adapted to birds. Broiler immunization may also be limited because it has to be efficient within a short period of time and be efficient all along the rearing period. Vaccination of broilers is only advised in flocks with recurrent botulism outbreaks, and considering the time and cost of such vaccination, a cost analysis should be conducted before immunization. This could also be advised in other avian production systems of high economic value, such as pheasants and ostriches.

Recombinant subunit botulism vaccines have also been developed recently, avoiding the drawbacks of toxoids, such as potential hazards during detoxification, expensive and time-consuming production, and side effects. These recombinant subunit vaccines show fewer adverse reactions and induce a similar or superior protective level of neutralizing antibody titers.

Regardless of the production system, the most important management measure to prevent further botulism cases consists of the collection and disposal of carcasses. This is particularly important to prevent cases of avian botulism. Quick removal of carcasses during outbreaks is effective in slowing down the rate of avian outbreaks. This has been demonstrated to be effective in reducing botulism losses for wild birds but it is labor intensive and, thus, costly and inefficient in very large wetlands. In poultry production, it is advised to quickly separate healthy birds from sick ones.

Nutritional management is also important to control botulism outbreaks. Administration of a diet low in energy and rich in cellulose should be given to animals; supplementation with sodium, selenium, and vitamins A, D3, and E is also helpful. Removal of suspected sources of BoNTs and/or *C. botulinum*, such as potentially contaminated feed or water, is highly recommended.

Manure or litter should be managed with great care, as, during botulism outbreaks, it is usually highly contaminated by *C. botulinum* spores and this could be a potential source of dissemination. Burning of manure from farms with botulism outbreaks is often recommended.

Treatment

Treatment of botulism is usually not successful in the advanced stages of the disease and euthanasia is frequently advised. For mammalian species, antitoxin can be administered to affected animals but this has to be done when the toxin is circulating before it is bound to the neuromuscular junction. Antitoxins are not commercially available in some countries.

For cattle, vaccination can be effective in an outbreak situation.

When possible, waterfowl should be provided with fresh water and shade or injected with antitoxin; recovery rates of 75–90 % have been reported. Treatment of shorebirds, gulls, American coots, and grebes is usually not successful.

In cases of toxico-infection, antibiotics have also proven useful. Use of beta-lactams is usually effective to treat poultry botulism, and administration of ampicillin in drinking water is efficient in reducing the mortality rate in poultry production. However, symptoms often reappear at the end of the treatment.

Diagnosis

Diagnosis of animal botulism mainly due to group III *Clostridium botulinum* types C, D, and their mosaic types C/D and D/C is first based on clinical signs that are indicative but not specific, and laboratory confirmation to rule out differential diagnosis including several neuroparalytic diseases or toxicosis, among others. A botulism outbreak can typically be suspected when there is a quick rise in mortality, the presence of flaccid paralysis, or a prior history of botulism, and when post-mortem examinations of dead animals are found negative for specific evidence. The definitive confirmation for botulism diagnosis requires detection and identification of the neurotoxin type. This could be achieved by detecting the neurotoxin itself or the producing bacteria after a culture-enrichment step. Confirmation of suspected animal botulism can be provided by (Figure 26.4):

- Detection of BoNTs in samples collected from the suspected animal;
- Detection of BoNTs producing clostridia in samples collected from the suspected animal;
- Detection of BoNTs or BoNT-producing clostridia in samples collected in the close environment of suspected animals;
- An antibody response in suspected animals.

Samples of serum (10 ml), ruminal or gastrointestinal contents, fecal matter, and tissue (notably liver) have to be taken as soon as symptoms are observed or just after the animal's death to be sure that free toxin is still present in the sample. For example, a serum sample has to be taken when the toxin is circulating and not blocked at the neuromuscular junction, otherwise the analysis will be negative. Environmental samples collected near to suspected animals could also be analyzed when all samples collected on animals are negative. For cattle, gastrointestinal contents and the liver are the best samples. For birds, serum, intestinal contents, or tissue samples are recommended. Cloacal swabs have also recently been suggested as being relevant samples for botulism confirmation. Regarding sample transport conditions, as BoNT is sensitive to heat but stable at low temperatures, and the spores are resistant to environmental conditions, samples can be transported within 24 hours (recommended), under the applicable rules regarding "infectious substances transport", at a temperature between 4 °C and 8 °C and stored for several weeks at −20 °C prior to analysis.

BoNT detection

Diagnosis of botulism is performed by testing for the presence of BoNTs. Serum and gastrointestinal contents are used to detect the presence of active BoNTs. Different methods are available for toxin detection. The gold standard is still the mouse bioassay, but several others, such as immunological, enzymatic, or cell-based techniques have also been developed and used.

The gold standard: the mouse bioassay

The mouse bioassay (MBA) is still considered the benchmark method for BoNT detection and identification, and it is the most common method used by European laboratories (more than 80%). Mice are injected intraperitoneally for each suspected sample. BoNT presence in suspected animals is tested by analyzing serum, gastrointestinal or ruminal contents, fecal matter, or feed material. The injected mice are monitored for up to four days for botulism symptoms. Botulism signs occur generally within 6 to 24 hours. In mice, typical symptoms are hind limb paralysis, a contracted abdomen (wasp waist), and labored breathing.

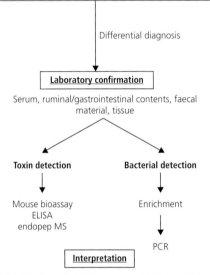

Figure 26.4 General botulism diagnostic workflow. Based on suspicion of botulism symptoms, diagnosis confirmation is achieved by detecting the botulism toxins with *in vivo* or *in vitro* assays prior to or following an enrichment step. A positive result for botulism toxins directly from suspected samples confirms the diagnosis. Detection of the neurotoxin or of a toxin-producing clostridium after an enrichment step strongly emphasizes the botulism diagnosis but should be interpreted within the epidemiological context, as it indicates that the organism might be naturally present in the environment.

Identification of the BoNT type is achieved by monitoring protected mice with neutralized antibody. The protected toxin type mouse survives and the others die. An alternative subcutaneous injection resulting in muscle paralysis avoids animal death. As little as 5–10 picograms of neurotoxin can be detected using these methods. The MBA is specific, sensitive, and could be used with different kinds of samples. Although the mouse test is considered the most sensitive test, false negatives are possible. Cattle, horses, and possibly some birds may be more sensitive to BoNTs than mice. Given the high sensitivity of cattle to BoNTs, use of the MBA for confirmation of bovine botulism is sometimes considered inappropriate. False negatives can also occur if toxins are degraded by other bacteria in the intestinal tract or if serum sampling is performed when the toxin is no longer circulating. The period of time during which BoNT is detectable in blood before being internalized at the neuronal junction is actually quite short. In foals with shaker foal syndrome, only 20% of suspicions are confirmed by the MBA. Another drawback of the MBA is the impossibility of discriminating between mosaic types and the partial cross-reactivity of type C or D antitoxin when diagnosing mosaic botulism. For example, BoNT C/D can be neutralized by both type C and type D antitoxin or sometimes only by type D antitoxin.

The MBA method is laborious, time-consuming, expensive, requires animal facilities, and presents ethical issues. Only a few laboratories worldwide, such as certain national reference laboratories, are fully equipped to perform the assay. Thus, there has been a great need for a faster, equally sensitive method that is not based on animal use, which has led the scientific community to develop other toxin detection methods.

Immunological, enzymatic, and cell-based detection methods as a replacement for the MBA

The development of an alternative analytical method comparable to the MBA has been a challenging problem owing to the extreme toxicity and chemical nature of the BoNTs. A substitute method for the MBA requires very high detection sensitivity and specificity, and the ability to measure the active toxin exclusively. A variety of techniques to detect BoNTs has been developed, including enzyme-linked immunosorbent assays (ELISAs), enzymatic methods based upon BoNT cleavage of synthetic peptides followed by different detection of the specific product or cell-based assay. These methods are used by 19.2% of European laboratories to confirm botulism.

Immunoassays using specific antibodies to detect targeted toxins are routinely used methods. Many ELISA detection methods have been developed to detect BoNTs; these are easy, rapid to use, and, with the development of signal amplification methods, are as sensitive as the MBA. Samples presumed to contain BoNT are added to toxin-specific polyclonal or monoclonal antibodies. The toxin–antibody complexes are then revealed using a second toxin-specific antibody linked to a specific enzyme (phosphatase or peroxydase) producing a light signal through enzymatic cleavage of a chromogenic substrate. However, these detection methods are limited due to the difficulty in obtaining high-quality antibodies. Furthermore, they are not able to differentiate between active and inactivated toxins that may cause false positive results. Genetic variation within toxin serotypes may also result in decreased test affinity, causing false negative results. Despite these drawbacks, use of the ELISA has been widely reported for rapid diagnosis of animal botulism. Microplates are generally used, but given the size of samples taken from animals (blood and tissue), antigen-capture ELISAs utilizing immunosticks as the solid substrate have been developed. This test was successfully used for the diagnosis of type C botulism in birds and in mammals.

ELISA is also used to demonstrate the presence of BoNT-producing clostridia. The presence of BoNTs is detected after an enrichment step performed on the the gut contents of suspected animals (five days under anaerobic conditions).

A new approach based on monitoring the zinc protease cleavage activity of BoNTs on a specific substrate (synaptic protein SNARE), and using the specificity of the unique peptide products, has been developed to overcome immunoassay issues. Specific substrate peptides for each toxin serotype are incubated with BoNTs, followed by serotype-specific revealing peptide products by Matrix Assisted Laser Desorption Ionization (MALDI) and/or Electrospray Ionization (ESI) Mass Spectrometry (MS). This method has proved to be highly sensitive and specific. An Endopep-MS method has been successfully tested on clinical animal samples (liver and serum). Detection of the activity of BoNTs by FRET has been tested for type D and E toxins but does not work for type C toxins at the moment. This method has notably been used to quantify BoNT/E in avian samples. These approaches allow detection of active toxin by measuring their enzymatic activity located in the light chain of the toxin but fail to determine the binding capacity of the heavy chain, and cannot differentiate between types C, D, and their mosaic variants C/D and D/C.

To further improve the methods presented above, developments have been made in enzymatic activity detection methods which, to date, have only been applied to human botulism. Functional enzymatic activity receptor-binding assays using brain synaptosomes have also been developed. However, like most enzymatic assays, it is quite sensitive to interference from matrix components. An alternative toxin-detection method that detects fully functional toxin is the cell-based assay. It offers a sensitive model based on cell-surface binding, endocytosis, translocation into the cellular cytosol, and enzymatic activity on SNARE substrates of BoNTs. The assays require incubation of the cells with BoNTs, followed by quantitative endpoint toxin activity determination, achieved by Western blot ELISA, or live-cell quantitative immunofluorescence methods using cleavage-specific antibodies.

BoNT-producing clostridia detection method

As previously mentioned, botulism is due to BoNT contamination by BoNT-producing clostridial strains. In parallel to neurotoxin detection, a diagnostic alternative is to detect the BoNT-producing bacteria. Although detecting the presence of the bacteria does not mean that the toxin was produced in the sample analyzed, isolation of these microorganisms coupled with clinical signs suggestive of botulism is considered by some authors evidence enough to confirm a botulism diagnosis. PCR-based methods are used by 42.3% of European laboratories to confirm botulism.

C. botulinum responsible for animal botulism shares cultural, biochemical, and physiological characteristics with other clostridia such as *Clostridium novyi*, *Clostridium haemolyticum,* and *Clostridium septicum.* As there are no proper selective media available, it is currently not possible to detect or isolate *Clostridium botulinum* by classical microbiological methods. The number of *C. botulinum* organisms in naturally contaminated samples is often very low (10 to 1000 spores/kg) and with the ability to form resistant spores, detection of the target organism directly from sample materials can be difficult. Anaerobic enrichment is thus a prerequisite to germinating spores and increasing vegetative cell concentration in the sample.

To demonstrate the presence of BoNT-producing clostridia, there are two main strategies:

- Reveal the presence of BoNTs after sample culturing using the methods presented above;
- Detect the encoding BoNT genes by molecular methods.

Bonts are distinct genes located on a specific genetic locus situated on the chromosome, a plasmid, or a phage. The *bont* genes for *Clostridium botulinum* involved in animal botulism are located on unstable phages. The botulinum locus is made up of the *bont* neurotoxin-encoding gene, a non-toxic, non-hemagglutinin gene (NTNH), several hemagglutinin genes (*HA33, HA70, HA17*), other regulatory elements (botR, p21), and yet-uncharacterized genes (*p47, OrfX1, X2, X3*). This genetic locus is specific to *C. botulinum* and necessary to produce the toxin. Thus, it is the perfect genetic target for detection using DNA-based methods.

Polymerase chain reaction (PCR) DNA amplification methods have been democratically used in many laboratories for the detection of botulinic genetic targets. *Bont* PCRs for botulism detection of bont/type C and D associated with animal botulism, or environmental investigation have been developed. But a post-PCR gel migration step is required to visualize the PCR products. Thus, real-time PCR has been the step forward for detection assay development. Monitoring amplification of the target gene after each PCR cycle enables rapid interpretation and quantification of the target sequences, reflecting the level of contamination by the organism. Real-time PCRs for bont/C, D, and their mosaic variants C/D and D/C have been readily developed. The introduction of fluorogenic probes increases specificity and allows the possibility of simultaneously detecting different targets in the same assay by multiplexing them. Using DNA intercalate chemistry, it is possible to calculate the melting temperature of the amplified target DNAs, and to differentiate between specific and unspecific PCR products. *Bont* genes are the preferential targets for botulism detection, as they confirm the presence of *bont*-producing bacteria. The NTNH gene is also a good candidate for molecular detection, as the gene is associated with the botulism genetic locus. Use of PCR methods to confirm animal botulism has been successfully validated on different animal species including cattle, broiler chickens, coots, dogs, guinea fowl, gulls, horses, mink, turkeys, pochards, and other ducks. Evidence of a toxin gene does not mean that the toxin is actively produced. Another approach consists of detecting expression of *bont* genes using reverse transcriptase real-time PCR. However, detection of mRNA related to *bont* genes is not necessarily associated with production of functional neurotoxin. Thus, positive detection results using these molecular methods indicate the presence of the *Clostridium botulinum* organism only. Furthermore, as environmental and feed samples may harbor PCR inhibitors, internal amplification controls as well as an internal positive control should be implemented for routine diagnostic PCR to control potential inhibition by the sample material or contamination.

In summary, demonstration of BoNTs and of BoNT-producing clostridia in samples collected from affected animals is the best alternative to confirm a presumptive clinical diagnosis. Concordance of results obtained by both methods or a positive result obtained by at least one of the two approaches allows confirmation of the diagnosis. Unfortunately, false negative results are common, notably when trying to demonstrate the presence of BoNTs. In this case, the diagnosis is based on the clinical symptoms, the history, and the exclusion of an alternate diagnosis by laboratory tests.

Conclusion

Despite having been reported worldwide for a long time, animal botulism is still poorly understood. It seems that there has been a rise in the number of outbreaks, especially in Europe, but as this disease is not reportable, data about its incidence are only estimated and probably underestimated. Prevention of the disease is a more effective strategy than controlling an outbreak after it begins. Development of knowledge about the epidemiology of the disease is now crucial to suggest efficient strategies to better prevent outbreaks and to be able to explain the rise in the number of outbreaks observed in European countries in production systems of several animal species.

Botulism is a life-threatening disease caused by the most potent toxin known to date. In animals, the disease is encountered frequently, particularly in poultry and in cattle. Diagnosis of the disease requires monitoring specific botulism symptoms associated with identification of the toxin type involved. To date, the reference method remains the mouse bioassay. Great efforts have been made, and certain successes achieved, in the development of other botulism toxin-detection assays and molecular methods for the identification of toxin-producing clostridia. Major review articles, notably Lindström *et al.*'s "Laboratory diagnostics of botulism" (2006), and Dorner *et al.*'s "Complexity of botulinum neurotoxins: Challenges for detection technology" (2013), summarize these methods. Thanks to the alternative strategies of this type currently under development or validation, and especially due to the ethical issues surrounding the mouse bioassay, this test is destined to disappear within the next few decades.

Bibliography

Abbasova, S.G., *et al.* (2011) Monoclonal antibodies to type A, B, E and F botulinum neurotoxins. *Bioorg. Khim.*, **37**: 344–353.

Anniballi, F., *et al.* (2012) Multiplex real-time PCR SYBR Green for detection and typing of group III *Clostridium botulinum*. *Vet. Microbiol.*, **154**: 332–338.

Anniballi, F., *et al.* (2013) Multiplex real-time PCR for detecting and typing *Clostridium botulinum* group III organisms and their mosaic variants. *Biosecur. Bioterror.*, **11**: S207–S214.

Anniballi, F., *et al.* (2013) Management of animal botulism outbreaks: From clinical suspicion to practical countermeasures to prevent or minimize outbreaks. *Biosecur. Bioterror.* **11**: S191–S199.

Anonymous (2002) *Rapport sur le botulisme d'origine aviaire et bovine.* Agence française de sécurité sanitaire des aliments, Alfort, France.

Anonymous (2012) *Animal botulism in Europe: Current status of an emerging disease. Abstracts of reports of botulism in animals over the last decade written by participants of the animal botulism workshop.* AniBio.Threat. Uppsala, Sweden.

Anza, I., *et al.* (2014) New insight in the epidemiology of avian botulism outbreaks: Necrophagous flies as vectors of *Clostridium botulinum* type C/D. *Environ. Microbiol.,* **6**: 738–743.

Anza, I., *et al.* (2014) The same clade of *Clostridium botulinum* strains is causing avian botulism in southern and northern Europe. *Anaerobe,* **26**: 20–23.

Arimitsu, H., *et al.* (2004) Vaccination with recombinant whole heavy chain fragments of *Clostridium botulinum* Type C and D neurotoxins. *Clin. Diag. Lab. Imm.,* **11**: 496–502.

Auricchio, B., *et al.* (2013) Evaluation of DNA extraction methods suitable for PCR-based detection and genotyping of *Clostridium botulinum. Biosecur. Bioterror.,* **11**: S200–S206.

Barash, J.R., *et al.* (2014) A novel strain of *Clostridium botulinum* that produces type B and type H botulinum toxins. *J. Infect. Dis.,* **209**: 183–191.

Bennetts, H., *et al.* (1938) Botulism of sheep and cattle in Western Australia: Its cause and its prevention by immunization. *Aust. Vet. J. Ag. Food Chem.,* **14**: 105–118.

Böhnel, H., *et al.* (2001) Visceral botulism – a new form of bovine *Clostridium botulinum* toxication. *J. Vet. Med. A Phys. Path. Clin. Med.,* **48**: 373–383.

Böhnel, H., *et al.* (2008) Tonsils – Place of botulinum toxin production: Results of routine laboratory diagnosis in farm animals. *Vet. Microbiol.,* **130**: 403–409.

Boyer, A.E., *et al.* (2005) From the mouse to the mass spectrometer: Detection and differentiation of the endoproteinase activities of botulinum neurotoxins A–G by mass spectrometry. *Anal. Chem.,* **77**: 3916–3924.

Brooks, C.E., *et al.* (2011) Diagnosis of botulism types C and D in cattle by a monoclonal antibody-based sandwich ELISA. *Vet. Rec.,* **168**: 455.

Bruckstein, S., *et al.* (2001) Food poisoning in three family dairy herds associated with *Clostridium botulinum* type B. *Israel J. Vet. Med.,* **56**: 95–98.

Chaffer, M., *et al.* (2006) Application of PCR for detection of *Clostridium botulinum* type D in bovine samples. *J. Vet. Med. Series B: Infect. Dis. Vet. Pub. Health,* **53**: 45–47.

Chatla, K., *et al.* (2014) Zebrafish (*Danio rerio*) bioassay for visceral toxicosis of catfish and botulinum neurotoxin serotype E. *J. Vet. Diagn. Invest.,* **26**: 240–245.

Chun, C.L., *et al.* (2013) Association of toxin-producing *Clostridium botulinum* with the macroalga Cladophora in the Great Lakes. *Environ. Sci. & Tech.,* **47**: 2587–2594.

Cunha, C.E.P., *et al.* (2014) Vaccination of cattle with a recombinant bivalent toxoid against botulism serotypes C and D. *Vaccine,* **32**: 214–216.

Dahlenborg, M., *et al.* (2001) Development of a Combined Selection and Enrichment PCR Procedure for *Clostridium botulinum* Types B, E, and F and Its Use to Determine Prevalence in Fecal Samples from Slaughtered Pigs. *App. Environ. Micro.,* **67**: 4781–4788.

Dahlenborg, M., *et al.* (2003) Prevalence of *Clostridium botulinum* types B, E and F in faecal samples from Swedish cattle. *Int. J. Food Microb.,* **82**: 105–110.

Deprez, P.R. (2006) Tetanus and botulism in animals. In: Duchesnes, C. *et al.* (eds) *Clostridia in Medical, Veterinary and Food Microbiology*, pp. 27–36. European Commission, Brussels, Belgium.

Divers, J.T., *et al.* (2011) Clinical Neurology. *Vet. Clin. N. Am.: Equine Practice,* **27**: ix–x .

Döbereiner, J., *et al.* (1992) Epizootic botulism of cattle in Brazil. *Deutsche Tierarztliche Wochenschrift,* **99**: 188–190.

Dohms, J.E., *et al.* (1982) Cases of type C botulism in broiler chickens. *Avian Dis.,* **26**: 204–210.

Dohms, J.E., *et al.* (1982) The immunization of broiler chickens against type C botulism. *Avian Dis.,* **26**: 340–345.

Dorner, M.B., *et al.* (2013) Complexity of botulinum neurotoxins: Challenges for detection technology. *Curr. Top. Microbiol. Immunol.,* **364**: 219–255.

Duncan, R.M., *et al.* (1976) A relationship between avian carcasses and living invertebrates in the epizootiology of avian botulism. *J. Wildl. Dis.,* **12**: 116–126.

Eklund, M.W., *et al.* (1984) Type E botulism in salmonids and conditions contributing to outbreaks. *Aquacult.*, **41**: 293–309.

Eklund, M.W., *et al.* (2004) Susceptibility of coho salmon, *Oncorhynchus kisutch* (Walbaum), to different toxins of *Clostridium botulinum*. *Aqua. Res.*, **35**: 594–600.

Elad, D., *et al.* (2004) Natural *Clostridium botulinum* type C toxicosis in a group of cats. *J. Clin. Microbiol.*, **42**: 5406–5408.

Evans, E.R., *et al.* (2009) An assay for botulinum toxin types A, B and F that requires both functional binding and catalytic activities within the neurotoxin. *J. Appl. Microbiol.*, **107**: 1384–1391.

Fach, P., *et al.* (1996) Investigation of animal botulism outbreaks by PCR and standard methods. *FEMS Immunol. Med. Microbiol.*, **13**: 279–285.

Forrester, D.J., *et al.* (1980) An epizootic of avian botulism in a phosphate mine settling pond in northern Florida. *J. Wildl. Dis.*, **16**: 323–327.

Franciosa, G., *et al.* (1996) PCR for detection of *Clostridium botulinum* type C in avian and environmental samples. *J. Clin. Microbiol.*, **34**: 882–885.

Frey, J., *et al.* (2007) Alternative vaccination against equine botulism (BoNT/C). *Eq. Vet. J.*, **39**: 516–520.

Galey, F.D., *et al.* (2000) Type C botulism in dairy cattle from feed contaminated with a dead cat. *J. Vet. Diagn. Invest.*, **12**: 204–209.

Galey, F.D. (2001) Botulism in the horse. *Vet. Clin. North Am.: Eq. Prac.*, **17**: 579–588.

Gerber, V., *et al.* (2006) Equine botulism and acute pasture myodystrophy: New soil-borne emerging diseases in Switzerland? *Schweizer Archiv für Tierheilkunde*, **148**: 553–559.

Gil, L.A., *et al.* (2013) Production and evaluation of a recombinant chimeric vaccine against *Clostridium botulinum* neurotoxin types C and D. *PLoS One*, **8**: e69692.

Gismervik, K., *et al.* (2014) Invasive slug populations (*Arion vulgaris*) as potential vectors for *Clostridium botulinum*. *Acta Vet. Scand.*, **56**: 65.

Gross, W.B., *et al.* (1971) Experimental botulism in gallinaceous birds. *Avian Dis.*, **15**: 716–722.

Hardy, S.P., *et al.* (2011) Risk of botulism for laying hens and broilers. *Vet. Rec.*, **169**: 133.

Hardy, S.P., *et al.* (2013) Type C and C/D toxigenic *Clostridium botulinum* is not normally present in the intestine of healthy broilers. *Vet. Microbiol.* **165**: 466–468.

Hatheway, C.L. (1988) Botulism. In: Balows, A. *et al.* (eds) *Laboratory Diagnosis of Infectious Diseases: Principles and practice*, pp. 111–133. Springer-Verlag, London.

Hedeland, M., *et al.* (2011) Confirmation of botulism in birds and cattle by the mouse bioassay and Endopep-MS. *J. Med. Microbiol.*, **60**: 1299–1305.

Heider, L.C., *et al.* (2001) Presumptive diagnosis of *Clostridium botulinum* type D intoxication in a herd of feedlot cattle. *Can. Vet. J.*, **42**: 210–212.

Hill, B.J., *et al.* (2010) Universal and specific quantitative detection of botulinum neurotoxin genes. *BMC Microbiol.*, **10**: 267.

Hill, K.K., *et al.* (2007) Genetic diversity among botulinum neurotoxin-producing clostridial strains. *J. Bacteriol.*, **189**: 818–832.

Hinkle, N.C., *et al.* (2008) External parasites and poultry pests. In: Saif, Y.M. *et al.* (eds) *Diseases of Poultry*, 12th edition, pp. 1011–1024. Iowa State University Press, Ames, IA.

Hofer, J.W., *et al.* (1972) Survival and dormancy of Clostridia spores. *Tex. Med.*, **68**: 80–81.

Holdeman, L.V. (1970) The ecology and natural history of *Clostridium botulinum*. *J. Wildl. Dis.*, **6**: 205–210.

Holzhauer, M., *et al.* (2009) Botulism in dairy cattle in 2008: Symptoms, diagnosis, pathogenesis, therapy, and prevention. *Tijdschr. Diergeneeskd.*, **134**: 564–570.

Hoorfar, J., *et al.* (2003) Diagnostic PCR: Making internal amplification controls mandatory. *Lett. Appl. Microbiol.*, **38**: 79–80.

Hunter, L.C., *et al.* (1999) The association of *Clostridium botulinum* type C with equine grass sickness: A toxicoinfection? *Eq. Vet. J.*, **31**: 492–499.

Huss, H.H., *et al.* (2007) The incidence of *Clostridium botulinum* in Danish trout farms: I. distribution in fish and their environment. *Int. J. Food Sci. Tech.*, **9**: 445–450.

Jean, D., *et al.* (1995) *Clostridium botulinum* type C intoxication in feedlot steers being fed ensiled poultry litter. *Can. Vet. J.*, **36**: 626–628.

Johnson, A.L., *et al.* (2014) Quantitative real-time PCR for detection of neurotoxin genes of *Clostridium botulinum* types A, B and C in equine samples. *Vet. J.*, **199**: 157–161.

Kirchner, S., *et al.* (2010) Pentaplexed quantitative real-time PCR assay for the simultaneous detection and quantification of botulinum neurotoxin-producing clostridia in food and clinical samples. *Appl. Environ. Microbiol.*, **76**: 4387–4395.

Kiris, E., *et al.* (2011) Embryonic stem cell-derived motoneurons provide a highly sensitive cell culture model for botulinum neurotoxin studies, with implications for high throughput drug discovery. *Stem Cell Res.*, **6**: 195–205.

Klarmann, D. (1989) The detection of *Clostridium botulinum* in fecal samples of cattle and swine and in the raw material and animal meal of different animal body rendering plants. *Berliner und Münchener tierärztliche Wochenschrift*, **102**: 84–86.

Kouguchi, H., *et al.* (2006) Quantitative detection of gene expression and toxin complex produced by *Clostridium botulinum* serotype D strain 4947. *J. Microbiol. Meth.*, **67**: 416–423.

Krüger, M., *et al.* (2013) Efficacy of *Clostridium botulinum* types C and D toxoid vaccination inDanish cows. *Anaerobe*, **23**: 97–101.

Krüger, M., *et al.* (2013) Glyphosate suppresses the antagonistic effect of Enterococcus spp. on *Clostridium botulinum*. *Anaerobe*, **20**: 74–78.

Lindberg, A., *et al.* (2010) Real-time PCR for *Clostridium botulinum* type C neurotoxin (BoNTC) gene, also covering a chimeric C/D sequence – application on outbreaks of botulism in poultry. *Vet. Microbiol.*, **146**(1–2): 118–123.

Lindstrom, M., *et al.* (2004) Type C botulism due to toxic feed affecting 52,000 farmed foxes and minks in Finland. *J. Clin. Microb.*, **42**: 4718–4725.

Lindstrom, M., *et al.* (2006) Laboratory diagnostics of botulism. *Clin. Microbiol. Rev.*, **19**: 298–314.

Locke, L., *et al.* (1989) *Avian Botulism: Geographic expansion of a historic disease*. Waterfowl Management Handbook Fish and Wildlife Leaflet 13.2.4.

Macdonald, J.W., *et al.* (1978) An outbreak of botulism in gulls on the Firth of Forth, Scotland. *Biolog. Conserv.*, **14**: 149–155.

Maksymowych, A., *et al.* (1999) Pure botulinum neurotoxin is absorbed from the stomach and small intestine and produces peripheral neuromuscular blockade. *Infect. Immun.*, **67**: 4708–4712.

Malcolm, J.M. (1982) Bird collisions with a power transmission line and their relation to botulism at a Montana wetland. *Wildl. Soc. Bull.*, **10**: 297–304.

Martin, S. (2003) *Clostridium botulinum* type D intoxication in a dairy herd in Ontario. *Can. Vet. J.*, **44**: 493–495.

Matveev, K.I., *et al.* (1974) The role of migrating birds in disseminating the agent of botulism. *Gigiena i Sanitariia*, **12**: 91–92.

Mitchell, W.R., *et al.* (1987) Type C botulism: The agent, host, susceptibility and predisposing factors. In: Eklund, M.W. and Dowell, V.R. Jr (eds) *Avian Botulism: An international perspective*, pp. 55–72. Thomas CC, Springfield, IL.

Moeller, R.B. Jr, *et al.* (2003) Determination of the median toxic dose of type C botulinum toxin in lactating dairy cows. *J. Vet. Diagn. Invest.*, **15**: 523–526.

Moriishi, K., *et al.* (1996) Molecular cloning of the gene encoding the mosaic neurotoxin, composed of parts of botulinum neurotoxin types C1 and D, and PCR detection of this gene from *Clostridium botulinum* type C organisms. *Appl. Environ. Microbiol.*, **62**: 662–667.

Myllykoski, J., *et al.* (2006) The detection and prevalence of *Clostridium botulinum* in pig intestinal samples. *Int. J. Food Microbiol.*, **110**: 172–177.

Myllykoski, J., *et al.* (2009) Type C bovine botulism outbreak due to carcass contaminated non-acidified silage. *Epidemiol. Infect.*, **137**: 284–293.

Myllykoski, J., *et al.* (2011) Fur animal botulism hazard due to feed. *Res. Vet. Sci.*, **90**: 412–418.

Nakamura, K., *et al.* (2010) Characterization of the D/C mosaic neurotoxin produced by *Clostridium botulinum* associated with bovine botulism in Japan. *Vet. Microbiol.*, **140**: 147–154.

Nakamura, K., *et al.* (2012) Unique biological activity of botulinum D/C mosaic neurotoxin in murine species. *Infect. Immun.*, **80**: 2886–2893.

Neimanis, A., *et al.* (2007) An outbreak of type C botulism in herring gulls (*Larus argentatus*) in southeastern Sweden. *J. Wildl. Dis.*, **43**: 327–336.

Nol, P., *et al.* (2004) Prevalence of neurotoxic *Clostridium botulinum* type C in the gastrointestinal tracts of tilapia (*Oreochromis mossambicus*) in the Salton Sea. *J. Wildl. Dis.*, **40**: 414–419.

Notermans, S., *et al.* (1981) Persistence of *Clostridium botulinum* type B on a cattle farm after an outbreak of botulism. *Appl. Environ. Microbiol.*, **41**: 179–183.

Notermans, S.H., *et al.* (1985) Incidence of *Clostridium botulinum* on cattle farms. *Tijdschrift voor diergeneeskunde*, **110**: 175–180.

Nuss, J.E., *et al.* (2010) Development of cell-based assays to measure botulinum neurotoxin serotype A activity using cleavage-sensitive antibodies. *J. Biomol. Screen.*, **15**: 42–51.

Ortolani, E.L., *et al.* (1997) Botulism outbreak associated with poultry litter consumption in three Brazilian cattle herds. *Vet. Human Tox.*, **39**: 89–92.

Payne, J.H., *et al.* (2011) Emergence of suspected type D botulism in ruminants in England and Wales (2001 to 2009), associated with exposure to broiler litter. *Vet. Rec.*, **168**: 640.

Peck, M.W. (2009) Biology and genomic analysis of *Clostridium botulinum*. *Adv. Microb. Physiol.*, **55**: 183–265.

Peck, M.W., *et al.* (2011) *Clostridium botulinum* in the post-genomic era. *Food Microbiol.*, **28**: 183–191.

Pellett, S., *et al.* (2011) Sensitive and quantitative detection of botulinum neurotoxin in neurons derived from mouse embryonic stem cells. *Biochem. Biophys. Res. Commun.*, **404**: 388–392.

Piazza, T.M., *et al.* (2011) *In vitro* detection and quantification of botulinum neurotoxin type E activity in avian blood. *Appl. Environ. Microbiol.*, **77**: 7815–7822.

Popoff, M. (1989) Revue sur l'épidémiologie du botulisme bovin en France et analyse de sa relation avec les élevages de volailles. *Revue Scientifique et Technique de l'Office Internat des Epiz*, **8**: 129–145.

Quinn, P. (1984) A two-year study of botulism in gulls in the vicinity of Dublin Bay. *Irish Vet. J.*, **38**: 214–219.

Quinn, P. (1994) *Clinical Veterinary Microbiology*. p. 198. Wolfe, London.

Radostits, O.M., *et al.* (2000) Diseases caused by *Clostridium* spp. In: Radostits, O. *et al.* (eds) *Veterinary Medicine: A textbook of the diseases of cattle, sheep, pigs, goats and horses*, 9th edition, pp. 753–777. W. B. Saunders, London.

Raphael, B.H., *et al.* (2007) Real-time PCR detection of the nontoxic nonhemagglutinin gene as a rapid screening method for bacterial isolates harboring the botulinum neurotoxin (A–G) gene complex. *J. Microbiol. Meth.*, **71**: 343–346.

Rebhun, W. (1995) *Diseases of Dairy Cattle*. Lippincott Williams & Wilkins, Philadelphia.

Reed, T. (1992) The role of avian carcasses in botulism epizootics. *Wildl. Soc. Bul.*, **20**: 175–182.

Rocke, T.E., *et al.* (1998) Preliminary evaluation of a simple *in vitro* test for the diagnosis of type C botulism in wild birds. *J. Wildl. Dis.*, **34**: 744–751.

Rocke, T. (1999) Avian botulism. In: Friend, M. and Franson, J.C. (eds) *Field Manual of Wildlife Diseases: General Field Procedures and Diseases of Birds*, pp. 271–281. Biological resources division information and technology report 1999–2001.

Rocke, T. (1999) Environmental characteristics associated with the occurrence of avian botulism in wetlands of a northern California refuge. *J. Wildl. Mgmt*, **63**: 358–368.

Rocke, T. (2000) Efficacy of a type C botulism vaccine in green-winged teal. *J. Wildl. Dis.*, **36**: 489–493.

Rocke, T.E. (2004) Type C botulism in pelicans and other fish-eating birds at the Salton Sea. *Stud. Av. Biol.*, **27**: 137–140.

Rocke, T. (2006) The global importance of avian botulism. In: Boere, G.C. *et al.* (eds) *Waterbirds Around the World*, pp.422–426. The Stationery Office, Edinburgh, UK.

Rocke, T.E. (2007) Avian botulism. In: Thomas, N.J. *et al.* (eds) *Infectious Diseases of Wild Birds*, pp. 377–416. Blackwell Publishing Ltd., Oxford, UK.

Sakaguchi, Y. (2005) The genome sequence of *Clostridium botulinum* type C neurotoxin-converting phage and the molecular mechanisms of unstable lysogeny. *Proc. Nat. Acad. Sci.*, **102**: 17472–17477.

Sasaki, Y., *et al.* (2002) Phylogenetic analysis and PCR detection of *Clostridium chauvoei*, *Clostridium haemolyticum*, *Clostridium novyi* types A and B, and *Clostridium septicum* based on the flagellin gene. *Vet. Microbiol.*, **86**: 257–267.

Sato, S. (1987) Control of botulism in poultry flocks. In: Eklund, M.W. and Dowell, V.R. (eds) *Avian Botulism: An international perspective*, pp. 349–356. Charles C. Thomas, Springfiled, IL.

Schmid, A. (2013) Occurrence of zoonotic Clostridia and Yersinia in healthy cattle. *J. Food Prot.*, **76**: 1697–1703.

Seyboldt, C., *et al.* (2015) Occurrence of *Clostridium botulinum* neurotoxin in chronic disease of dairy cows. *Vet. Microbiol.*, **177**: 398–402.

Shayegani, M. (1984) An outbreak of botulism in waterfowl and fly larvae in New York State. *J. Wildl. Dis.*, **20**: 86–89.

Shin, N. (2010) An outbreak of type C botulism in waterbirds: Incheon, Korea. *J. Wildl. Dis.*, **46**: 912–917.

Simpson, L.L. (2004) Identification of the major steps in botulinum toxin action. *Ann. Rev. Pharmacol. Toxicol.*, **44**: 167–193.

Skarin, H. (2010) Molecular characterization and comparison of *Clostridium botulinum* type C avian strains. *Avi. Pathol.*, **39**: 511–518.

Skarin, H., *et al.* (2011) *Clostridium botulinum* group III: A group with dual identity shaped by plasmids, phages and mobile elements. *BMC Genom.*, **12**: 185.

Skarin, H. (2013) The workshop on animal botulism in Europe. *Biosecur. Bioterror.*, **11**: S183–S190.

Skarin, H., *et al.* (2013) Botulism. In: Swayne, D.E. (ed.) *Diseases of Poultry*, 13th edition, pp. 953–957. Wiley-Blackwell, Ames, IA.

Skarin, H., *et al.* (2014) Plasmidome interchange between *Clostridium botulinum*, *Clostridium novyi* and *Clostridium haemolyticum* converts strains of independent lineages into distinctly different pathogens. *PLoS One*, **9**: e107777.

Smart, J. (1977) An outbreak of type C botulism in broiler chickens. *Vet. Rec.*, **100**: 378–380.

Smith, G. (1976) Botulism in waterfowl. *Wildfowl*, **27**: 129–138.

Smith, L.D.S. (1977) *Botulism, the Organism, its Toxins, the Disease*. Charles C. Thomas, Springfield, IL.

Smith, T.J., *et al.* (2007) Analysis of the neurotoxin complex genes in *Clostridium botulinum* A1–A4 and B1 strains: BoNT/A3, /Ba4 and /B1 clusters are located within plasmids. *PLoS One*, **2**: e1271.

Souillard, R. (2013) Recherche de *Clostridium botulinum* neurotoxinogène par PCR temps réel dans des élevages de volailles atteints de botulisme et des élevages indemnes. In: *Dixièmes Journées de la Recherche Avicole et Palmipèdes à Foie Gras*, La Rochelle, France, 26–28 March 2013.

Stahl, C. (2009) Immune response of horses to vaccination with the recombinant Hc domain of botulinum neurotoxin types C and D. *Vaccine*, **27**: 5661–5666.

Sugiyama, H. (1970) *Clostridium botulinum* type E in an island bay (Green Bay of Lake Michigan). In: Herzberg, M. (ed.) *Proceedings of the First U.S.–Japan Conference on Toxic Micro-organisms, Mycotoxins, Botulism*, pp. 287–291. U.S.–Japan Cooperative Program in Natural Resources and U.S. Department of Interior, Washington, DC.

Swift, P., *et al.* (2000) Desert bighorn sheep mortality due to presumptive type C botulism in California. *J. Wildl. Dis.*, **36**: 184–189.

Takeda, M. (2005) Characterization of the neurotoxin produced by isolates associated with avian botulism. *Avian Dis.*, **49**: 376–381.

Tevell Åberg, A., *et al.* (2013) Mass spectrometric detection of protein-based toxins. *Biosecur. Bioterror.*, **1**: S215–S226.

Thomas, R.J. (1991) Detection of *Clostridium botulinum* types C and D toxin by ELISA. *Aust. Vet. J.*, **68**: 111–113.

Trueman, K. (1992) Suspected botulism in three intensively managed Australian cattle herds. *Vet. Rec.*, **130**: 398–400.

Tsukamoto, K. (2005) Binding of *Clostridium botulinum* type C and D neurotoxins to ganglioside and phospholipid. Novel insights into the receptor for clostridial neurotoxins. *J. Biol. Chem.*, **280**: 35164–35171.

Van Der Lugt, J. (1995) Two outbreaks of type C and type D botulism in sheep and goats in South Africa. *J. S. Afri. Vet. Assoc.*, **66**: 77–82.

Vidal, D., *et al.* (2011) Real-time polymerase chain reaction for the detection of toxigenic *Clostridium botulinum* type C1 in waterbird and sediment samples: Comparison with other PCR techniques. *J. Vet. Diagn. Invest.*, **23**: 942–946.

Vidal, D., *et al.* (2013) Environmental factors influencing the prevalence of a *Clostridium botulinum* type C/D mosaic strain in nonpermanent Mediterranean wetlands. *Appl. Environ. Microbiol.*, **79**: 4264–4271.

Webb, R. (2007) Protection with recombinant *Clostridium botulinum* C1 and D binding domain subunit (Hc) vaccines against C and D neurotoxins. *Vaccine*, **25**: 4273–4282.

Whitemarsh, R.C., *et al.* (2012) Novel application of human neurons derived from induced pluripotent stem cells for highly sensitive botulinum neurotoxin detection. *Toxicol. Sci.*, **126**: 426–435.

Whitlock, R.H. (2002) Botulism (Shaker foals; Forage poisoning). In: Smith, B.P. (ed.) *Large Animal Internal Medicine*, 3rd edition, pp. 1003–1008. Mosby, St. Louis, MI.

Whitlock, R. (2006) Equine Botulism. *Clin. Tech. Eq. Prac.*, **5**: 37–42.

Wilder-Kofie, T.D., *et al.* (2011) An alternative *in vivo* method to refine the mouse bioassay for botulinum toxin detection. *Comp. Med.*, **61**: 235–242.

Williamson, J.L., *et al.* (1999) *In situ* detection of the *Clostridium botulinum* type C1 toxin gene in wetland sediments with a nested PCR assay. *Appl. Environ. Microbiol.*, **65**: 3240–3243.

Wobeser, G.A. (1983) Avian botulism during late autumn and early spring in Saskatchewan. *J. Wildl. Dis.*, **19**: 90–94.

Wobeser, G.A. (1987) Occurrence of toxigenic *Clostridium botulinum* type C in the soil of wetlands in Saskatchewan. *J. Wildl. Dis.*, **23**: 67–76.

Wobeser, G.A. (1997) Avian botulism – another perspective. *J. Wildl. Dis.*, **33**: 181–186.

Wobeser, G.A. (1997) Botulism. In: *Diseases of Wild Waterfowl*, 2nd edition, pp.149–162. Springer Science, New York.

Woo, G. (2010) Outbreak of botulism (*Clostridium botulinum* type C) in wild waterfowl: Seoul, Korea. *J. Wildl. Dis.*, **46**: 951–955.

Work, T. (2010) Avian botulism: A case study in translocated endangered Laysan Ducks (*Anas laysanensis*) on Midway Atoll. *J. Wildl. Dis.*, **46**: 499–506.

Woudstra, C., *et al.* (2012) Neurotoxin gene profiling of *Clostridium botulinum* types C and D native to different countries within Europe. *Appl. Environ. Microbiol.*, **78**: 3120–3127.

Yamakawa, K. (1992) *Clostridium botulinum* type C in healthy swine in Japan. *Microbiol. Immunol.*, **36**: 29–34.

Yeruham, I. (2003) Outbreak of botulism type B in a dairy cattle herd: Clinical and epidemiological aspects. *Vet. Rec.*, **153**: 270–272.

Yule, A. (2006) Toxicity of *Clostridium botulinum* type E neurotoxin to Great Lakes fish: Implications for avian botulism. *J. Wildl. Dis.*, **42**: 479–493.

Diseases Caused by Other Clostridia Producing Neurotoxins

John F. Prescott

Introduction

There are no well-described reports of clostridia other than *Clostridium botulinum* and *Clostridium tetani* causing neurologic diseases in animals, with the exception of epsilon toxin-producing type D *Clostridium perfringens*.

Neurologic disease associated with *Clostridium perfringens* type D

Disease produced by *Clostridium perfringens* type D has been described in Chapter 13. Neurologic disease is often noted if affected animals (sheep, goats, and rarely cattle) do not die suddenly; the clinical signs of aimless wandering and isolation, central blindness, opisthotonus or "star gazing" and head pressing, are attributed to brain edema in acute and sub-acute cases and, in some sub-acute and chronic cases, to multifocal, bilateral, and symmetrical encephalomalacia resulting from initial perivascular edema in the brain and hypoxic injury.

Botulism caused by *Clostridium baratii* and *Clostridium butyricum*

In humans, botulism has rarely been associated with intoxication by some strains of *Clostridium baratii* (type F neurotoxin) and *Clostridium butyricum* (type E neurotoxin) (Chapters 7 and 26). These strains are, in other respects, typical members of their species. In humans, the rare cases of botulism due to neurotoxigenic *C. baratii* and *C. butyricum* have mainly been associated with infant botulism and

Clostridial Diseases of Animals, First Edition. Francisco A. Uzal, J. Glenn Songer, John F. Prescott and Michel R. Popoff.

adult intestinal botulism (that is, infectious *C. botulinum*-producing toxin *in vivo*) although food-borne intoxication has also been described, more notably for *C. butyricum*. Type E infant botulism acquired from *C. butyricum* and toxin-laden water in a tank holding pet "yellow-bellied" terrapins has been described. Further details about all aspects of botulism are presented in Chapter 26.

Diagnosis of cases of *C. baratii* and *C. butyricum* infection or intoxication has been made on the basis of identification of toxin type in serum or feces of patients by mouse bioassay or by real-time PCR identification of the toxin gene in feces, and by isolation of the organism from feces.

Bibliography

Fach, P., *et al.* (2009) Development of real-time PCR tests for detecting botulinum neurotoxin A, B, E, F producing *Clostridium botulinum, Clostridium baratii and Clostridium butyricum. J. Appl. Microbiol.,* **107**: 465–473.

Filho, E.J.F., *et al.* (2009) Clinicopathologic features of experimental enterotoxemia *Clostridium perfringens* type D enterotoxemia in cattle. *Vet. Pathol.,* **46**: 1213–1220.

Hannett, G.E., *et al.* (2014) Two cases of adult botulism caused by botulinum neurotoxin-producing *Clostridium baratii. Anaerobe,* **30**: 178–180.

Peck, M.W. (2009) Biology and genomic analysis of *Clostridium botulinum. Adv. Microb. Physiol.,* **55**: 183–265.

Rings, M.D. (2004) Clostridial disease associated with neurologic signs: Tetanus, botulism, and enterotoxemia. *Vet. Clin. N. Am.,* **20**: 379–391.

Shelley, E.B., *et al.* (2015) Infant botulism due to *C. butyricum* type E toxin: A novel environmental association with pet terrapins. *Epidemiol. Infect.,* **143**: 461–469.

Uzal, F.A., *et al.* (2008) Diagnosis of *Clostridium perfringens* intestinal infections in sheep and goats. *J. Vet. Diagn. Invest.,* **20**: 253–265.

Uzal, F.A., *et al.* (2010) *Clostridium perfringens* toxins involved in mammalian veterinary diseases. *Open Toxin J.,* **2**: 24–42.

Index

abomasitis, clostridial
  braxy (*C. septicum*), 205–208
  calves, 211–215
  control, 218–219
  diagnosis, 217
  etiology general, 209
  goats, 211–213
  lambs, 211–213
  predisposing factors, 218
  prophylaxis, 217
  Sarcina spp., 4, 208, 210, 217
  treatment, 219
Agr-like quorum-sensing system for CPB, 49
alpha toxin *see Clostridium perfringens* alpha
    toxin
amyloid precursor protein, 167
APP *see* amyloid precursor protein
aquaporin-4, 165

bacillary hemoglobinuria, *Clostridium*
    haemolyticum, 265–273
Bacillus piliformis see Tyzzer's disease
beta toxin *see Clostridium perfringens* beta toxin
bighead, 246
black disease *see* infectious necrotic hepatitis
blackleg, 231–241
BoNT *see* botulism
botulinum locus
  general characteristics, 80–81
  genomic localization, 81–83
botulinum toxins *see* botulism
botulism *see also Clostridium botulinum*
  cell-based diagnostic methods, 321–322
  clinical signs, 314–316
  Clostridium baratii, 331–332
  Clostridium butyricum, 331–332
  control, 316–318
  diagnosis, 318–324
  disease in different species, 305–308
  environmental conditions, 310

enzymatic diagnostic methods, 321–322
epidemiology, 308–313
etiology, 303–304
general characteristics, 303
gross changes, 316
healthy carriage, 308
immunological diagnostic methods,
    321–322
microscopic changes, 316
molecular epidemiology, 312–313
mouse bioassay, 319–321
pathogenesis, 304
prophylaxis, 316–318
risk factors, 311–312
sources of contamination, 308
treatment, 318
vaccination, 317–318
braxy, 205–208

canine
  Clostridium perfringens type A enteric
      infection, 114–115
  hemorrhagic gastroenteritis, 114–115
  NetF-canine hemorrhagic gastroenteritis,
      114–115, 118–119
CDAD *see Clostridium difficile*-associated
    disease
CDT *see Clostridium difficile* ADP-ribosylating
    toxin
cerebellar vermis herniation, 161, 162,
    169, 170
clostridial abomasitis, 205–218
clostridial neurotoxins
  mode of action, 93–96
  structure, 92–93
Clostridium aminovalericum see Tyzzer's disease
Clostridium argentinense
  general characteristics, 75
  neurotoxins *see Clostridium botulinum*
      group IV

Clostridial Diseases of Animals, First Edition. Francisco A. Uzal, J. Glenn Songer,
John F. Prescott and Michel R. Popoff.
© 2016 John Wiley & Sons, Inc. Published 2016 by John Wiley & Sons, Inc.